P9-AZW-278

Also by Kurt Brungardt

THE COMPLETE BOOK OF ABS

THE COMPLETE BOOK OF BUTT AND LEGS

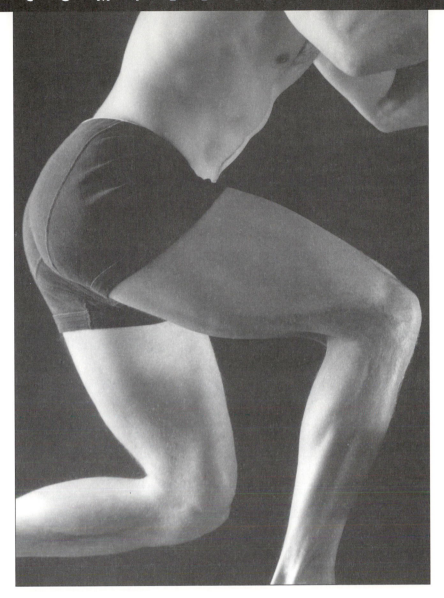

Butt and Legs

KURT, MIKE, AND BRETT BRUNGARDT

VILLARD BOOKS
NEW YORK
1995

Copyright © 1995 by Kurt Brungardt

All rights reserved under International and Pan-American Copyright
Conventions.
Published in the United States by Villard Books, a division of Random
House, Inc., New York, and simultaneously in Canada by Random House
of Canada Limited, Toronto.

Villard Books is a registered trademark of Random House, Inc.

Library of Congress Cataloging-in-Publication Data
Brungardt, Kurt.
The complete book of butt and legs / by Kurt, Mike, and Brett Brungardt.
p. cm.
Includes index.
ISBN 0-679-75481-4
1. Exercise. 2. Buttocks. 3. Legs. I. Brungardt, Mike. II. Brungardt, Brett. III. Title.
GV508.B787 1994
613.7′1—dc20   94-29524

Design by Beth Tondreau Design / Mary A. Wirth

Manufactured in the United States of America
on acid-free paper

9 8 7 6 5 4 3

This book is dedicated to those who embrace the ideal of the journey. Although the goal is important, those who accept *the journey* are the ones most likely to succeed and enjoy what the goal has to offer. The process of accepting each day, even with its repetitious actions and encounters, makes the journey worthwhile and more glorious. Taking responsibility for its successes and failures is itself a step toward fulfillment.

Those who adhere to this belief will embrace fond memories of the experience, whether it be in life or a fitness goal, for true fitness is indeed a lifetime journey. Those who don't follow this path aren't likely to repeat the steps necessary for success. Those who have things handed to them will never truly appreciate any goal or the rewards of accomplishment.

You can wallow in your fears and anger, or you can take this task of life and savor each step and breath—but the journey is inevitable. Ultimately, whether one encounters success or failure, the goal is not as important as the joy of the journey.

ACKNOWLEDGMENTS

There are many people and organizations that have made this book possible. We would especially like to thank Doug Stumpf of Villard, without whom this book would not have been possible. His vision, help, and guidance were irreplaceable. In addition we would like to extend a special thanks to the owners and staff of Snowmass Lodge and Club of Snowmass Village, Colorado, for their exceptional hospitality and help during the photo shoot.

We would also like to thank Kenneth E. Salyer, M.D., F.M.D., F.A.C.S., and director of the International Craniofacial Institute and Cleft Lip and Palate Treatment Center of Dallas, Texas, for his assistance in research.

Thanks also to the Little Nell Hotel and Bleeker Street Gym, both of Aspen, Colorado, the Bulldog Gym of Grand Junction, Colorado, and to the numerous professionals who contributed routines, especially Becky Chase, Bryan Holmes, and Deb Holmes, for adding their expertise to this book.

CONTENTS

Part Four: The Routines

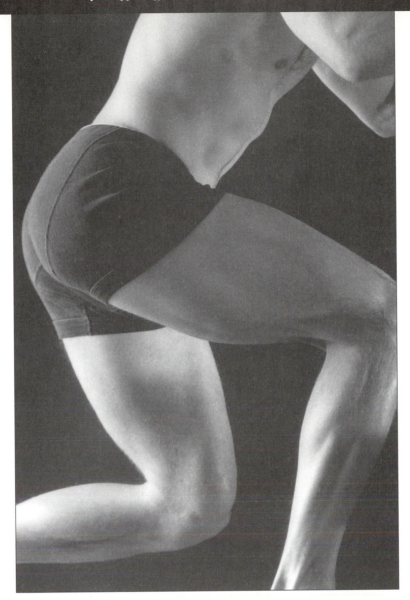

PART ONE

The Foundation

Working Out: The Truth

Why a Book on Lower Body Training

It's impossible to create a universal hierarchy of body parts, because everyone is different. If you had to prioritize what areas were most important to you, you would choose specific areas and have different reasons for your choices than someone else would. We chose to focus on the lower body after abs because of its significance in everyday wellness, because the subject is often filled with misconceptions and confusion, and because the butt and thighs are a major area of concern aesthetically. Almost everybody wants a great butt and great legs. There are thousands of aerobics classes, hundreds of exercises, and a score of routines that come out every month in health and fitness magazines attesting to this fact. It's hard to know where to begin, which classes to take, which exercises to do, and which routine to follow. The aim of this book is threefold: First, it compiles all the major lower body exercises in a single volume so you have a complete resource. Second, it compiles and organizes a comprehensive battery of routines to fit the needs of almost every exerciser. And finally, it teaches the exerciser the principles behind complete lower body development.

The Truth

The truth is: There are no shortcuts. The only way to strengthen and tone your butt, thighs, and calves is through a combination of consistent, focused exercises, a disciplined diet, and regular cardiovascular work such as running, biking, or rowing. The bright spot in the middle of this harsh reality is that once you know the truth, you can get what you want. A good plan is half the battle. *The Complete Book of Butt and Legs* maps out a step-by-step process to help you achieve your goals.

Your part of the bargain is to make the commitment. This shouldn't scare or intimidate you: Commitment doesn't mean signing away your life. A holistic workout program doesn't have to change your lifestyle. It doesn't have to turn you into a workout freak. But at some level it has to become a positive part of your lifestyle. The key to exercise is consistency over time. *You must be consistent.* It makes no sense to exercise three months and then take three months off. Set realistic goals and then follow them. You will be surprised at the benefits you receive from spending a small amount of time, three times a week, on your lower body. Your muscles will start to firm up, your posture will improve, and you will have more energy. Once the workout habit is established, you naturally will want to move to the next level of fitness. *Focus on how you feel and the aesthetics will follow.*

Myths and Facts

There are many misconceptions surrounding the lower body. Some of the devices that have been marketed over the years promising to trim the butt and thighs include plastic suits, the Thighmaster, girdles that you wear to the office, and machines that jiggle your butt. Here are some commonly believed myths surrounding the butt and thighs:

1. *If I stop exercising, all my muscle will turn to fat.*
   Muscle cannot turn into fat. Molecularly the two are as different as gold is to fool's gold (pyrite). If you stop exercising, your muscles will atrophy and decrease in size. They will not change to fat or anything else. However, when you stop working out you will burn fewer calories and you will store more fat. In other words, the muscles will shrink and you will gain weight.

2. *Using the butt machines at the gym will help me specifically reduce fat in my glutes (butt).*
   To an extent this statement is true. Such exercises will help decrease body fat—but not just in that area. Current theory shows that exercise stimulates fat reduction throughout the entire body, not in localized spots. You can't spot reduce specific areas. Tests done on tennis players show that their dominant arm (the arm they swing the racquet with) is bigger, with more muscle mass than their inactive arm, but has the same fat percentage. Similarly, if you focus your workout on your butt, that area will get stronger and firmer. You may have a firm butt, but no one will see it until you reduce the fat throughout your entire body. This is best accomplished through a combination of diet and well-rounded exercise.

3. *If I work out hard and often enough, I can get a butt and legs like a professional bodybuilder.*
   Professional bodybuilders are the exception rather than the rule. They are genetically predisposed for their sport, much like someone who is seven feet tall is genetically advantaged in basketball. Even bodybuilding champions don't look like Mr. or Ms. Olympia 365 days a year. They go through a strict precompetition routine that is extreme and may involve questionable health practices that can include the use of steroids, diuretics, excessively low-calorie diets, as well as extensive and dedicated workouts (up to six hours a day). Extreme dieting and dehydration give the "ripped" competition look that is nearly impossible to achieve without such measures. This look can be maintained for only short periods of time without severe health risks.

4. *I'm too old to have a firm butt and shapely legs.*
   Although studies indicate you may lose muscle mass as you become older, you can slow or reverse the process through exercise. There is no reason why you cannot improve the strength, flexibility, and overall appearance of your butt and legs no matter how old you are. The old adage "Use it or lose it" applies here. Most peo-

ple lose muscle mass because they stop exercising, not because they're old. They become sedentary. Depending on your present level of fitness, you can add muscle mass to some degree or another. Many dedicated athletes and bodybuilders who are now in their sixties still have the bodies of thirty-year-olds. You're never too old to receive the health benefits of exercise and to look great.

5. *The only way I can burn calories is in aerobics class or on the StairMaster.*
Although cardiovascular work is one of the most efficient ways to burn calories, you also burn calories by just existing. You may not receive a digital readout of how many calories you've burned after doing your squats or lunges, but you are still burning calories at an increased rate. The more muscle mass you have, the more calories you will naturally expend, because muscle is an active tissue. So, having more muscle mass will enable you to burn up more calories whether you are working out or just doing everyday activities. This doesn't mean you should neglect your cardio training; rather, you should aim for a balanced workout.

7. *My leg workout is really tough. I spend two hours at the gym working them out. And I still don't see the results I want.*
Although there are many variables involved in effective training, quantity (total volume) may be the least important. The most important concept is quality. The components that make up quality include: intensity of exercise, proper exercise technique, and correct training principles. This boils down to doing the right exercise the right way. It means being focused on each and every repetition, feeling every contraction. It *does not* mean doing your workout on automatic pilot.

8. *If I train my lower body with weights I will get muscular like a man.*
The possibility of a female developing large muscle mass is unlikely because women do not produce enough of the hormone (testosterone) and/or enzymes responsible for producing mus-

cle enlargement. On the other hand, improved tone and firmness cause the muscle to become slightly larger. This combined with a reduction in body fat will produce a more sleek and trim lower body. The look that female bodybuilders attain is the result of extreme training habits like those discussed earlier.

9. *If I bike, run, walk, use the StairMaster, etc., I don't need to do any additional leg training.*
Strength training is necessary for a complete fitness program. The specific advantages of leg training include: improved performance (increased strength both neuromuscular and structural), increased flexibility, and reduced potential for injury (improved bone density, increased strength in connective tissue, and joint integrity). All recreational activities and cardiovascular work are beneficial, but this alone will not bring you to your full fitness potential. Any successful program incorporates aerobic work, specific strength training, and diet for the best results.

10. *It's a waste of time for me to work out because I'll never look like a model.*
There are many benefits that can be gained from exercise other than a beautiful body, the most important being improved health. The latest longevity studies show that doing a little exercise can mean a lot. Research from the Adult Fitness Program at San Diego State University, which has been conducted over the last thirty-seven years, indicates that those who exercise two to three times a week (walking, jogging, biking, circuit training) have improved quality of life. This is measured by increased cardiovascular efficiency, increased muscular efficiency, and lower body fat. When you exercise, the most important thing to focus on is how you feel, not how you look. In short, doing a little exercise will improve your quality of life.

11. *I don't squat because it's bad for my knees.*
This exercise has a bad reputation because it is usually done incorrectly. The truth is (and recent studies support this) that, when done correctly, squatting is one of the most beneficial

exercises for leg development and joint (knee) integrity. The section on the squat (see pages 161–75) teaches the correct techniques and principles in detail. Unless you have a specific medical problem that prohibits it, you should be able to do one of the squat variations in this book. Squatting is an intense exercise, but a safe one. If it were easy, we'd all be squatting fools.

12. *I was born with cellulite, so I will never get rid of it.*

 Although an ounce of prevention is worth a pound of cure, cellulite can be controlled and reduced. The effects of this therapy are much more beneficial if administered before an individual is forty (because the skin is more responsive then), but benefits can be derived at any age. Therapy for cellulite reduction is a matter of fat reduction. The most effective way to lower body fat is proper diet and exercise.

13. *High-impact aerobics are the only way to trim my butt and thighs.*

 The most efficient way to burn fat is by doing low- to moderate-intensity activities over a longer period of time. When resting, the body's fuel of choice is fat. It just doesn't burn it at a high rate. Higher-intensity activities are going to burn stored carbohydrate calories (muscle glycogen and blood glucose) instead of metabolizing fat for energy. So doing low- to moderate-aerobic exercise, which can be safer, combined with specific resistance work for your butt and thighs, is an excellent way to achieve your goals.

The Complete Lower Body Philosophy

When surrounded by myths and misconceptions, what you need is a comprehensive program that fits your lifestyle. You need a complete lower body training program that will give you the results you want. The chapters that follow outline everything you need to know about training your lower body and give you a variety of routines and exercises to fit your individual requirements and goals, regardless of your fitness level. The concept of complete lower body training may sound intimidating. You might think you have to hire a personal trainer or have to be an expert in exercise physiology to use this system. Not true. This book is like having a personal trainer. It breaks down the process step-by-step, educating you along the way.

Body Basics: Anatomy

This chapter gives you an overall view of the structural components that make up the lower body and will help you understand how the muscles of the lower body work, thus improving your ability to successfully train.

There are numerous muscle groups that make up the butt and the lower body. These muscles control the movement of the lower body and either work independently or in some assisting capacity. Some of the exercises in Part 3 of this book will help you to train and isolate each of these muscle groups in order to strengthen areas of weakness or imbalance. Other exercises train two or more muscles at the same time so as to produce between the muscles a synergistic relationship that mimics daily movements or athletic endeavors.

Movement/Anatomy Guidelines

This chapter is divided into three basic sections: structural (skeletal), kinesiology (movement), and muscular. Each section includes descriptions and anatomical drawings to refer to when you embark on your workout routines.

STRUCTURAL (SKELETAL)

Osteology is a science that focuses on the study of the structural or skeletal system. The skeletal system of the lower body can be divided into the following three areas: hip, thigh, and shin. Each bone in the lower body is an organ that plays an integral part in the functioning of its immediate area as well as in the functioning of the overall skeletal system.

Functions: The skeletal system has five basic functions:

Support—Provides the structure and framework to which the muscles and organs of the body are attached.

Protection—Protects the essential components of the body (heart, lungs, brain, central nervous system, etc.).

Movement—Bones act as levers and joints as axes when the muscles contract.

Hemopoiesis—Bone marrow produces white blood cells, red blood corpuscles, and platelets.

Mineral storage—Bones and teeth store about 99 percent of the calcium and 90 percent of the phosphorus in the body.

HIP

The skeletal makeup of the hip consists of the pelvic girdle (see picture). The pelvic girdle and the ligaments associated with it support the mass of the body through the vertebral column and also protect vital organs.

Gender Difference: There are two significant characteristics that make the female pelvic girdle differ from the male and that may need to be addressed when considering workout technique:

• A female's whole pelvic girdle is tilted forward.
• A female's pelvis is wider.

Joint Type: The hip joint is a ball and socket joint formed by the head of the femur, or thighbone, joining the acetabulum— the cup-shaped socket—of the os coxa. This type of joint allows for the greatest range of movement. The joint is supported by a strong joint capsule, many ligaments, and several powerful muscles.

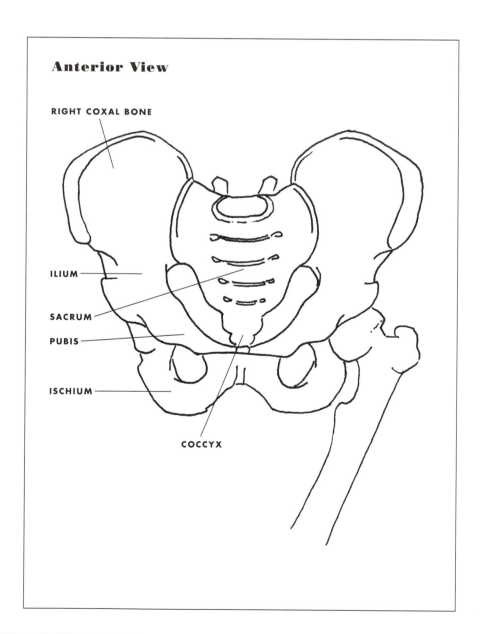

Anterior View

RIGHT COXAL BONE

ILIUM

SACRUM

PUBIS

ISCHIUM

COCCYX

THIGH

The femur, or the thighbone, is the longest, strongest, and heaviest bone in the body. The femur (see picture) unites with the acetabulum—the cup-shaped socket at the hipbone—at the proximal (closest) head of the bone, and with the tibia at the distal (farthest) end.

Gender Difference: In both sexes the femur is slightly curved inward in the middle so that it moves closer to the opposite thigh and the body's center of gravity. This convergence (moving together) is greater in the female because of the wider pelvis.

PATELLA

The patella—more commonly known as the kneecap—is positioned on the front (anterior) side of the knee joint (see picture). The main purposes of the patella are to protect the knee joint and to strengthen the quadriceps tendon.

Joint Type: The knee joint is classified as a hinge joint. This type of joint allows a large range of movement in one direction. Created by the juncture of the femur and the tibia, the patella is the largest and most complex joint in the body. In addition, it is probably the most vulnerable joint in the body. This is something you must consider when learning technique and when performing exercises. You can greatly reduce the potential for injury to the knee joint by following the guidelines set forth in this book.

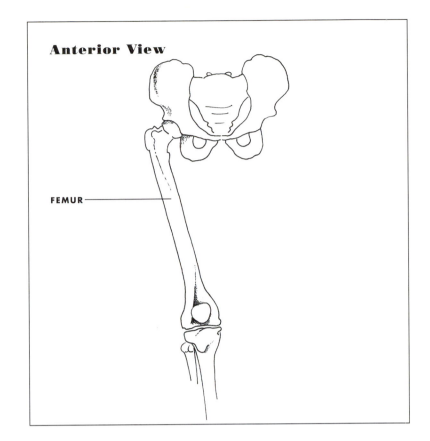

Anterior View

FEMUR

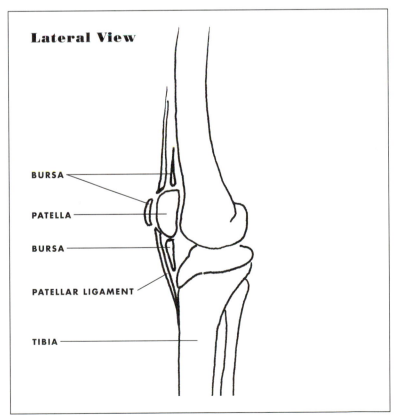

Lateral View

BURSA

PATELLA

BURSA

PATELLAR LIGAMENT

TIBIA

SHIN

The fibula and the tibia constitute the skeletal makeup of the lower leg, or shin (see picture). The tibia is located medially (inside) and is the larger of the two bones. The tibia also functions as the major load bearer. The fibula, located laterally (outside), is better suited for muscle attachment.

Joint Type: The ankle joint is actually made up of two joints, both of which are hinge joints. The basic movements of the ankle joint are plantar flexion (pointing your toes down) and dorsi flexion (flexing your toes up).

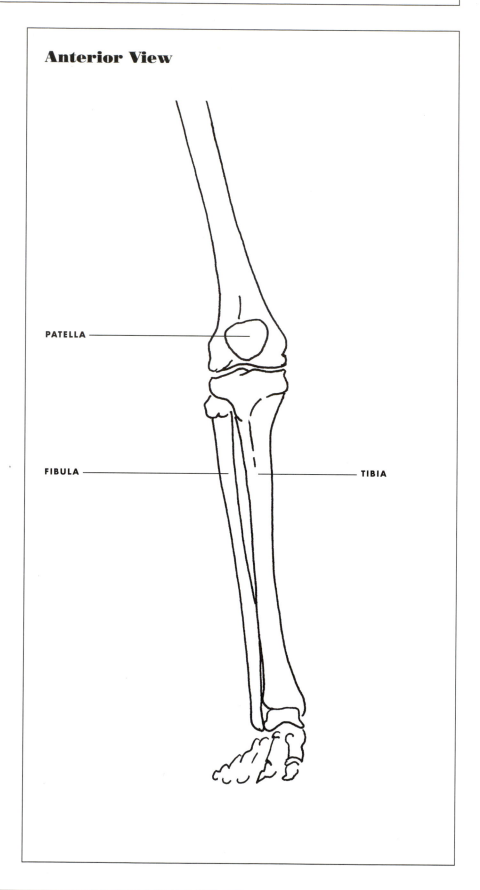

Anterior View

PATELLA

FIBULA — TIBIA

KINESIOLOGY

Kinesiology is the science of human movement. Understanding how your body moves—that is, which muscles contract and move specific lower body segments—will help you better visualize, and therefore enhance, the mind-muscle link.

Movement Terminology: Below are some basic definitions of various joint and muscle movements as they apply to lower body training:

Flexion—action of two adjacent body segments approaching each other; the angle of the joint decreases (e.g., Leg Curls).

Extension—opposite of flexion; the angle of the joint increases (e.g., Leg Extension).

Hyperextension—movement beyond normal extension (e.g., Knee Hyperextension).

Abduction—movement in the frontal plane away from the midline of the body (e.g., Leg/Hip Abduction).

Adduction—opposite of abduction; movement toward the midline of body (e.g., Leg/Hip Adduction).

Circumduction—movement of a body segment in a conelike or circular motion (e.g., Leg Circumduction).

Rotation—movement of a body segment in a rotary action around its longitudinal axis (e.g., internal and external rotation of the thigh).

Inversion—turning toe inward with weight on the outside of the foot.

Eversion—turning toe outward with weight on the inside of the foot.

Directional Terminology: Below are some directional terms that are used throughout this and other workout books.

Superior—the top; toward the top.

Inferior—the bottom; toward the bottom.

Anterior (ventral)—the front; toward the front.

Posterior (dorsal)—the back; toward the back.

Medial—toward the midline of the body.

Lateral—away from the midline of the body; the side of the body.

Proximal—nearer the principal mass of the body.

Distal—away from the principal mass of the body.

For positional terminology (i.e., foot positions) see pages 111–12.

The Muscular System: Skeletal, or striated, muscle comprises all of the muscles attached to the skeleton. It provides the force of movement for the bony, leverage system; or put more simply, striated muscle allows the bones of the body to move. Unlike muscles such as the heart, striated muscle acts voluntarily; it requires purposeful, conscious use. An example would be the rectus femoris (see illustration, page 13).

Skeletal Muscle Contractions: When following your exercise program there will be basically two types of muscle contractions:

Isometric—involves no joint movement, permitting maximum muscular contraction. Strength development is specific to 20 degrees on either side of the angle rather than through a full range of motion. Although tension does develop, no mechanical work is performed. This is also referred to as a "static" contraction.

Isotonic—involves limb or body movement throughout a full range of motion. The muscle either shortens or lengthens, resulting in mechanical work. There are three different types of isotonic contractions. (1) Concentric (positive) contractions involve a shortening of the muscle as resistance is overcome. An example of this would be the "ascending" phase of the Leg Extension (see page 138). (2) Eccentric (negative) contractions occur when the muscle lengthens. An example of this would be the "descending" phase of the Leg Extension. (3) Isokinetic contractions are contractions in which the speed of movement is controlled.

Muscle Action Terminology:

Prime mover—a muscle that is directly responsible for performing a movement (e.g., soleus during Seated Heel Raises).

Agonist—a concentric contraction resulting in joint action (e.g., rectus femoris during Leg Extension).

Antagonist—a muscle contracting in opposition to the agonist (e.g., biceps femoris during Leg Extension).

Synergist—a muscle that contributes to movement, but isn't the prime mover; a secondary mover (e.g., pectineus during Hip Adduction).

Fixator—a muscle that holds, or "fixes," a body part so that other muscles can function (e.g., hip flexors during Leg Extension or Leg Flexion).

Basic Properties of Muscle Function: Understanding the following basic properties of muscle function will help you train successfully as you read through this or any other workout book.

1. *Strength*—the ability of a muscle to exert and resist force; it is a measure of the amount of effort that a muscle can apply to a single contraction. Strength can be divided into two categories:

   a. Dynamic Strength—involves the application of force through a full range of motion. Strength of this nature predominates in most skills, and is achieved only through application of the S.A.I.D. and Overload principles (see pages 278 and 22).

   b. Static Strength—the maximum amount of resistance that may be overcome involving little or no joint movement. An example would be isometric training.

2. *Power*—the rate at which work is performed, combining strength and velocity. It is sometimes referred to as "explosive strength." An example would be the act of jumping.

3. *Muscular Endurance*—the ability to exert force submaximally—that is, not at maximum intensity—repeatedly over time. This is a very important component in that most training sessions involve repeated bouts of exercise.

4. *Hypertrophy*—an increase in size of muscle tissue.

5. *Hyperplasia*—when muscle fibers actually split and multiply in number.

6. *Atrophy*—the opposite of hypertrophy. It results from submaximal training levels (below 30 percent intensity) and from disease. An example of this would be the decrease in size of a limb that has been immobilized in a cast.

As mentioned, there are numerous muscles involved with the movement of the lower body. To simplify the potentially complex endeavor of training, we identify muscles in relationship to location (front, back, inside, outside, and lower) and to anatomical movement. This will also allow you to visualize how each muscle relates to its movement.

For each of the five areas of the lower body we include a picture of the muscles involved, a description of the muscles, and analysis of the muscle movement (refer to pages 13–19), as well as examples of exercises that train those specific muscles.

FRONT

Hip Flexion: Hip flexion involves the front/anterior portion of the thigh (see picture). It is the movement of the thigh toward the pelvis: lifting the leg, lifting the leg while running.

a. Rectus femoris.*
   Performance: flexion of the hip, knee extension: running, jumping.
b. Iliopsoas.
   Performance: hip flexion, lateral rotation of the thigh: leg lifts, running.
c. Sartorius.*
   Performance: flexion of the hip, flexion of the knee, slight lateral rotation of the thigh as it flexes the knee and hip: alternating straight leg raises, straight leg cable hip flexion.
d. Pectineus.
   Performance: flexion of the hip, hip adduction: straight leg cable hip flexion.
e. Tensor fasciae latae.
   Performance: flexion of the hip, horizontal abduction, inward rotation of the hip: leg raises with medial rotation of the thigh.

*Two-joint muscle, the knee and the hip.

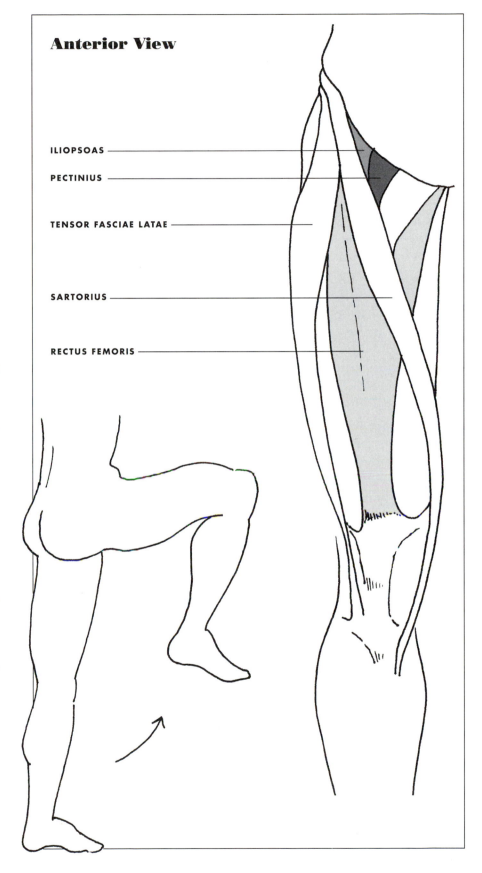

Anterior View

ILIOPSOAS

PECTINIUS

TENSOR FASCIAE LATAE

SARTORIUS

RECTUS FEMORIS

BACK

Hip Extension: Hip extension involves the back/posterior portion of the thigh and butt. It is the opposite of or return from flexion, ascending during the squat.

a. Biceps femoris.*
   Performance: extension of the hip, knee flexion, lateral rotation of the hip and knee: jumping, leg curls.
b. Semimembranosus.*
   Performance: extension of the hip, knee flexion, medial rotation of the hip and knee: stiff leg dead lift, leg curls.
c. Semitendinosus.*
   Performance: hip extension and knee flexion: walking.
d. Gluteus maximus.
   Performance: extension of the hip, outward rotation of the hip: lunge, squat, back extensions.

*Two-joint muscle, the knee and the hip.

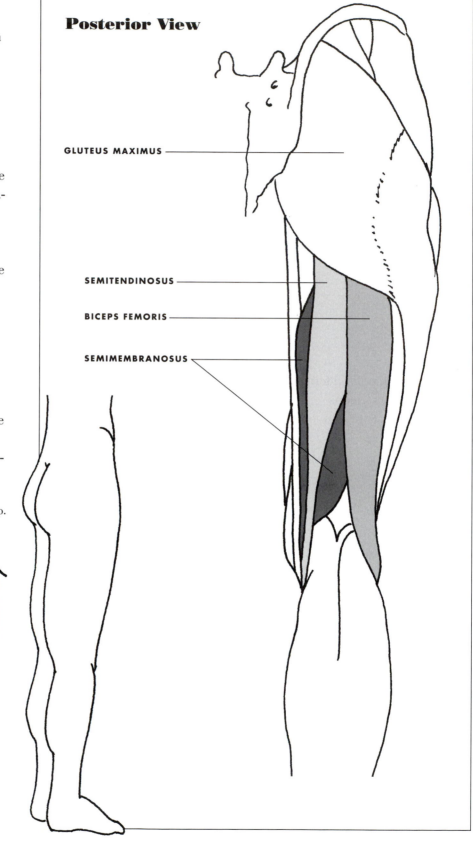

Posterior View

GLUTEUS MAXIMUS

SEMITENDINOSUS

BICEPS FEMORIS

SEMIMEMBRANOSUS

OUTSIDE

Leg Abduction: Leg abduction involves the outer/lateral portion of the thigh and butt. The leg moves away from the midline of the body in the frontal plane: abduction movement on four-way hip machine.

a. Gluteus medius. Performance: leg/hip abduction, medial rotation of the thigh: lateral changes in direction.

b. Gluteus minimus. Performance: hip/leg abduction, outward rotation of femur: speed skating.

c. Outward rotators— pyriformis, gemellus superior, gemellus inferior, obdurator externus, obdurator internus, and quadratus femoris. Performance: outward rotation of the hip: swinging a bat.

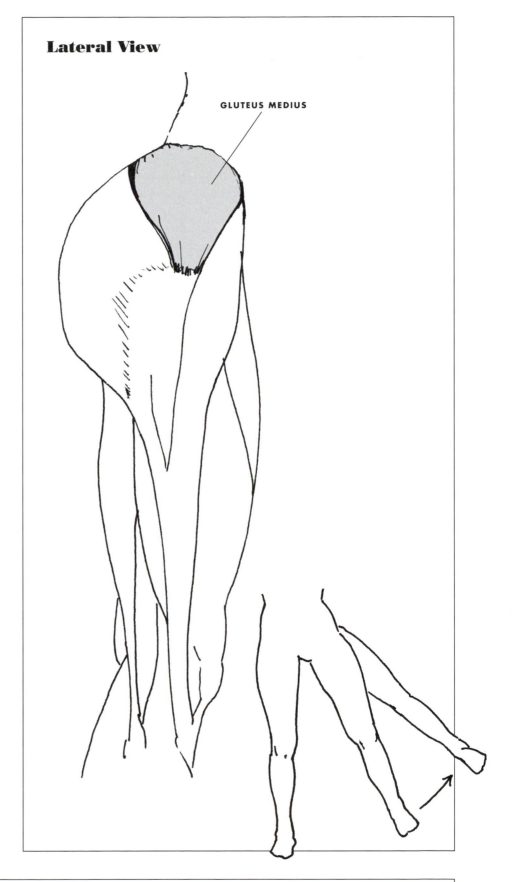

Lateral View

GLUTEUS MEDIUS

INSIDE

Leg Adduction: Leg adduction involves the inner part of the thigh. The leg moves toward the midline of the body (in the frontal plane), opposite of leg abduction: adduction movement on the four-way hip machine.

a. Adductor longus.
   Performance: hip/leg adduction, helps in hip flexion, cable leg adduction.
b. Adductor brevis.
   Performance: hip/leg adduction, rotation of the thigh outward: soccer-style kick.
c. Adductor magnus.
   Performance: hip/leg adduction.
d. Gracilis.
   Performance: crisscross stride.

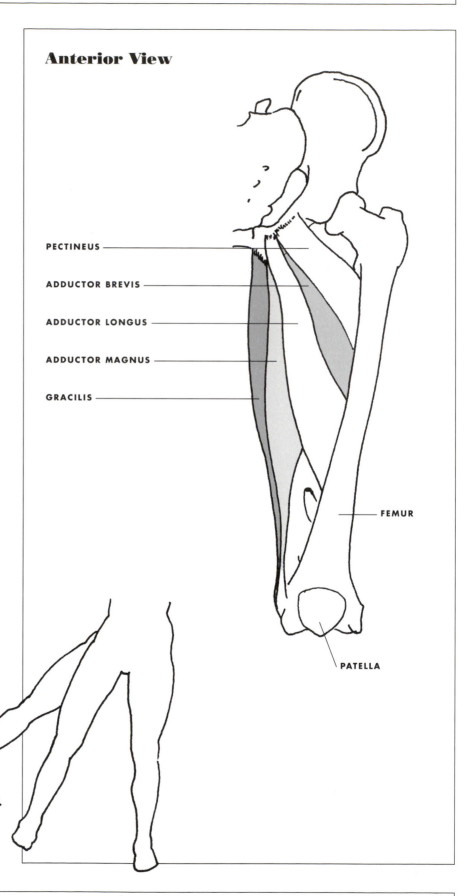

Anterior View

PECTINEUS

ADDUCTOR BREVIS

ADDUCTOR LONGUS

ADDUCTOR MAGNUS

GRACILIS

FEMUR

PATELLA

FRONT

Knee-Leg Extension: This movement involves the front part of the thigh to the knee. It is the straightening of the lower leg:

a. Rectus femoris.
   Performance: knee extension, hip flexion, kicking.
b. Vastus medius.
   Performance: extension of the knee, leg extension machine.
c. Vastus intermedius.
   Performance: jumping, lunge.
d. Vastus lateralis.
   Performance: running, squat.

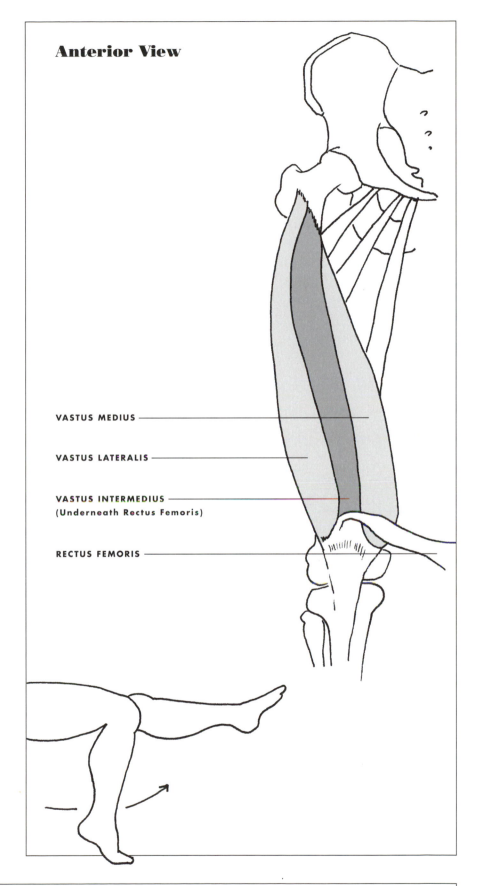

Anterior View

VASTUS MEDIUS

VASTUS LATERALIS

VASTUS INTERMEDIUS
(Underneath Rectus Femoris)

RECTUS FEMORIS

BACK

Knee-Leg Flexion: Knee-leg flexion involves the back part of the thigh. It is the movement of the heel toward the butt.

a. Biceps femoris.*
   Performance: knee flexion, extension of the hip, lateral rotation of the hip and knee: leg curls, running.
b. Semimembranosus.*
   Performance: knee flexion, extension of the hip, medial rotation of the hip and knee: standing leg curls.
c. Semitendinosus.*
   Performance: knee flexion, hip extension: walking.

*Two-joint muscle, the knee and the hip.

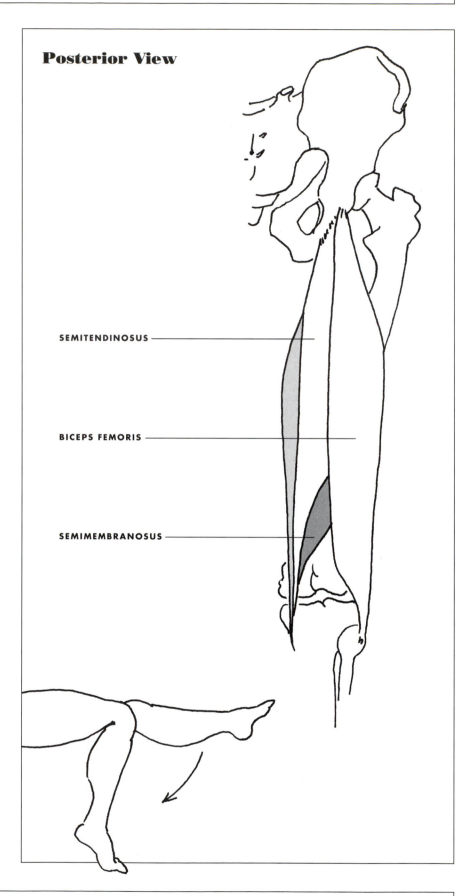

Posterior View

SEMITENDINOSUS

BICEPS FEMORIS

SEMIMEMBRANOSUS

LOWER

Plantar Flexion: Plantar flexion involves pointing your toes away from your shin (back part of the lower leg): heel raises.

a. Gastrocnemius.
   Performance: plantar flexion, knee flexion, jumping.
b. Soleus.
   Performance: plantar flexion, walking.

Dorsi Flexion: Dorsi flexion involves pulling your toes toward your shin (front part of lower leg): toe raises.

c. Tibialis anterior.
   Performance: dorsi flexion, toe raises.

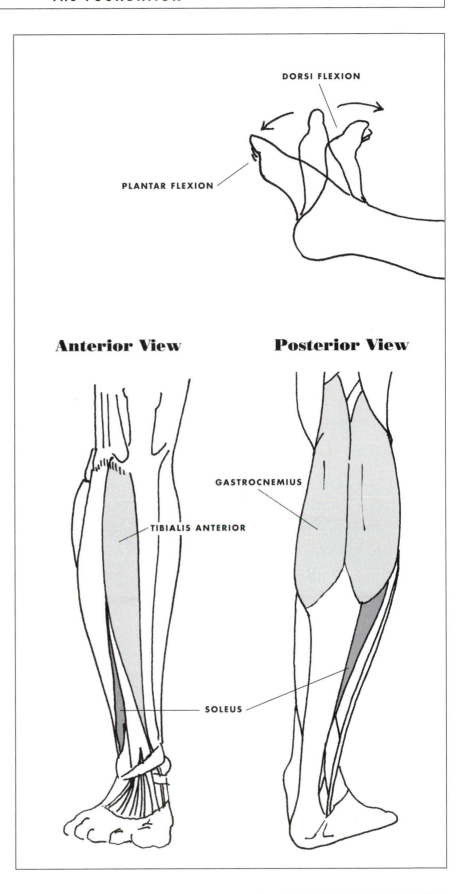

Anterior View   **Posterior View**

References

Abrian, Marlene, John M. Cooper, and Ruth B. Glassow. *Kinesiology.* 5th ed. St. Louis: C. V. Mosby Co., 1982.

O'Bryant, Harold, and Mike Stone. *Weight Training: A Scientific Approach.* 1st ed. Minneapolis: Burgess Publishing Co., 1984.

Proper Technique: The Body

Proper technique is essential to have a successful training program. It is important for two reasons: First, it provides the optimum results in the least amount of time. Second, proper technique decreases the chance of injury during training. This chapter contains important training principles essential for complete lower body development.

The Complete Butt and Leg Philosophy

To achieve successful lower body development, you need to train and condition all the muscles in your lower body. An unbalanced approach in lower body training will cause muscular imbalance and/or weakness. This can lead to structural problems and can also increase chance of injury during sports, exercise, and other favorite activities.

The lower body is a system that works synergistically. In most movements, one muscle group acts as the prime mover, another group works in an assisting capacity (secondary mover), while a third provides stabilization. If you don't train for development, one or two of the muscle groups will not perform optimally and overall performance will suffer. To achieve your full potential you must train not only the entire lower body, but the whole body, with a balanced program.

STARTING OUT

The most frequently asked questions when beginning a training program are: "What should I do?", "How much should I do?", and "Where should I start?" There is no single, correct answer to these. Every person is different. *You must intelligently experiment to find the answers.* Let's address these questions separately.

"What should I do?" You should include exercises that will train all the muscle groups in the body. This book targets the lower body but by no means should you limit your training to the legs and butt only.

"How much should I do?" When starting out you should do just enough to promote fatigue, no more. Your total exercise volume (sets and reps) should be minimal, perhaps no more than one set with fifteen to twenty repetitions for each selected exercise. This will eliminate the negative physical and mental effects of excessive muscular soreness and will decrease the potential for injury from fatigue and lack of concentration.

"Where should I start?" The following two principles will help you determine a proper starting place:

• When learning a new exercise, use minimal intensity (if possible) and perform it while you are fresh.
• Once you have mastered the exercise technique, increase the intensity (weight) gradually until you can no longer perform the movement for the prescribed number of repetitions, or until you have a breakdown in proper technique. After this happens, drop back to the previous, lighter weight. This will be your starting point. When experimenting with finding a starting weight, perform no more than three sets per exercise, per session.

This may sound tedious, but remember that technique is the key to success. Be patient; proper execution of your exercises is not only safer, but the results will be greater in the long run.

The Basic Principles

OVERLOAD AND PROGRESSION

For a muscle to get stronger it must be overloaded. Overloading means subjecting your muscles to more stress than they are accustomed to. Overloading muscles can be accomplished in two ways, both progressive. First, add volume. This is done by increasing the repetitions per set, adding sets, or by adding additional exercises for that muscle group. Second, increase the intensity of training: this can be accomplished by increasing the resistance (adding weight or doing a more difficult exercise) or by decreasing the rest time between sets and exercises. These forms of progressive overloading should be done separately (*either* increase volume *or* intensity), but may on occasion be done simultaneously. When both are done simultaneously, you increase the chance of overtraining.

FULL RANGE OF MOTION

It is important to perform all exercises with the prescribed full range of motion. This is especially true for sports performance. Most performance skills are dynamic (in motion); therefore your muscles need to be strengthened throughout their full range of motion. To do this you must maintain resistance on the muscles throughout the prescribed range of motion.

SPEED OF MOVEMENT

The speed at which you do an exercise is an important part of a successful training program. Generally, movement should be slow and controlled through the negative (eccentric) phase. The positive, or concentric, phase of the movement should be as explosive as possible without creating momentum, keeping constant tension on the muscles.

As you reach advanced levels of training, it is important to vary the speed of the exercise to achieve peak development. The basic concepts behind speed of movement are described on pages 107–08.

CONSTANT TENSION

During a movement you must maintain constant tension on the muscle, feeling its contraction throughout the full range of motion. Do not let momentum take over; feel the muscle do the work at every phase of the movement. In addition, when using a machine do not allow the weight stacks to touch, as this would eliminate constant tension.

CHOICE OF EXERCISE

Selecting exercises is a key component in the design of any training program. The following criteria are essential when considering which exercise to choose:

- Specificity (training for specific results)
- Injury prevention, or muscle balance
- Available equipment
- Goals
- Time

WORKOUT LENGTH

The length of a training session is dependent on sets and reps, what type of exercise you do, how much rest time you take, and what your goals are. Another variable that determines workout length is intensity. High-intensity work will increase the need for recovery time, possibly increasing total workout length. Depending on your goals you may spend anywhere between ten minutes to two hours working out your legs. Part 4 ("The Routines") offers a wide variety of routines to fit your needs and goals.

FREQUENCY OF TRAINING

Frequency of training is dependent upon many variables, including your recovery time, your level of experience, your work or competition schedule, and your goals. Recovery time is important because strength gains and muscle growth occur during these periods. If recovery time is not adequate between workouts, your strength gains will not be optimal, and the result could be overtraining.

EXERCISE ORDER

There are many factors to consider when choosing exercise order. Your individual weak areas, sport-specific routines, and personal level of fitness are some of the considerations.

Generally, exercises are completed in an order that moves from the highest energy expenditure to the lowest, especially when starting out. Or another way of explaining it: Work from the largest muscles to the smallest muscles.

THE ROUTINES

To a large extent, the problems of exercise order are already worked out for you in the routines in part four. But as you progress, you will reach a stage when you must decide what variations you need in order to get peak results. You will have to determine your own genetic strengths and weaknesses, how you want to look, and then will have to choose the exercises that will accomplish this fine-tuning. As with everything else in life, at some point you will be left alone to face the truth about your butt and legs. But have no fear, you won't fall into the butt abyss. Chapter 26, "Creating Your Own," will guide you safely through this existential experience!

WARM-UP

It is always important to warm up your body before exercising. This prepares your body for action in two main ways:

1. Warming up increases muscle blood flow and increases general muscle metabolism. This makes the muscles perform more efficiently.
2. Warming up allows the muscles to contract with more force and with greater speed due to an increase in muscle temperature. If the muscles are warm, contraction will be optimal. This reduces the chances of injury and positively affects performance.

When a warm-up for strength training is undertaken it should proceed from general to specific. For a specific warm-up routine, refer to pages 99–102.

BREATHING

As in all exercise, proper breathing is essential. The breathing technique to use for resistance training is as follows:

1. Inhale before the start of the negative contraction, when you are moving against the least resistance.
2. Exhale during the last two-thirds of the positive contraction.

For example, when performing the Squat you would inhale before you lower your body and exhale as you raise back up.

INTENSITY

Intensity is a complex subject. For our purposes, intensity means the amount of energy output it takes to complete an exercise. Intensity can be increased or decreased by choosing easier or more difficult exercises and by adding or subtracting weight. In each workout you should aim for an intensity level that will produce muscular exhaustion in the prescribed number of repetitions.

VARIETY

Variation is often the most neglected training principle. People get comfortable in a routine and don't want to change. We are creatures of habit. But the body thrives on both structure and change. You will start on a routine and get hooked into the structure of it. This will be a growth period. You will see gains in one or more of the following areas: strength, endurance, and/or body appearance. But after a period of time, your body will adapt to this routine and plateau. This means it's time for a change. The body wants something new. It needs a new routine for challenge, adaptation, and growth.

Variation also removes the boredom and monotony in training. And hitting the muscles from a variety of angles gives better overall development. The routines in Part 4 have variety built into them and you can use them as a model when you are ready to create your own routine.

REPETITIONS

A repetition is the completion of an entire movement of an exercise. If an athlete performs ten squats, he or she has completed ten repetitions. Repetitions are commonly referred to as reps.

SET

A set is a series of consecutive repetitions. If you perform ten repetitions of Leg Curls, then rest, and then perform another ten repetitions, you have performed two sets of ten repetitions (2×10).

HOW MUCH DO I AIM FOR?

The number of repetitions and sets you do depends on your fitness level and your goals. There are no hard-and-fast rules. Professional bodybuilders and top athletes get results using a wide variety of routines, differing numbers of sets, reps, and exercises. Train as hard and as frequently as you can without overtraining.

Chapter 26, "Creating Your Own," will give you intelligent guidelines for achieving these goals and for meeting your individual needs.

Overtraining: As mentioned, overtraining simply means doing too much and not giving yourself enough rest. It means you have worked the muscle too often and too intensely without giving it enough time to repair itself. It is the same as being overworked at the office. You become less efficient and start to burn out. Sometimes less is more. It is easy to push yourself too hard, to become critical, always wanting more and more. Training shouldn't become an unhealthy obsession. Remember, the purpose of exercise is to improve the quality of your life (mentally and physically), not just your physical appearance. Be patient, train wisely, and enjoy every repetition. Get into the process, not just the results.

QUALITY OF THE REP

The most important element in training is not quantity but quality. Don't sacrifice technique for more weight. Concentrate on quality and technique; keep your technique strict and go through the prescribed range of motion on each repetition. Feel the contraction of each rep, keeping constant tension on the muscles throughout the movement. *Indulge* in each and every repetition.

REST PERIODS DURING WORKOUTS

The purpose of a rest period between sets is to recover for the next set. In general, you should keep your rest time as short as possible. But again, this depends on your goals and your fitness level. Beginners need more rest time. High-intensity training generally requires more rest time.

PAIN

An important aspect of working out is getting in touch with your body. Part of this journey is learning to distinguish between "good" pain and "bad" pain; so be smart and listen to your body.

Good pain is the feeling of being pumped, of having the muscle fill with blood. And yes, even that burning sensation that comes from lactic acid buildup is a good pain. This signals fatigue in the muscle or muscles you are working, which is the goal of exercise. These are feelings you will learn to thrive on and may even come to regard as pleasurable.

Bad pain is a warning sign. It means you've injured yourself. When you feel bad pain, stop immediately. If you have any doubts, it's better to play it safe and stop the workout. Don't risk injury. If you have lower back problems, this is something you must be very careful about. Be aware of your lower back at all times. Warning signs are sharp pains, spasms, and periphery pain that moves into your legs, arms, feet, and hands. Don't push yourself through bad pain. Rather, take time off, see a doctor if the pain persists, or switch to exercises that won't cause such problems. See Chapter 6 for more about the lower back and preventing injury.

SORENESS

Muscle soreness is common after a workout. Don't worry if you're a little sore (good pain). Soreness may be caused by microscopic tears in muscle tissue. These need recuperation time and proper nutrition for repair. If you are too sore to train during your next session, you have overdone it. Most of the time it is good to train lightly through soreness, as increased blood flow will help the area. Train hard and train smart. Exercise is for a lifetime.

References

Brungardt, Brett. "Spring and Summer Four Week Mini Cycles." *National Strength & Conditioning Association Journal,* vol. 7, no. 5 (December/ January 1986), 34–35.

O'Bryant, Harold, and Mike Stone. *Weight Training: A Scientific Approach.* 1st ed. Minneapolis: Burgess Publishing Co., 1984.

CHAPTER FOUR

Proper Technique: The Mind

Medicine and academia separate the world into specializations and subjects. We separate the body into parts: abs, butt and legs. This is not the truth. Such separation is done for emphasis and is, to a degree, arbitrary and subjective. The body is whole. It works synergistically (the whole is greater than the sum of its parts). It works as a system, each part interdependent with another. The goal is balance and synchronicity. But sometimes the body falls out of balance. So you need to isolate and train weak areas. Ultimately, the goal is understanding how your body works as a whole.

Two important aspects of the whole that are often neglected when training the body are the brain (intellect) and the mind (consciousness). These two elements create the triad of training: body, brain, and mind. This chapter gives you techniques to exercise the brain, and mind, marshaling their powers for the training of your body. This chapter will be broken down in the broad categories of brain (what your linear intellect must do), body (how the physical system works), and mind (how your consciousness can help you achieve your goals).

The Brain

For our purposes, there are three key roles of the brain when working out. The first role is planning or creating the proper routine (most of that work is done for you in this book). The second role is goal setting. Ultimately you alone are responsible for setting your goals, because only you know what you want. The good news is that we're not asking you to make a difficult life choice. More simply, you only need to choose the butt and legs you want. The third role of the brain is its relationship to motivation. Motivation often comes from deep emotional places where the intellect doesn't dare go. But motivation is so central to your success that you need to use your brain and seek it out.

GOAL SETTING

You must have a goal. What do you want to look like? How do you want to feel? Do you have a time frame in which to accomplish these aspirations? You must write these goals down. Remember, *a goal is not a goal unless it is written down.* Reread your goals every day. There's no use writing them down if you don't read them daily. Read them on days when you're excited about working out. And especially, read them on days when you're dragging, when the last thing you want to do is work out. Voice them out loud. Own your goals; take responsibility for them.

When making goals, you will find the following format useful. It is important to have long-term, intermediate, short-term, and daily goals.

Long-Term Goals: Write down where you would like to be a year from now. Be specific. For example, one goal might be having more defined thighs or buns of steel. You might have a picture from a magazine of how you want to look. Cut it out and paste it next to the written goal.

Intermediate Goals: Write down goals for where you want to be six months from now. If you consistently work your butt and legs for six months, you can accomplish some very noticeable improvements, so set high goals.

Short-Term Goals: Write down goals for where you want to be one month from now. Every month you need to update these goals, always keeping in mind the end result you want in six months or a year. Examples of short-term goals you might wish to attain would be: losing a certain amount of weight or body fat, achieving a certain degree of firmness and definition, developing a certain amount of strength and endurance.

Daily Goals: For each day set at least two goals. You can plan the night before or in the morning before you start your day. Take a few minutes to write down your daily goals. These tasks should be geared toward helping you to achieve your overall goals. Be specific about each task. You should not only include what the task is, but at what time it will be performed. For example, on Monday your daily tasks might be: (1) Work out legs: lift and StairMaster (specific program) at 6 P.M., and (2) Salad and a whole wheat roll for lunch. This strategy will give you a specific plan designed to help you accomplish your short-term, intermediate, and long-term goals.

Setting goals is one thing; following through is another. Many times people get discouraged and lose interest. If things don't progress as quickly as you want, there is a tendency, often subconscious, to quit. The rest of this chapter gives you tools to fight this tendency.

MOTIVATION

Motivation is a key component for the success of an exercise program. It is the primary reason most people hire personal trainers. They just can't do it by themselves. There are hundreds of motivational self-help books and infomercial gurus with celebrity endorsements and money-back guarantees.

All that we will say on this subject is, Take your motivation wherever you can get it. Order the infomercial tapes; read the books; let sports heroes push you to the next level; cut out pictures in magazines (movie stars and models); be inspired by old loves or new loves; use anger (lift it and run it right out of your body); train for an upcoming vacation; or just indulge in exercise as a good in itself.

You need constant motivation because there are no shortcuts. Your only hope is in developing a work ethic. Never give up. Love the struggle. It may be the only lifelong friend you'll ever have.

The Body

It is not necessary to read an exercise physiology text to get the most out of your workout. Instead, it is helpful to have a general insight as to what takes place from a neuromuscular standpoint when you perform a resistance exercise. Understanding how your body operates should enhance your ability to integrate the physical and mental processes involved in exercise into a single, mind-body effort.

If we were to take a particular exercise for the butt and legs and analyze it from a neuromuscular standpoint, it would obviously be a very complex sequence of events. So, we will analyze the Squat (in a simplified manner), giving you a basic idea of the main principles that are involved in the movement.

In the downward phase of the Squat your neuromuscular system tells the motor units that form the knee extensors and hip extensors to perform an eccentric contraction (lengthening of the muscle). The lower portion of the hamstrings are told not to contract so as not to inhibit the motion.

On the upward phase of the lift, the neuromuscular system tells the motor units of the knee extensors and hip extensors to perform a concentric contraction and at the same time tells the motor units of the upper hamstrings to perform a concentric contraction to assist you upward. The knee flexors are told not to contract. There are numerous other things taking place in the neuromuscular system while all of this is happening. The sensory nerves are sending feedback to the central nervous system, which in turn monitors and controls such things as balance and posture.

In performing the Squat, realize that the mind has a vision of that particular movement and therefore will initiate and monitor the movement. If, however, you have performed this movement before, you have already created motor pathways in your neuromuscular system to duplicate this movement. Therefore, the blueprint, or circuitry, already exists to fire the appropriate motor units at the appropriate times; this completes the lift correctly (or incorrectly if you have performed it wrong in the past). Just like a computer, what you program is what you get. The old adage "garbage in, garbage out" is true. If you program correctly you will get the desired results. However, it is common for people to program for failure. Many times this is because there are so many experiences of failure recorded in our brain. To avoid this, always practice and visualize perfection. Practice doesn't make perfect. Perfect practice makes perfect.

The Mind

We have discussed above the principles involved with the body to give you a better understanding of what takes place from a neuromuscular standpoint when you perform an exercise. Knowing this, you can better perform visualization techniques and develop mind-body strategies to improve your movements.

At George Williams College a series of experiments were performed to determine the "psychologic" influences on human strength. In these experiments arm strength was measured under normal conditions. It was also measured while the subject screamed loudly, after a loud noise, under the influence of alcohol and amphetamines, and under hypnosis (in which the subjects were told they were stronger). All of these cases generally increased strength above normal levels. The greatest increases resulted from hypnosis, which was the inducement most focused on the mind, or consciousness. This is similar to what can happen using visualization techniques.

In another experiment, which involved free-throw shooting in basketball, sixty novice basketball players were divided into three groups of twenty each. Each group was tested in shooting free throws. Over the next two weeks one group practiced shooting a specified number of free throws for a specified time every day; another group avoided basketball over the next two weeks; and the third group visualized shooting free throws in the same manner that the first group actually practiced shooting for those two weeks. At the end of the two-week period all three groups were retested. The group that neither visualized nor practiced free throws did not improve, but the group that visualized improved almost as much as the group that actually practiced shooting free throws. What does this tell us? It doesn't tell us that we will improve our strength or muscle tone by visualizing, but it does indicate that we can improve our exercise abilities and performance by utilizing visualization techniques. This, of course, can be used in all of our activities, not just in exercise.

RELAXATION

It is common knowledge that there are many benefits to be derived from relaxation. It reduces stress and rejuvenates the body. It is also necessary for effective visualization. You will learn two basic relaxation skills in this section: controlled breathing and progressive relaxation.

Controlled Breathing: One way to achieve a relaxed state is by concentrating on your breathing. Settle into a comfortable position—lying down or sitting—and focus on inhaling and exhaling for approximately one minute. Then start to inhale on a count of five and exhale on a count of five, until you feel that your breathing pattern is smooth and regular. Next, focus on feeling the air coming into your lungs and imagine it being transported and suffused into every cell of your body. Every time you breathe out, let any negative thoughts or feelings you might have leave your body with the breath. And each time you breathe in, imagine the air purifying and energizing your body. If it helps, imagine the air entering your body as a white cleansing light. Continue this process until you feel a release of muscular tension, a decreased heart rate, rhythmic, calm breathing, and a feeling of being "centered." Now you are ready for visualization and positive programming.

Progressive Relaxation: Using this technique is a way to consciously program your body to relax. Settle into a comfortable position, either lying or sitting, take a couple of deep breaths, and slowly exhale, giving your body the message to relax. Next, feel where your body is making contact with the floor or the chair. If you're lying down, feel your heels, buttocks, shoulders, and head touching the floor. Then move your focus down to your feet. Send a message of relaxation to the little muscles on the soles of your feet and across the top of your feet. Move up to your calves, and tell your calf muscles to relax. Move up to your thighs and hamstrings and tell them to relax. Go to the muscles of your buttocks, telling them to relax. Then move to your lower back, middle back, and upper back, giving each portion of your back the message to relax. Then send the message one by one to your shoulders, arms, hands, chest, and stomach. Relax your neck, head, face, and throat. Tell all the little muscles around your eyes, cheeks, and jaws to relax. Finally, tell your forehead and scalp to relax. After you have given your entire body, part by part, the message to relax, allow yourself to enter deeper and deeper into a state of relaxation with each breath, giving in to gravity and melting into the floor.

When you have reached a desired level of relaxation you are ready for visualization and positive programming.

To bring yourself out of this state, simply say, "On a count of three I will open my eyes, feel relaxed and have a reserve of energy, and be ready to go on with my day." This technique is also good to practice with a partner; have him or her talk you through the process.

In practicing this technique it is important that you tune in to your body; thus you become more aware of when you are tense, which often leads to the discovery of hidden tension. Consciousness is the first step toward change. Start to become aware of specific and habitual tension areas so you can consciously relax them.

CUE WORDS

After you feel totally relaxed, give yourself a cue that you can use later when you need to relax more quickly. The cue can be something physical such as making a circle with your thumb and index finger, or a phrase such as "be, be, be." This cue can be used at any time to help you relax. Eventually, with practice, you will be able to get the full effect of the progressive relaxation by just saying or thinking the cue words.

VISUALIZATION

In a nutshell, visualization is the creation of mental pictures. At an unconscious level you are constantly creating images. These pictures program and create your self-image. The goal of visualization is to consciously create positive images that will help you achieve the goals you want.

To get the butt and legs you want, you must be able to see them in your mind's eye. Your model could be a picture from a magazine, the way you looked a few years ago, someone you saw on the beach, or any combination of these images. What's important is that you create a specific image of the way you want your lower body to look. It is important to keep an element of truth and realism in your picture. Create an image that fits your genetic type and potential. Create a picture you can believe in, not one that is impossible. Your picture can change and evolve and refine itself. You are not locked in to one image forever.

When you create an image, picture, or scene it is important to see everything with vivid detail. The more vivid the visualization, the more effective it will be. It is essential to use sensory details. Imagine the definition in your lower body. What do your butt and legs look like? See the separation of the muscles. See the color of your skin. Make the snapshot of your ideal butt and legs as clear as possible.

It is also important to imagine how this new body will make you feel. Feel the tightness in your butt and legs, the hardness of the muscles. See how others react to them. Walk down the beach with them. In your mind's eye, see your lover's response.

To effectively visualize, you must practice every day (or night), not just when you feel like it. Any negative aspects existing in the subconscious have taken years to formulate and cannot be changed overnight. However, with a consistent visualization strategy you can begin to change these negative aspects and program for success and the body you want.

Preworkout Visualization: A preworkout visualization is a way to get you into your body, leaving behind the stresses and the thoughts of the day. This is your time to be self-indulgent and to focus in on your body. It is a time to motivate yourself and push toward a second wind with focus. This visualization can take two to five minutes depending on how rough your day was.

Just as you have to warm up the body before you work out, you also have to warm up the mind. This visualization is a mental warm-up. Lie on the floor or sit in a chair and practice a breathing and relaxation technique of your choice. Then take a quick inventory of how you want your body to look, in order to hook your mind in to your goals and to psych yourself up for a workout. Tune in to your body by hearing the sound of your heart beating and by feeling your blood push through your veins. The body makes a lot of noise if you listen. Then start to imagine a power surging up in your body. Imagine yourself leaping up in the air with the explosion of Michael Jordan or Mikhail Baryshnikov. Feel the power in your legs. Then imagine a few of the exercises you have in your workout. Feel your body drive and explode through the weight. Feel your muscle, like coiled springs, driving the weight. See yourself performing the exercise with perfect form. Then imagine your body with the power and sleekness of an animal whose prowess impresses you. Feel that power in your body. Stay in the body and feel the power and energy surge. Then on a count of three open your eyes; you are ready to push through an amazing workout!

Visualization Technique to Improve Your Lifting Performance: When working out you don't have a lot of time to do an extensive relaxation. The following technique can be used to achieve a degree of relaxation.

Let us take the Squat and apply a technique to help you improve your performance. This technique can be especially helpful when trying to perform a one-rep max or to lift more weight than you have before. The visualization can be used with any exercise, but remember: Always use proper technique with any lift to prevent injury.

Close your eyes and perform your cue (physical or phrase). Inhale deeply for a count of five. As you inhale through your nose, imagine a beam of light entering your head and emitting energy. On the fifth count lift your chin and try to breathe in a little more into the upper chest. Hold for two counts. Exhale slowly through the nose for a count of five. As you exhale imagine all negativity leaving your body.

Now imagine that you are walking over to the bar and taking ten pounds off each side of the bar. "See" yourself take the weight off. "Feel" yourself take the weight off. The bar is now twenty pounds lighter! Now imagine yourself approaching the bar and taking it off the rack. Notice how light it feels. "See" and "feel" yourself setting your feet and performing the number of repetitions you wish to perform—perfectly. When you have completed this visualization tell yourself you are relaxed, energized, and ready to perform. Count to five and open your eyes. Shake out your arms and legs to energize your body. Now go and perform what you just visualized.

LETTING GO

One problem that many people have in performing a physical activity is that they often become immersed in trying to think themselves through the activity while they are actually performing the activity. Thinking so often destroys a person's timing. It also can destroy the relaxation needed for the body to perform optimally. Tension can often create a situation where the antagonist muscles (muscles on the other side of the joint being exercised) work against the agonist muscles (the actual muscles we wish to use). This obviously hinders performance. To avoid this you must develop a habit of letting go and trusting your ability. You have visualized success. You have programmed yourself for success. You must now allow what you have programmed to take over. Remember: Once the action starts, the thinking stops. This is not easy. We tend to want to analyze ourselves as we perform, but you must overcome the habit of trying to think yourself through the movement. This is as important as any principle we have discussed. *Don't worry about success when in action.* Even if you fail, the sun will still come up tomorrow, and you can always correct mistakes in the future.

PROGRAMMING POWER PHRASES

Power programming is the creation of an affirmation phrase that will help push you to achieve your goals. This phrase doesn't have to be detailed. But it must be evocative enough to eliminate negative thoughts. Phrases such as "I will prevail" or "I am right on track" are examples of power phrases. Get into the habit of using them extensively, especially when you feel doubts or negative thoughts creeping into your mind. Everyone experiences these doubts. People who succeed fight through their doubts, no matter how extreme they may be. They continue to move forward. Every person has the ability to overcome these negative thoughts and doubts, but many people give in to them. Applying visualizations and affirmations will greatly enhance your chances of overcoming this negative programming.

Putting the Mind in the Muscle in Your Workout

If we are to accept the premise that the mind and the body are essentially one, then it becomes imperative that we put the mind in the muscle to improve our workout. Bodybuilders tend to be particularly adept at

focusing on the exact muscles they are working and feeling those muscles in their contractions. This is important because it allows you to more effectively use and develop that muscle. This also improves your kinesthetic awareness of your body in motion, thus improving coordination.

When you exercise you need to feel the exact muscle you are emphasizing go through its concentric (shortening) and eccentric (lengthening) contraction. Before you exercise visualize that muscle. Make it burn. Feel it burn. When you have completed this visualization tell yourself you are relaxed, energized, and ready to perform. Count to five and open your eyes.

You have now programmed the proper movement. Now perform the exercise and focus on making the exact muscle you visualized burn. Put your mind in the muscle. Like anything else it will take practice to perfect your ability to make this mind-muscle link. Some people seem to have a natural kinesthetic awareness and therefore make the link easily, but if you consistently work at it, you too will make the mind-body link. Be consistent. Try to make the link in every exercise, every time you work out.

Pushing For and Through Good Pain

As stated in Chapter 3, there is a difference between good pain and bad pain. To have the most effective workout possible you must exercise through the good pain. This is difficult for many people because it is not a comfortable experience; yet it is the essence of moving into the principles of progression and overload (see page 22). You must fatigue the muscle to get maximum results. Of course, the amount of fatigue you are striving for depends on several variables such as your goals, your present state of physical health, and sometimes what your body is telling you on that particular day. Ideally, you want to be able to push yourself into good pain on every exercise without forfeiting proper technique. This requires a mental toughness on your part to continue to exercise even though you are experiencing fatigue.

In order to motivate yourself through good pain it is wise to begin each exercise session with a quick relaxation (as described above) and then to program yourself with power phrases. Repeat your power phrase every time you feel fatigue or good pain. Once again, consistency in this approach will help you to establish good habits and the toughness you desire.

Closing Out Your Workout

It is important to acknowledge your victories after every exercise session. At the end of each session, go through your relaxation technique and then acknowledge your accomplishments. Even if you feel you've had a bad workout it is important to realize that you still worked out and that, in and of itself, is a victory. Recognize that fact and pat yourself on the back for at least pushing through the workout even though it wasn't exactly what you had hoped for. Also pat yourself on the back for taking a day off when you feel like it, for listening to your body, and not pushing yourself, in a type A manner, into the common syndrome of over-training. Tomorrow's another day and the only way to prepare for success is to set yourself on a positive path. Remember, you can succeed, you will succeed, you have prepared yourself to avoid failure.

The mind is the great motivator. The power of the mind will allow you to push past your preconceived limits. This is what will take you to the next level. You have to create a vision and work toward it every day. The power of the mind allows you to harness your untapped potential, taking you to the next level, and to push to places you have never been. First, create a vision. Then work toward it, step-by-step, every day. The most effective way is to have the body, the brain, and the mind in harmony.

References

Huang, Chungliang Al, and Jerry Lynch. *Thinking Body, Dancing Mind.* New York: Bantam Books, 1992.

Kellner, Stan. *The Strength Kit.* 2nd ed. Aspen, Co.: Strength Advantage, 1990.

McArdle, William D., Frank I. Katch, and Victor L. Katch. *Exercise Physiology.* 2nd ed. Philadelphia: Lea & Febiger, 1986.

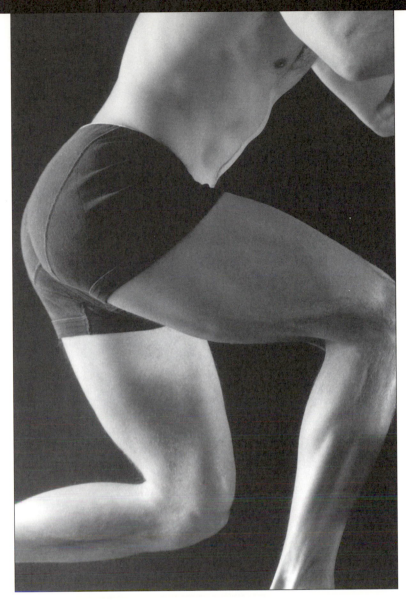

PART TWO

Wellness

CHAPTER FIVE

Power Nutrition

BY BECKY CHASE, M.S., R.D.

Nutrition can mean the difference between having enough energy to get by and feeling really good. There are no magical foods or nutritional supplements that will give you a strong, lean body, but eating well will maximize your efforts in the gym. To achieve the shape you want, you have to *work off what you eat* and *eat what you work off*. This simply means working off excess calories and body fat and replacing the essential nutrients used during those workouts.

The information that follows applies to all exercisers. Whatever your sport or fitness goal, you have to follow nutrition basics to achieve lasting results. Remember, *food is fuel*. Choosing the right fuels, in the right proportions, will enhance your exercise effectiveness and help you achieve a healthy, fit body—that's the power of Power Nutrition. The six-week Power

Nutrition Plan at the end of this chapter will help you get started *and* stay on track.

Water—The Single Most Important Nutrient

Sixty percent of an adult's body weight is water. Every metabolic reaction in the body involves water, including the burning of body fat and other fuels for energy. The body's dependence on water is reflected in the fact that a person can live only three days without it, whereas it is possible to survive many days without food. When a person is low on water—dehydrated—all body functions suffer, including the ability to exercise. Losing as little as 1 to 2 percent of your body weight through sweat can cause a 10 percent decrease in aerobic capacity—your ability to use oxygen for energy production. As a result, your stamina goes down. You can easily lose that much water in one hour of hard exercise. Severe dehydration, of course, has fatal consequences. But even mild levels will cause you to feel sluggish and "not your best."

HOW MUCH IS ENOUGH?

The average adult uses 6 to 12 cups of water daily to take care of essential tasks such as removing waste products, transporting nutrients and oxygen throughout the body, and maintaining normal body temperature. This water is lost through urine, breath, sweat, and stool. Exercisers lose even more water, especially if working out in high altitudes or in hot, humid weather. Remember the advertisements for sweat suits in the back of magazines and on late-night TV? "Lose an inch a day while walking your way to slimness in our new exercise-enhancement suits." Well, the term *sweat suit* is appropriate. Such heavy suits trap water, preventing the body from cooling itself through sweat evaporation. The body then produces more sweat in an effort to compensate. The inches lost were inches of water! A dehydrated body *appears* slimmer, right up to the moment it collapses from lack of water.

So be good to yourself and drink plenty of water daily to replace normal fluid losses and to replace the water used during exercise. Most people need 8 to 10 cups of water daily. This may sound like you will be drowning yourself. However, once you get used to drinking plenty of water, you won't mind because the reward is feeling more energetic.

FLUID OPTIONS

While it is important to drink several glasses of plain water each day, you can use other beverages too—juices, soups, skim milk, herbal tea, decaffeinated coffee, seltzer water, and sports drinks. Even juicy foods help, such as oranges, tomatoes, and cucumbers. Caffeine and alcohol have a *diuretic* effect on the body, meaning they cause you to make more urine and lose more water. If you drink caffeinated or alcoholic beverages, do so in moderation and do not count them as part of your water intake.

How can you be sure you are getting the fluids you need? Your sense of thirst is not always reliable, so monitor your urine output. You should make frequent

FLUID REPLACEMENT GUIDELINES

MODERATE TO HEAVY WORKOUTS (1 TO 1½ HOURS LONG)

BEFORE: Drink 1 to 2 cups of plain cool water 30 minutes before exercise.

DURING: Drink ½ cup of water every 15 minutes.

AFTER: Drink 1½ to 3 cups of water after exercising, over a 1- to 2-hour period of time.

ENDURANCE EVENTS

BEFORE: Weigh yourself before the event!

            Drink 2 to 4 cups of plain cool water during the 2 hours before the event.

DURING: Drink ½ cup of water every 15 minutes.

            Also drink ½ cup of carbohydrate sports drink after 1 hour of exercise and every 20 to 30 minutes.

AFTER: Drink 1 cup of water, fruit juice, or sports drink every 20 minutes until your preevent weight is reached, about 2 cups per pound lost.

trips to the bathroom and have clear urine, except for first thing in the morning. Note: Vitamin supplements may cause your urine to be yellowish-green in color, whatever your hydration status. Follow the guidelines on page 36 for water intake during exercise.

The Energy Nutrients—Your Body's Fuel Source

Energy from food is measured in the form of calories. Fat, carbohydrate, protein, and alcohol all contain calories in varying amounts, as shown in Table 1.

Fat and alcohol provide more than twice the calories of carbs or protein. Also, current research is telling us that all calories are not created equal. It appears the body is far more efficient at storing fat calories than carbohydrate calories. If you eat 100 calories of extra fat—say a tablespoon of margarine—the body stores about 97 of those calories in your fat cells. The other 3 are lost as heat. (This process is called the TEF, or thermal effect of food.) However, if you eat 100 calories of extra carbs—about 2 tablespoons of jam—the body stores only 77 calories as fat and loses 23 as heat. And those extra carbs are first stored in the muscle and liver as glycogen. Only when the glycogen stores are full will the carbs be stored as fat. Any food eaten to excess can be stored as fat, but fat calories are more fattening than carbohydrate calories. Even if you are not eating any

extra calories, a low-fat, high-carbohydrate diet allows for a leaner body. So instead of *buttered* toast, eat *jammed* toast.

Burning Fats and Carbs

As you sit and read this book, 50 to 80 percent of the calories you are using come from fat and the rest are mostly carbohydrate. Of course, you aren't burning enough of either one to produce weight loss, which is why the read-books-and-lose-weight diet was never a success. Now, if you jump up and sprint to the corner, your body shifts into burning mostly carbs. Should you then decide to walk briskly to the store four miles away, you will start to burn significant amounts of fat, too, after about the first mile and a half. If you sprint hard the last quarter mile, you switch back to using mostly carbs for energy.

Carbohydrates inside the body are in the form of glycogen, stored in the muscles and liver, and glucose (blood sugar). We can store pounds and pounds of fat, but glycogen stores are limited to one pound for the average adult and up to two to three pounds for highly trained athletes. Brain cells and nerve tissue rely almost exclusively on glucose for energy. And since carbs are stored in the muscle, they are the most readily available source of energy. So they get used in large amounts during the early stages of exercise, such as in

	CALORIES/GRAM	CALORIES/TABLESPOON	SOME FOOD SOURCES
TABLE 1. WHERE CALORIES COME FROM			
FAT	9	120 (oil)	Oil, butter, mayonnaise, cream, bacon, fatty meat, and margarine
CARBOHYDRATE	4	46 (sugar)	Grains, vegetables, fruits, legumes (beans and peas)
PROTEIN	4	*	Meats, fish, milk, cheese, legumes, nuts, grains
ALCOHOL	7	*	Wine, beer, spirits

*Because foods are usually not pure protein or pure alcohol, tablespoon measurements do not apply.

FIGURE 1. FUELS BURNED DURING EXERCISE

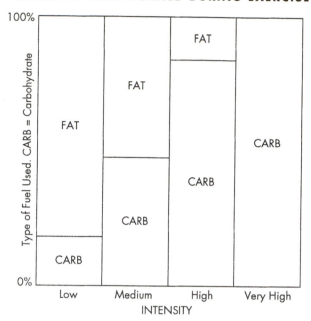

the sprint to the corner. After the body gets revved up (the four-mile walk to the store), fat stores begin to break down for energy also. If you continue to increase the intensity of the exercise—another sprint—you would have to use your reserve of carbs (glycogen). As shown in Figure 1, as the intensity of an exercise increases, you tend to burn proportionately more carbohydrate and less fat. Of course, as intensity increases, you tend to burn more total calories too!

BURNING BODY FAT

As mentioned earlier, you are always using fat for a part of your energy, although you never burn fat exclusively. Fat burning requires oxygen, so aerobic exercises involving continuous movement—bicycling, walking, running, cross-country skiing, skating—burn a higher percentage of fat than nonaerobic exercises—weight lifting, horseback riding, short and fast sprints.

Though not aerobic, weight training is a critical part of improving the body's lean-to-fat ratio. Weight training builds muscle. Muscle tissue burns more calories than fat tissue. The more muscle you have, the more calories you will burn, even while sitting. Since half or more of those calories are fat, you will burn more total fat. So the way to burn more fat is to become more fit, with a combination of weight training and aerobic exercise.

A Few Words About Cellulite: Everybody especially hates cellulite, but it is really just ordinary body fat. Cellulite looks different due to the way it is trapped by tight connective tissue, forcing the fat to bulge out in a lumpy pattern. Most likely, cellulite is an inherited pattern of fat. It cannot be treated externally or targeted specifically with exercise or nutrition. The way to attack cellulite is the same way you attack any other body fat—exercise and well-balanced, low-fat meals. There are no credible *magic* solutions.

Carbohydrates

Carbohydrates, since we don't store them in large amounts, have to be eaten daily to meet energy demands and keep active muscles primed. A minimum of 50 grams of carbohydrate is required to feed the brain, to spare protein from being used as a fuel source, and to allow for fat to be oxidized for energy. *The minimum, however, is not at all ideal!* Eating only 50 grams (200 calories' worth) of carbohydrates would force you to eat far too much protein and fat to meet your energy needs. For optimum health and energy levels, eat 400 to 600 grams, or 55 to 60 percent, of your total calories from carbs. A training diet for an endurance athlete should consist of 3½ to 4 grams of carbohydrate for every pound of body weight, daily. Table 2 (opposite) lists the carbohydrate content of various common foods.

There are two kinds of carbohydrates in food—simple and complex. Simple carbs are found predominately in sugars, milk, and fruit. They are simple in their chemical structure, just two molecules hooked together. Simple carbs are digested and absorbed into the bloodstream quickly, which is why people talk about getting an *energy high* from sugary foods. The blood sugar rises quickly, giving the body *quick* energy. One downside to simple carbs is that some people also get a corresponding *energy low* (from a drop in blood sugar) if they eat too many simple carbs or eat them without other foods.

Sugars are basically devoid of any nutritional value other than the carbohydrate, making them *empty calories.* Too many empty calories spell DEMISE to a well-balanced diet. A little sugar is okay if you are active enough to afford the empty calories, say one serving of sugary junk food a day. More than that can compromise nutrient intake.

Complex carbs consist of long strings of molecules, often referred to as *starch*. In spite of everything your old diet books may have said about starch, complex carbs should dominate your diet. The old *bread is fattening* myth began with studies done on rodents in the 1970s. It appears that high-carbohydrate diets do lead to fat storage—in rats. But as it turns out, humans are not like rats! As mentioned previously, in humans carbohydrates are used immediately as energy or stored as glycogen. Only when glycogen stores are completely full will the body convert carbs to fat, and then inefficiently.

So eat plenty of starch! You will find complex carbs in breads, noodles, cereals, potatoes, corn, beans, and peas. Plenty of grains, vegetables, and legumes should fill your plate. Fruits are important too because even

though they are mostly simple carbs, they provide necessary fiber, vitamins, and minerals.

Oh yes, did I mention fiber? Dietary fiber, undigestible carbohydrate, is essential for a healthy gut. Some types of fiber (oat bran, for instance) aid in lowering blood cholesterol levels. Other types, such as wheat bran, make it easier to pass stool and have been associated with lowering the risk of developing colon cancer. Whole grains, vegetables, and fruits all contribute dietary fiber. It is recommended that you eat 20 to 35 grams per day. See Table 2 for the fiber content of various foods.

Fats—A Little Dab'll Do Ya!

Now that you are working hard to have a lean body, the last thing you want to do is refeed your fat cells. Any

TABLE 2. CARBOHYDRATE CONTENT OF FOODS

| FOOD ITEM | CARBOHYDRATE CONTENT IN GRAMS | | | |
	TOTAL	COMPLEX	SIMPLE	FIBER
Bagel	31.0	27.8	2.0	1.2
Spaghetti, 1 cup, cooked	39.0	35.2	1.7	2.1
Baked potato, medium, with skin	26.7	22.9	0.8	3.0
Carrot, medium, raw	7.3	0.2	4.8	2.3
Apple, medium, with skin	21.1	0.3	17.8	3.0
Banana, medium	26.7	7.1	17.8	1.8
Grape-Nuts, ½ cup	46.8	40.1	4.0	2.7
Raisin Bran, ½ cup	21.4	9.8	8.6	3.0
Oatmeal, 1 cup, cooked	25.3	22.3	0.9	2.1
Raisins, 2 tablespoons	14.4	1.6	11.8	1.0
Orange juice, ½ cup	13.4	0.2	13.0	0.2
Acorn squash, ½ cup, cooked	15.0	8.9	3.9	2.2
Pumpkin, canned, ½ cup	9.0	0	4.0	5.0
Whole wheat bread, 1 slice	11.3	7.5	1.0	2.8
White bread, 1 slice	12.2	10.5	1.0	0.7
Broccoli, ½ cup, cooked	3.9	0.8	1.1	2.0
Black beans, canned, ½ cup	19.0	12.0	0	7.0
Brown rice, ½ cup, cooked	22.9	21.2	0	1.7
English muffin, 1 whole	29.8	26.3	2.0	1.5

Data taken from N-Squared Computing, programs NIII, 7.0 and NIV, 2.0, and from product labels.

extra calories can become stored fat, but remember that fat calories get stored most readily. Many people have the mistaken idea that they should not eat *any* fat. This is simply not true! Fat is a necessary part of a well-balanced diet, but a little does go a long way.

BODY FAT

Fat has such a bad reputation these days; perhaps it would be helpful for you to understand why fat is important for good health. A certain amount of body fat is essential to live. Body fat protects internal organs, helps to maintain body temperature, and is a vital component of all body cells.

Although estimates vary, men probably require a minimum of 5 percent body fat and women require 12 to 15 percent body fat to sustain life and good health. Optimum fitness is likely achieved with body fat levels higher than the minimum, 10 to 25 percent for men and 15 to 30 percent for women. These may seem like pretty liberal ranges. However, people vary greatly in how healthy they are at certain body weights and body fats. We tend to forget this fact in our fat-phobic society. I have known exercisers who feel too lethargic and get sick more often when their body fat gets lower than optimum for them. As you work to achieve the look you want, pay attention to how your body feels. You may be more comfortable at a slightly higher body fat level than shooting for the lowest level you can achieve.

HOW MUCH FAT AND WHAT KIND OF FAT SHOULD YOU EAT?

We need some food fat to supply essential fat-soluble vitamins and fatty acids required to make hormones and other compounds necessary for life and optimum health. Technically, we can meet our need for fat with a diet of only 5 percent fat calories. Practically speaking, a diet that low in fat would create problems. It would eliminate many nutritious foods from the diet. Food fat also helps you feel satisfied after eating and, because it slows down digestion, fat keeps you from being hungry all the time. Fat contributes a lot of flavor to food too.

Fat is present in most foods. You will find it in nearly all foods except pure sugars—honey, table sugar, molasses, etc. So every piece of whole-grain bread and every ounce of lean tuna will provide some fat. For good health and disease prevention, limit fat intake to no more than 30 percent of total calories. If you need to lose body fat, shoot for about 20 percent fat calories. I don't recommend going lower than 10 percent fat calories because of the difficulty in complying with this very low fat level.

FIGURING YOUR RECOMMENDED FAT INTAKE

Knowing what percentage of fat calories to eat is not as helpful as knowing how many fat *grams* to eat. Food labels and calorie charts list grams of fat in foods, so you can count your fat intake easily. Table 3 (opposite) provides a quick method for estimating how many grams of fat you can eat and still be within the percentage of fat calories you want.

TYPES OF FOOD FAT

After learning the amount of fat to eat, your next consideration is the *type* of fat. Three types of fatty acids give us calories: saturated (SAT), polyunsaturated (POLY), and monounsaturated (MONO). The chemical difference between the three has to do with the amount of hydrogen ions attached. If a fat has all the hydrogens it can handle, it is considered *saturated*. If only one hydrogen is missing, it is a *monounsaturated* fat and if several hydrogens are missing it is *polyunsaturated*.

HEALTH ISSUES

The significance, healthwise, is that SATs tend to increase blood cholesterol, especially LDL-cholesterol—the harmful kind. SATs are found predominately in fatty animal products, such as cheese, whole milk, and fatty meats. The recent good news about fat is that the predominant saturated fatty acid in beef and chocolate, stearic acid, does not seem to affect LDL-cholesterol. So feel free to enjoy lean beef and the occasional chocolate bar.

POLYs are the type of fat in most plants, except coconut and palm oil, which are saturated. When saturated fats in the diet are replaced with polyunsaturated ones, LDL-cholesterol declines. The same is true if MONOs replace SATs. Olive oil and canola oil are two predominant sources of MONOs.

You have probably seen the term *hydrogenated* on labels of shortening, margarine, peanut butter, and

TABLE 3. HOW MUCH FAT CAN I EAT?

First, estimate your total calorie needs and the number of fat calories. Then figure grams of fat to eat daily. It is best to calculate a range of intakes instead of a single number.

EXAMPLE

1. Multiply your present weight by the appropriate factor to estimate baseline calorie needs.

Men: 11 _____ pounds × 11 = _____

Women: 10 _____ pounds × 10 = _____

135-pound female who is normal weight and moderately active.

135 pounds × 10 = 1,350 baseline calories

2. Multiply your weight by the appropriate *activity factor** to estimate calories needed for activity.

	Sedentary	Light	Moderate	Heavy
Men:	3.2	6	7.2	10.5
Women:	3.0	5	6	9

_____ pounds × _____ (factor) = _____

135 pounds × 6 = 810 activity calories

3. Add together the calories from steps 1 and 2 to estimate *total calorie needs* per day.

_____ + _____ = _____

(Add 500 calories to total if currently underweight. Subtract 200 calories from total if currently overweight.)

1,350 + 810 = 2,160 total calories

4. Multiply the total calories by .20 or .30 for 20 or 30 percent fat calories.**

_____ × .20 = _____

_____ × .30 = _____

2,160 × .20 = 432 fat calories (20 percent)

2,160 × .30 = 648 fat calories (30 percent)

5. Divide the calories from fat by 9 to get your *daily fat gram allotment.*

20 percent = _____ /9 = _____

30 percent = _____ /9 = _____

432/9 = 48 fat grams for 20 percent

648/9 = 72 fat grams for 30 percent

*Sedentary = little exercise and sit-down job; Light = some exercise or standing job; Moderate = exercise three to five times a week and/or moderately active job; Heavy = exercise five or more times a week or very active job (construction work).
**Eat approximately 20 percent fat calories to help lose excess body fat.

TABLE 4. PRIMARY SOURCES OF FOOD FAT		
SATURATED	MONOUNSATURATED	POLYUNSATURATED
Bacon, Sausage	Canola Oil	Corn Oil
Beef	Olives	Fish Oil
Butter	Olive Oil	Peanut Oil
Cheese		Safflower Oil
Cream		Soybean Oil
Coconut Oil		Sunflower Oil
Hydrogenated Oils		Walnuts
Lamb		
Lard		
Palm Oil		
Pork		
Poultry Skin		
Whole Milk		

other foods. *Hydrogenated* is the term used when manufacturers *saturate* a plant oil by adding hydrogens. Controversy exists about the health effects of hydrogenated fats. It is probably a good idea to use oil instead of shortening when possible, but the most important point is to use very little of either.

This fatty acid stuff can get pretty technical. The important thing for you to know is that too much of any fat is too much. The fats that you do eat should be about half MONOs and a quarter each from POLYs and SATs. This means use small amounts of olive or canola oil in cooking and salad dressings, eat only lean animal products, and the POLYs will take care of themselves through the fat found in whole grains and vegetables.

CHOLESTEROL

Cholesterol is another type of fat that affects heart health but does not provide calories. Many experts consider total fat in the diet more important than total cholesterol, but limiting cholesterol intake to 300 milligrams per day is still recommended. This is especially important if you already have a high blood cholesterol level or if it runs in your immediate family. Cholesterol is made in the liver of animals, including humans. Since plants do not have livers, they have no cholesterol. It is possible for a food to be high in fat and low in cholesterol—oil for example. It is also possible to have a high-cholesterol, low-fat food—boiled

shrimp. Shrimp, calamari (squid), organ meats, and egg yolks are some of the biggest contributors of cholesterol in our diet, so go easy on them.

Protein Builds Muscle, Right?

You've seen the advertisements. An extremely well-developed man with a perfect body is touting protein powder as the reason for his incredible physique. Everyone knows muscle is made of protein, so it is logical to assume you need to eat more protein if you want to build muscle. The logic has some merit, but *the amount of extra protein needed is actually very small.*

Although still debated among sports nutritionists, exercisers probably do require more protein than nonexercisers, with endurance athletes and bodybuilders requiring the most. Sedentary adults need 0.4 gram of protein per pound of body weight and exercisers, especially during the early stages of training, require 0.6 to 0.9 gram per pound. If you are a 150-pound bodybuilder, your maximum protein requirement is 135 grams. I often see men eat that much protein without even trying! As you become more fit, your body becomes more efficient in using protein, so your requirement drops again, assuming you eat plenty of carbs for energy. Virtually all foods, except pure sugars and pure fats, contain some protein. Table 5 (opposite) gives the protein content of some common foods.

TABLE 5. PROTEIN CONTENT OF SELECTED FOODS

FOOD	PROTEIN (GRAMS)
Canned tuna, 6.5-ounce can	45.5
Chicken breast, 4 ounces	36.0
Refried beans, 1 cup	15.8
Broccoli, cooked, 1 cup	5.8
Brown rice, 1 cup	4.9
Whole wheat bread, 2 slices	4.8
Green beans, 1 cup	2.4
Baked potato, 1 medium	2.0

Although we burn a little protein to supply energy, the body has to spare most of its protein for more important functions, such as the building and repair of tissue and the formation of enzymes, hormones, and other important compounds. At rest, the body only uses protein for 2 to 5 percent of its calories. Endurance activities will increase protein's usage to 5 to 10 percent of energy because protein can be converted into glucose. If an exerciser fails to eat adequate carbohydrate, his or her usage of protein for energy will increase. This takes protein away from its other duties and can lead to dehydration and calcium losses. Generally, protein intake is safe and adequate if it makes up no more than 10 to 20 percent of total calories.

PROTEIN SUPPLEMENTS

Rarely does someone need a protein supplement to meet protein needs. Protein powders are expensive for the amount of protein you get. In spite of marketing claims to the contrary, the right foods will supply plenty of lean protein and all the necessary amino acids.

Some bodybuilders swear by eating large quantities of protein, up to 1⅓ grams per pound body weight. But the dangers of excessive protein make the indiscriminate use of protein supplements or high-protein diets unwise. Excess protein can be stored as body fat. But,

more important, excess protein causes the body to lose calcium. You then have to eat more calcium, and more phosphorus, to maintain calcium balance. Because there is no known benefit to eating a high-protein diet, it isn't worth upsetting your calcium balance.

PROTEIN—MEAT EATERS VERSUS VEGETARIANS

The debate is lively and often heated. Should humans eat meat or not? Research indicates many of the life-threatening diseases in the United States could be diminished if we ate fewer animal products, both animal fats and animal proteins. The key word here is *fewer*, not *none*. Since the Stone Age, humans have been omnivorous, able to digest and absorb nutrients from animals as well as plants. (Of course, there were no processed foods then, so diets were lower in fat, sugar, and salt.) A healthy diet can be achieved *with or without* animal flesh or animal milk. The key is knowing how to choose a nutrient-rich diet.

Body protein is made by putting together various amino acids according to specific directions from DNA. Your body is programmed to do this, assuming all the necessary amino acids are available. Most amino acids can be produced by the body, but there are several that have to be supplied from food, the so-called *essential amino acids* (EAA). The advantage of animal protein is that it contains all of the EAA, in optimum proportions, and is therefore known as *complete protein*. Some plant foods, such as corn, are missing one or more essential amino acid and are known as *incomplete proteins*. Other plants, like rice, contain all the essentials, but in very small quantities and less optimum proportions. The body does not utilize the protein in these plants as well as a complete protein. However, the limitations of plant proteins are easily overcome by combining plants in specific ways to create complete proteins. You will read more about *combining* below.

You do not have to eat a complete protein in order for your body to make the proteins it needs. After eating any protein food, be it steak or beans, the process of digestion breaks apart the protein and you absorb individual amino acids and pairs of amino acids. These enter the body's amino acid pool. When you need a protein built, the body will draw the necessary amino acids from this pool. As long as you obtain all the essential amino acids in enough quantity over the course of a few hours, it doesn't matter if they originally came from an animal or a plant.

Combining Proteins: Is it important to eat a complete protein, whether from animals or a combination of plants, at each meal? The answer depends in part on how much total protein you eat. Of course, it isn't an issue for meat eaters. If you eat no animal protein and limited amounts of vegetable sources, protein combining with plants becomes very important. You need to insure that all the essential amino acids are not only present, but present in the right amounts to support optimum protein metabolism.

Protein combining has developed spontaneously in places where animal protein is limited. It is very easy to combine proteins, so if you are a vegetarian, you might as well make it a habit. Any combination of grains and legumes, legumes and seeds, or dairy protein and plant protein make a complete protein. Table 6 lists examples of complete protein dishes common to the vegetarian diet.

TABLE 6. COMPLETE VEGETARIAN PROTEINS

Black Beans and Rice

Peanut Butter Sandwich

Bean Taco

Hummus on Pita Bread

Macaroni and Cheese

Rice Pudding

Noodles with Tofu Sauce

Lentil Curry on Rice

Cereal and Milk

Noodles with Peanut Sauce

Pros and Cons of Plant and Animal Proteins: Plant proteins, except for nuts and seeds, are usually very low in fat. However, today many red meats are also quite lean, as are certain fish, skinless poultry, and nonfat dairy products. Vegetarians are not guaranteed a low-fat diet; they have to select foods as carefully as meat eaters do.

An advantage to plant proteins, such as beans and whole grains, is that most of them are also high in complex carbohydrates. Of course, you have to eat 2 cups of beans to get the same amount of protein found in 4 ounces of chicken. So you have to consume more volume of plant protein than animal protein to meet your protein needs. This is not a handicap. We need lots of grains and vegetables to meet other nutritional needs anyway. Also, vegetarians are less likely to overdo it on protein unless they consume large amounts of eggs, milk, and cheese.

Let's not forget the nutritional advantages of *lean* animal protein. Red meat and dark poultry are excellent sources of iron. Also, animal flesh improves the absorption of iron from plant foods. Animal protein, especially meat, poultry, and fish, is also high in many B vitamins, zinc, and phosphorus. Ounce for ounce, lean beef contains four times as much zinc as tofu and eight times as much as pinto beans. Vitamin B_{12} is extremely limited in the plant world, but plentiful in animal foods.

Arguments can be made in favor of both vegetarian and meat diets. Both can be highly nutritious or disastrous, depending on food choices. The important thing is to eat an adequate, not excessive, amount of protein that provides all your essential amino acids.

Vitamins and Minerals

There are over forty essential nutrients that keep your body functioning. The scope of this chapter does not allow for an in-depth explanation of each of them. The majority of your vitamin and mineral needs can be met with the Power Nutrition Plan. We briefly discuss supplements later in this chapter.

Sodium—How Big an Issue Is It?

Clearly, most Americans eat far more sodium than our bodies require. Due to the prevalence and dangers of high blood pressure (HBP), many health experts recommend eating no more than 2,400 milligrams of sodium per day. That's just about the amount in 1 teaspoon of salt. Average sodium intakes are estimated to be 3,000 to 7,000 milligrams in this country.

The need for everyone to cut sodium intake is not supported by all researchers of HBP and heart disease. High-sodium diets do not cause or improve all cases of HBP. There are probably other dietary factors involved too, such as too little calcium, potassium, and magnesium in the diet. Perhaps we eat too much sodium *in relation* to these other minerals. This is an easy thing to do when one relies primarily on processed foods.

Sodium is widely used in the processing of foods, such as baked goods, frozen dinners, canned or dry soups, rice mixes, cured meats, and pickled foods. One cup of canned chicken noodle soup contains 1,107 mg of sodium! An estimated 75 percent of our sodium intake comes from processed foods. At the same time, processing often causes losses in other minerals, resulting in disproportionately high sodium content.

HBP is dangerous enough to warrant using sodium in moderation, even if your blood pressure is normally low. Begin by using fewer processed foods high in sodium. Look for low-salt soups and throw away the seasoning packets in packaged foods. Use herbs and spice blends, such as Mrs. Dash, for seasoning. Read food labels to become aware of sodium levels in foods. And don't salt your food until you've tasted it!

What About Alcohol?

Alcohol is a concentrated source of calories and has negative consequences when consumed in excess. When alcohol enters the body, it forces the liver to process it while other work comes to a standstill. As a result, fat metabolism slows down, leading to a buildup of fat in the liver. Also, alcohol metabolism ties up niacin and thiamin, B vitamins necessary for energy production. Carbohydrate metabolism is also affected by alcohol, leading to lower levels of muscle glycogen. This can make it difficult to exercise after a night of drinking. Also, muscle cells do not use alcohol for energy, so you cannot burn off a martini in the same way you can burn off a donut. And remember, alcohol has a *diuretic* effect on the body, forcing you to lose precious water.

A drink or two may help you feel calm and better able to handle the world. It might even decrease your risk of having a heart attack. But larger amounts can wreak havoc with your health and your intentions to exercise. If you are going to drink, don't do it right before or after exercise. When participating in a beer-sponsored sporting event, be sure to rehydrate your body with plenty of water before hitting the free beer!

The Caffeine High

Caffeine is a stimulant that, among other things, causes an increase in free fatty acids in the blood. With more free fatty acids available, exercising muscles can use them for energy, preserving glycogen for later. This improves endurance. Another potential benefit from caffeine is that it can make exercise *seem* easier.

These effects do not hold true for everyone, especially if coffee is the caffeine beverage of choice. Some people actually feel *worse* after drinking coffee due to stomach upset and nervousness. Coffee also acts as a laxative *and* the caffeine is a diuretic. Be forewarned! The caffeine high can turn out to be a real low. If you want to experiment with using coffee preexercise, the dose is 2 to 3 cups of brewed coffee one hour before your workout.

Putting It All Together— A Well-Balanced Diet

So what exactly is a well-balanced diet? There is so much conflicting information about nutrition, it can be difficult to get a clear grasp on the answer to that question. As more is learned about our nutritional needs in fighting disease, the message of exactly what to eat gets confusing for consumers. Well, you know the old adage, *Keep it simple.* It is applicable in nutrition, as in most things. The majority of the population could vastly improve their nutritional status by simply getting back to the basics, i.e., eating a variety of whole, unprocessed foods. This requires eating more baked potatoes instead of potato chips and more whole-grain bread instead of croissants.

GET THE BIGGEST NUTRITIONAL BANG FOR YOUR BUCK

We require fewer calories than our ancestors because we are less physical. However, our need for vitamins, minerals, and fiber has not decreased. This creates a situation where we need to get as many nutrients per calorie as possible, a principle known as *nutrient density*. But as our need for calories has decreased, our foods have become more processed. Processed foods typically provide fewer nutrients per calorie than whole foods. See Table 7 for examples. Eating foods that are close to their original form is the best way to increase nutrient density.

Surveys vary in their estimate of the percentage of the American population that eats a well-balanced diet, but by all accounts it is well below 50 percent. Some people complain that eating well is too compli-

cated and others say healthy foods don't taste good. As for the *how-to* part, follow this rule: *Choose more of the best and less of the rest*, meaning choose mostly wholesome, *real* foods and eat the processed junk food less often. Instead of instant macaroni and cheese, eat noodles topped with chicken and veggies. Have pudding made with skim or low-fat milk for dessert instead of creme-filled sandwich cookies.

As for good taste, you may have to reacquaint your taste buds with the flavor of real food. But what could taste better than a juicy peach, fresh steamed asparagus, a salad of mixed greens, or a bowl of pasta with spaghetti sauce? The spaghetti sauce can even contain meatballs and still be lean, healthy, and delicious. Use the Power Nutrition guidelines and the six-week plan to achieve a diet full of vital nutrients without a lot of unnecessary calories. The sample menus demonstrate how to create meals that add up to that elusive *well-balanced diet*.

BALANCED CALORIES EQUAL BETTER ENERGY

You now know where calories come from, but what is the best way to balance them for maximum energy levels? The body uses up more grams of carbohydrate than any other fuel. Since our storage volume of glyco-

TABLE 7. COMPARISON OF SELECTED NUTRIENTS PER 100 CALORIES

	FAT (gm)	POTASSIUM (mg)	ZINC (mg)	IRON (mg)	VITAMIN B_6 (mg)
Baked Potato	0.1	384	0.29	1.25	0.32
French Fries	5.2	232	0.12	0.24	0.07
Potato Chips	6.8	249	0.20	0.22	0.09
Corn on the Cob	0.8	315	0.70	0.70	0.18
Creamed Corn	0.5	185	0.70	0.50	0.09
Whole Wheat Bread	1.8	72	0.69	1.4	0.08
White Bread	1.4	42	0.23	1.1	0.01

Data adapted from *Food Values of Portions Commonly Used,* 15th edition.

gen is limited, we need to replace the glycogen used during exercise as well as to provide plenty of glucose to maintain optimum blood sugar levels. The only effective way to replace carbs is to eat carbs. We don't need to worry about replacing the fat we burned; we will always have plenty of fat onboard. Of course, as mentioned earlier, we need some fat in the diet for essential functions and satiety.

For better energy levels, the goal is to keep your blood sugar level within its optimum range. Your body works hard to do that by making you hungry when it needs glucose. After eating, hormones are stimulated to put the glucose where it is needed for immediate energy or into storage for later use. You can assist this process by not skipping meals and by selecting foods carefully.

I have found that most people feel more energetic and in better control of their appetite when they eat *mixed* meals, a combination of carbohydrates, protein, and a little fat. Mixed meals offer a longer-lasting supply of blood sugar. A currently popular approach to nutrition, called *food combining,* is not to combine starches and proteins, and to eat only fruit in the mornings. A few of my clients swear by this approach, but the majority do not, especially if they are exercising hard. Blood sugar levels are not well maintained by eating just fruit and the menu limitations with this approach are unnecessary.

GLYCEMIC INDEX—ADDITIONAL CONSIDERATIONS FOR EXERCISE AND WEIGHT MANAGEMENT

A phenomenon known as the *glycemic effect of foods* is gaining attention from sports nutritionists. *Glycemic effect* refers to the way a food affects one's blood sugar level—how quickly, how high, and how long it raises blood glucose. Scientists have managed to measure this effect and assign a *glycemic index* to various foods, mostly carbohydrates. A food with a high glycemic index (G-I) causes a rapid rise in blood glucose levels, providing an energy boost for exercising muscles. Those foods with a low G-I tend to offer a more gradual and sustained rise in blood sugar, which might be helpful if you plan to do a long workout or activity. Table 8 divides foods into high, moderate, and low G-I.

Many factors affect the G-I of a food, such as cook-

ing, density, and digestion. Also, if you eat a carbohydrate food along with fat or protein foods, its G-I will be lowered. Since very active people often eat meals or snacks made up of mostly carbohydrates, choosing foods according to the G-I may be useful. Theoretically, one should eat low- to moderate-G-I foods at the meal prior to a long workout. Eat moderate- to high-G-I foods during and after that workout to maintain blood glucose and to replace glycogen stores.

There is some evidence that eating foods with a low G-I can help suppress hunger and therefore decrease overall calorie intake. This will be useful if you need to lose excess body fat or if you suffer from food cravings that undermine your weight loss efforts. I know of no clinical trials using the G-I approach to weight management. But you can give it a try by eating low G-I foods versus high G-I foods at breakfast and at snacks. For example, eat the Spinach Omelette, a low G-I food (see Week 4, Menu One of the Power Nutrition Plan) instead of corn flakes, a high G-I food. Experiment with this method and see if it is helpful.

TABLE 8. GLYCEMIC INDEX OF SELECTED FOODS

HIGH G-I	MODERATE G-I	LOW G-I
Bagel	Grapes	Apples
Banana	Noodles	Applesauce
Chocolate bar	Oatmeal	Cherries
Corn	Orange	Chickpeas
Corn flakes	Potato, sweet	Coarse rye or
Corn syrup	Sponge cake	wheat bread,
Cracker, plain	Yam	European style
Honey		Dates
Molasses		Figs
Muesli		Fructose
Potato, white		Grapefruit
Raisins		Ice cream
Rice, brown		Milk
Rice, white		Navy beans
Rye bread		Peaches
Shredded wheat		Plums
Sucrose		Red lentils
White bread		Yogurt
Whole wheat bread		

When to Eat What—Timing Your Meal with Exercise

What you eat and when you eat it in relation to your workouts can make a big difference in how an exercise session goes. When exercising, your body shifts blood flow away from the digestive tract to the working muscles. Food digestion takes a backseat and you will want to time your meals accordingly.

FOOD BEFORE EXERCISE

Most of the energy used during a workout comes from your stores of glycogen and fat. However, if you exercise longer than one hour, a preexercise meal can contribute necessary glucose for long workouts. If you decide to take a run first thing in the morning, you will be low on glycogen stores from your overnight fast. A light, high-carbohydrate snack, perhaps a bagel with jam one hour before, will help abate hunger and prevent low blood sugar. If exercising at low to moderate intensity, you will probably feel fine on an empty stomach, provided you ate a high-carbohydrate meal the night before.

We used to think overweight people would burn more calories if they ate after, not before, exercising due to an increased thermal effect—that is, the increase in metabolism (rate of calories burned in response to food intake)—for the postexercise meal. More recent research indicates this is not true. However, exercise may decrease hunger for the following meal, especially if the exercise is rigorous.

The shorter the time period between food intake and exercise, the smaller and lighter the meal should be. You will want to minimize fat *and* fiber if eating less than three hours preexercise to avoid bloating and discomfort. Experiment with what works best for you. A general rule of thumb to follow for preexercise meals is:

- If eating less than one hour before exercising, choose a small snack, such as half a bagel, one slice of toast with jam, or a glass of skim or low-fat milk.
- If eating one to two hours before exercising, choose a liquid meal to provide calories in an easily digestible form. Liquids leave the stomach sooner than solids. A fruit-and-yogurt smoothie with a little cereal or wheat germ added should be enough.
- If eating two to three hours before exercising, choose a small meal, such as a small bowl of cereal with low-fat milk, toast with jam, and juice.
- If eating three to four hours before exercising, choose a larger meal, consisting of foods that have a low G-I (see Table 8). For example, a bowl of hearty bean soup with Ry-Krisp crackers, skim or low-fat milk, and an orange.

Remember, eat a high-carbohydrate diet *regularly* to maintain glycogen stores.

FOOD DURING EXERCISE

Exercise lasting longer than one and a half hours can be enhanced by consuming carbohydrates with a high G-I frequently throughout the exercise session. Small amounts of sugar help prolong exercise by providing a ready source of energy to the muscles and by maintaining blood sugar levels. Most sports drinks, candy, bananas, and raisins are all high G-I foods. Sports drinks vary in the source of carbohydrate. Fructose has a low G-I, so fructose-based beverages (Recharge) may not be as useful during exercise as a sucrose-based beverage (Gatorade). Glucose polymers (Exceed brand) may cause less stomach discomfort than other sugars. However, individual tolerance is the critical factor in choosing a sports drink. Use these drinks if they are helpful and only if you really need them; otherwise, they contribute unnecessary calories with the water you *definitely* need.

EATING AFTER EXERCISE

This is the time to feed your muscle cells; they like carbs! The first two hours after heavy exercise is the best time to replenish glycogen stores. The muscle cells are ravenous, as well as thirsty, if you have worked long and hard. The first meal following exercise should be primarily carbohydrates, especially the high-G-I variety. Eat a baked potato or rice with rolls and some grapes, for example, instead of a fatty cheeseburger and fries. Also, if you want a sugar fix, a soda or candy bar, this is the time to have it. All that sugar will be gobbled up by your muscle cells. Drinking fruit juice, a soda, or even a special *recovery* drink after exercise will replace needed water *and* carbs. A recovery drink is one that contains a higher concentration of carbohydrates than sports drinks in order to deliver lots of carbs to the muscles quickly. A brand name example is Carbo Fuel.

If you are an endurance athlete, eating carbs *immediately* after exercise is important in maximizing and maintaining your glycogen stores. This is known as *carbohydrate recovery*. Eat or drink about 1 gram of carbohydrate per pound of body weight within two hours, beginning within thirty minutes postworkout. The average exerciser probably doesn't run out of glycogen in a typical exercise session, but it is a good idea to *think carbs* the next time you are hungry after a workout.

The Power Nutrition Plan: A Six-Week Guide to Nutritional Fitness

What follows is a method for getting started on a nutritional fitness plan *and* strategies to help you stay on track. Healthy eating habits are not developed by good intentions alone. It takes time to change and a commitment on your part to stick with it. The plan begins with self-evaluation and goal setting. Then you will focus on your nutritional goals during each week of the plan. By the end of the six weeks, you will be well on your way to eating a fully *powered* diet.

This plan is for adults. It is not intended to take the place of a medical evaluation or prescribed medical/nutritional treatment. If you have any health problems, consult your physician.

STEP 1—SELF-EVALUATION OF BODY WEIGHT

Change begins with knowing your present nutritional status, both your weight status and your eating habits. Use the following assessment tools to evaluate your present body weight. DO NOT USE THIS INFORMATION TO BEAT YOURSELF UP! It's simply necessary to understand where you are in order to know where you need to go. If the thought of assessing your weight and body fat percentage is horrifying to you, then skip this part and move on to Step 2.

Body Weight: Weigh yourself on a *good* scale. Be sure the scale is balanced to zero before getting on it. Ideally, weigh early in the day, with no shoes and minimal clothing. This is the only time you need to weigh yourself during this plan! If you choose to weigh yourself regularly, do so no more than once a week and *only* if it is helpful. Do not obsess about your weight. Whatever the number on the scale, you are merely trying to evaluate your weight on the basis of health and fitness.

My weight on (date) _____ is _____.

Body Mass Index (BMI): The BMI is a more useful evaluation of weight than the standard height/weight tables. The BMI estimates your risk of developing a chronic, weight-related disease. Using the nomogram on page 50 and a ruler, draw a line from your weight to your height. The line will intersect the middle graph at your BMI. If your BMI is higher than desirable, use the nomogram to determine a healthier weight for you. Place the ruler at your height and within the desired BMI range. On the left, find your desirable weight.

DESIRABLE BMI	OVERWEIGHT
Women: 18.7 to 25	>27.3
Men: 20 to 25	>27.8

Health risk increases with increasing BMI over 25.

My BMI on (date) _____ is _____.

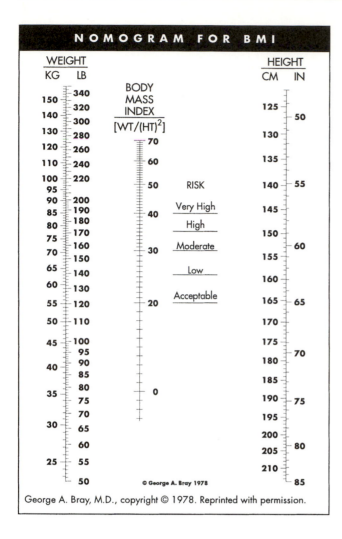

NOMOGRAM FOR BMI

WEIGHT		BODY MASS INDEX $[WT/(HT)^2]$		HEIGHT	
KG	LB			CM	IN
150	340	70			
140	320			125	
	300				50
130	280	60		130	
120	260				
110	240			135	
100	220	50	RISK	140	55
95	200				
90			Very High	145	
85	190	40			
80	180		High	150	
75	170				
70	160	30	Moderate	155	60
65	150				
	140		Low	160	
60	130				
55	120	20	Acceptable	165	65
50	110			170	
45	100			175	
	95			180	70
40	90				
	85			185	
35	80	0		190	75
	75			195	
30	70			200	
	65				80
	60			205	
25	55			210	
	50	© George A. Bray 1978			85

George A. Bray, M.D., copyright © 1978. Reprinted with permission.

Body Fat Percentage (BF%): It is difficult to measure on your own, but the BF% provides important information about whether or not you should lose weight. Someone can have a high BMI, yet be very lean—a football player or bodybuilder, for example. If you are overweight, but not over fat, then there may be no reason to lose weight.

The best way to determine your BF% is to seek out someone with the knowledge and expertise to measure it accurately. Registered dietitians, exercise physiologists, personal trainers, and even some physicians measure BF% using the skin-folds method—a method in which a professional uses calipers that grab the skin to measure its thickness in several places on the body—or electrical impedance—which utilizes mild electrical currents to estimate lean versus fat weight.

Health clubs and universities usually have someone on staff who can measure BF%. They might even offer the underwater weighing method, the gold standard of body fat measurements.

Waist-to-Hip Ratio (WHR): WHR is another way to assess health risk due to body fat. Fat around the abdomen is considered a greater health risk than fat in the hips and thighs. Using a tape measure, measure your waist (in the area of your navel) and your hips (at the hip bone). Divide the waist measurement by the hip measurement. For example, if your waist measurement is 32 inches, and your hip measures 38 inches, your WHR would be 32 ÷ 38, or 0.8.

LOWEST RISK

Women: <0.8
Men: <0.95

My WHR on (date) _____ is _____.

Based on your evaluations, do you need to lose weight (body fat)? If so, approximately how much? Use the exercise and eating guidelines in this book to tackle excess fat, five pounds at a time. DO NOT SEVERELY RESTRICT CALORIES OR OVEREXERCISE TO LOSE WEIGHT FAST. You will end up losing muscle mass instead of fat *and* overstressing your body, which leads to injury. Be sensible about this and you will have long-lasting results. See "Tips for Weight Loss," page 77.

STEP 2—SELF-EVALUATION OF EATING HABITS

Now let's look at what you eat. Don't assume you already know your habits; you may be surprised! First, write down *everything* you had to eat or drink over the last twenty-four hours. Do it now, even if you think yesterday's intake was unusual. And be honest with yourself. Evaluating a day when you didn't know anyone would be looking can be very telling.

How many servings of the following did you eat? Compare your intake with the servings recommended in the Goal column.

FOOD GROUP	SERVINGS EATEN	GOAL
Cereal, bread, grains (1 slice bread, ½ bagel, ½ cup cooked rice)	_____	6 to 11
Vegetables (½ cup cooked, 1 cup raw)	_____	3 to 5
Fruits (½ cup canned, 1 small piece, 6 ounces juice)	_____	2 or more
Protein (1 ounce meat, chicken, fish; ½ cup beans; 1 egg; 1 ounce cheese)	_____	3 to 6
Milk and Yogurt (1 cup of either)	_____	2 to 3
Fats (1 teaspoon margarine, butter, oil; 1 tablespoon mayonnaise, sour cream, half and half)	_____	0 to 3
Sugars (1 tablespoon sugar, honey, syrup; 2 cookies; small piece cake or pie; 12 ounces soda)	_____	0 to 2
Alcohol (12 ounces beer, 5 ounces wine, 1½ ounces liquor)	_____	0 to 2

Now, think about your typical or average food day. Consider weekends, late nights at work, restaurant meals, and snacks. With those in mind, take the Nutritional Fitness Quiz.

NUTRITIONAL FITNESS QUIZ

DO YOU EAT, ON AVERAGE:	YES	NO
meals or snacks in the morning, midday, *and* evening?	___	___
some sort of grain or bread at every meal?	___	___
100 percent whole wheat bread *more often than* wheat or white bread?	___	___
whole-grain or bran cereal *more often than* other cereals?	___	___
brown rice *more often than* white rice?	___	___
mostly low-fat crackers (saltines, Wasa, etc.) instead of regular snack crackers?	___	___
chips (potato, tortilla, etc.) less than twice a week?	___	___
muffins, donuts, croissants, and pastries less than twice a week?	___	___
at least 2 to 3 cups of vegetables every day?	___	___
deep yellow or green leafy vegetables every day?	___	___
at least two pieces of fruit or glasses of fruit juice every day?	___	___
berries, melons, citrus fruit, or other high–vitamin C foods every day?	___	___
mostly 100 percent fruit juices instead of fruit drinks?	___	___
mostly skim or 1 percent dairy products (milk, yogurt)?	___	___
milk (either cow, goat, or fortified soy) or yogurt daily?	___	___
fat-free or low-fat cheese more often than regular cheese?	___	___
packaged luncheon meats less than twice a week?	___	___
less than 8 ounces total of meat, chicken, and fish per day?	___	___
bacon, sausage, and hot dogs less than once a week?	___	___
beans, peas, or lentils at least twice a week?	___	___
skinless poultry most of the time?	___	___
four or fewer whole eggs a week?	___	___
only water-packed canned tuna?	___	___
deep-fried foods or gravy less than once a month?	___	___
mostly low-fat tub margarine instead of butter or stick margarine?	___	___
mostly low-fat or fat-free mayonnaise, sour cream, and salad dressings?	___	___
low-fat frozen desserts more often than regular ice cream?	___	___
less than two regular sodas or other sweets daily?	___	___
DO YOU DRINK, ON AVERAGE:		
3 or fewer cups of coffee per day?	___	___
at least eight glasses of water, including milk and juice, every day?	___	___
two or fewer servings of alcohol per day?	___	___
TOTALS	_____	

Total the number of answers in each column. The ideal answer to all of the questions is *Yes*. Although the quiz is not a scientific test, it is designed to help you see where you can make positive changes in your usual diet. The Power Nutrition Plan is aimed at helping you convert the *No* answers to *Yes* answers.

Scoring
Very fit: 28 to 31
Fit, but can do better: 24 to 27
Good intentions, now get serious!: 18 to 23
A nutritional disaster waiting to happen: <18

STEP 3—GETTING STARTED

Based on your self-evaluations, what do you want to change to improve your nutritional fitness? Maybe you need to lose body fat or reduce fat intake. Perhaps you want to improve your vegetable intake or start eating more whole grains. Whatever your goals, write them down. Be as specific as possible. For example, suppose you need more veggies in your diet. Your goal might be to eat three servings of vegetables every day. If you seldom eat vegetables now, eating three *every day* may be too ambitious to be realistic. You could start more slowly with something like adding V-8 juice or a salad to lunch three days a week.

MY GOALS FOR NUTRITIONAL FITNESS ARE:

1. _____
_____
2. _____
_____
3. _____
_____

Three is plenty to start with. Ready, set, go!

HOW THE PLAN WORKS

You will use the Power Nutrition Food Groups and the weekly menu guides to plan your meals and snacks. That's right, *you* do most of the meal planning. Why? Because you will be more successful that way! However, two preplanned menus and a few recipes are provided each week to help you out.

Each menu guide includes three meals and two to three snacks. The snacks are optional and should be eaten only if you are hungry. When you eat each meal or snack is up to you. The best time to eat is when you are hungry! You can also mix up the order in which you eat the meals or snacks to match your schedule.

You will notice there are *no calorie levels prescribed!* Counting calories is dieting and diets, typically, fail. Let's forgo that trauma. Portion sizes on the menu guides are listed only for proteins, milk, fats, and sugars. Other foods should be eaten in the amounts needed to satisfy your *physical* hunger. Eat slowly and only until satisfied, not stuffed. Most people need at least one snack a day. However, if you aren't hungry for the snacks, don't eat them, but *do not skip meals.*

Also, if you don't eat dairy products, you will need to concentrate on eating other foods high in calcium. In the Power Nutrition Food Groups, any food marked with a ** is a high-calcium food. Eat at least three of them daily.

It is important to be aware of how much fat you are eating. You can determine your daily fat gram allotment using Table 3, "How Much Fat Can I Eat?" on page 41. Now, estimate how much fat you are eating by referring to the fat grams listed in the following Power Nutrition Food Groups. If you want to be more precise, purchase any fat gram book, available at your local bookstore. I like *The T-Factor Fat Gram Counter* by Jamie Pope-Cordle and Martin Katahn. It is compact and includes fast foods.

No Forbidden Foods: There is absolutely no food you cannot eat in the Power Nutrition Plan. You simply strive to eat *more of the best and less of the rest.* To prove this to you, I included bacon in the first menu of Week 1. The total fat and saturated fat for the day are still within the guidelines. Bacon is not high on my list as a nutritious food, but I know how people love it. Telling a bacon lover to *never* eat the stuff again is not helpful because it doesn't work. Learning to allow for favorite, high-fat foods in your nutrition plan is an important ingredient for success. Humans typically do not do well with deprivation; it makes us defiant and determined to get what we want.

Counting fat grams gives you the flexibility to achieve nutritional fitness without feeling deprived. If you want a cheeseburger and fries, fine. You will be spending roughly 35 to 43 grams of fat, probably the biggest part of your daily fat gram allotment. So, eat very little fat the rest of the day. Whether it's bacon and eggs you crave or New York cheesecake, you can work any food in to the Power Nutrition Plan by counting fat grams and planning meals accordingly.

It will soon become obvious that you cannot eat a lot of high-fat foods on a regular basis and stay within your daily fat gram allotment. You will make food choices based on what you *really* want instead of overreacting to deprivation by overeating. Another plus to this plan, it gives you more flexibility when eating out. If the deli doesn't have low-fat mayonnaise for your turkey sandwich, and you really don't want mustard, you know you can eat the regular mayo and shave fat grams somewhere else.

Creating Success: To be most successful with the Power Nutrition Plan, keep daily records of everything you eat and drink. Are you groaning? Yes, it's a pain in the neck, but *record keeping is one of the most important things you can do to insure success!* And record as you go instead of trying to remember tomorrow what you ate today. That *never* works! Buy a small, pocket-sized spiral notebook you can carry with you. Record one day's food intake per page and list the fat grams next to each food. At the end of the day, count your fat grams and compare your intake to your daily allotment. Use the record to evaluate how you are doing toward your other goals as well. Use that information to plan menus for tomorrow. You will find weekly review forms at the end

of each week to help you evaluate overall progress. See the Troubleshooting Guide (pages 70–72) if you experience difficulty following the plan.

Who Is the Power Nutrition Plan For? Anyone needing to lose body fat or improve their nutritional fitness will benefit. This plan will especially be helpful for people who have been dieting and exercising, but can't seem to lose fat. It is helpful also for people who want to improve their diet, but either don't know how or don't want to give up their favorite foods. With the Power Nutrition Plan, you don't have to give them up! It's simply a matter of balancing all your food choices to meet your nutritional goals. The plan helps you make changes gradually and does not eliminate *any* foods.

POWER NUTRITION FOOD GROUPS
At the top of each food group (see charts on following pages), the recommended intake in *servings per day* is listed. Serving sizes are listed too. Foods are divided within each group by the *average* amount of fat present. Brands vary in fat content, so read food labels.

You won't find every food that exists in these food groups. That doesn't mean you have to limit your food choices to those on the lists. Just categorize your foods based on their ingredients. For example, pizza is not included in the food groups. However, if you choose to eat pizza, you know that it contains: grain (the crust), protein (cheese and meat toppings), a small amount of vegetables (tomato sauce and veggie toppings), and fat (in the crust, cheese, and olives).

GRAINS: BREADS, CEREALS, CRACKERS, COOKED GRAINS

6 TO 11 SERVINGS PER DAY	SERVING SIZES
0 to 1 gram of fat	
Breads:	
Whole-grain or enriched breads without egg or cheese	1 slice
Bagels, pita bread, **corn tortillas	1 each
English muffins, hard rolls, hamburger buns	½ each
Cereals:	
Dry cereals without nuts or oils, shredded wheat, Cheerios, etc.	1 ounce (½ to 1 cup usually)
Cooked cereals:	
Oatmeal, grits, Zoom, etc.	½ cup cooked
Crackers:	
Saltine or fat-free crackers	4 crackers
Whole-grain crackers without added fat: Ry-Krisp, Wasa, Kavli, etc.	2–4 crackers
Rice cakes	2 large
Baked tortilla chips	15 chips
Fat-free granola bars	1 bar
Grains:	
Whole-grain or enriched noodles, rice, millet, quinoa, buckwheat, couscous, etc.	½ cup cooked
Rice milk (Rice Dream)	½ cup
2 to 5 grams of fat	
Biscuit	1 biscuit
Croutons	½ to 1 ounce
Dinner roll, flour tortilla	1 each
Granola bar	1 bar
Muesli or granola cereal	½ cup
Muffin, small	1 small
Pancakes	4-inch pancake
Snack crackers	3 to 5
Soups: low-fat cream or vegetable soups	1 cup
Waffle, frozen	4-inch waffle
10 grams of fat	
Croissant	1
Tabbouleh (tabouli)	½ cup
Waffle, homemade	7-inch waffle

**Source of calcium

VEGETABLES

3 TO 5 SERVINGS OR MORE PER DAY	SERVING SIZES
0 to 1 gram of fat	
**Broccoli, kale, leaf lettuce, and seaweed	½ cup cooked
Spinach, carrots, squash, tomato, cauliflower, cabbage, okra, and other plain vegetables, except avocado	or 1 cup raw
V-8 or tomato juice	½ cup
**Winter squash and sweet potatoes	½ cup cooked
Potato, corn, plantain	½ cup cooked
3 to 5 grams of fat	
Baked french fries	10 fries
Candied sweet potatoes	½ cup
Coleslaw	½ cup
Marinara sauce, low-fat	½ cup
Mashed potatoes	½ cup
10 to 15 grams of fat	
Artichoke hearts, marinated in oil	¼ cup
Avocado (also listed in fat group)	½ medium
Fried french fries	10 fries
Hash brown potatoes	½ cup

**Source of calcium

FRUITS

2 OR MORE SERVINGS PER DAY	SERVING SIZE
0 to 1 gram of fat	
Citrus fruits, berries, and melons daily for vitamin C	1 medium or 1 cup
**Blackberries, pineapple juice, and fortified orange juice	½ cup
Bananas and other plain fruits	1 medium
Dried fruits, all **Figs and currants	2 tablespoons
Fruit juice (no sugar)	½ cup
**Source of calcium	

MILK/YOGURT

2 TO 3 SERVINGS PER DAY	SERVING SIZES
0 to 1 gram of fat	
Nonfat milk powder	¼ cup
Nonfat or skim milk	1 cup
Nonfat yogurt, plain or sweetened	1 cup
Evaporated skimmed milk	½ cup
Skim Lactaid milk	1 cup
Fat-free soy milk	1 cup
3 grams of fat	
1% milk	1 cup
Low-fat soy milk, some brands	1 cup
Low-fat fruited yogurt	1 cup
5 grams of fat	
2% milk	1 cup
Soy milk	1 cup
Low-fat yogurt, plain	1 cup
10 grams of fat	
Whole milk	1 cup
Yogurt, from whole milk	1 cup
Milk shake	1¼ cups
Goat's milk	1 cup

ANIMAL PROTEIN		PLANT PROTEIN	
3 TO 6 OUNCES TOTAL PER DAY	SERVING SIZES (3 ounces of cooked meat is about the size of a deck of cards)	USE 2 TO 3 TIMES/WEEK IN PLACE OF ANIMAL PROTEIN	SERVING SIZES ARE EQUAL IN PROTEIN TO 2 OUNCES OF MEAT
0 to 2 grams of fat		**0 to 2 grams of fat**	
1% or 2% cottage cheese	½ cup	**Legumes: beans, peas, and	1 cup cooked
Egg whites	2 whites	lentils, dried or canned and	
**Fat-free cheese	2 ounces	cooked without added fat	2 ounces
Flounder or sole, baked	3 ounces cooked	Seitan (White Wave or	
Oysters, raw	3 ounces	Meat of Wheat)	
Shrimp, boiled	3 ounces		
Tuna, packed in water	3 ounces	**6 to 9 grams of fat**	
		**Miso	½ cup
3 to 5 grams of fat		Tempeh	3 ounces
Regular cottage cheese	½ cup	Tofu, firm, raw	3 ounces
Chicken or turkey, no skin,	3 ounces		
baked or roasted		**25 grams of fat**	
Most fish and shellfish, grilled	3 ounces	Peanut butter (also listed in fat	3 tablespoons
or cooked without fat		group)	
Egg, whole	1 egg		
Low-fat luncheon meats	3 ounces		
**Salmon, pink, canned with	3 ounces		
bones			
8 to 12 grams of fat			
**Cheese, low-fat	2 ounces		
Chicken with skin, roasted	3 ounces		
Ham, lean, baked or canned	3 ounces		
Kippered herring	3 ounces		
Mackerel, canned	3 ounces		
Meatballs	2 to 3 ounces		
Oysters and scallops, fried	3 ounces		
Sardines	3 ounces		
Salmon, sockeye, grilled	3 ounces		
Shrimp and squid, fried	3 ounces		
Steak, broiled or grilled, fat	3 ounces		
trimmed			
15 to 25 grams of fat			
Beef, ground or roasts	3 ounces		
**Cheese	2 ounces		
Chicken, fried	3 ounces		
Hot dogs	2 to 3 ounces		
Lamb	3 ounces		
Luncheon meats	2 to 3 ounces		
Pork	3 ounces		
Sausages	2 to 3 ounces		
**Source of calcium			

FATS/OILS

USE IN MODERATION AND
WITHIN DAILY FAT GRAM ALLOTMENT   SERVING SIZES

0 to 3 grams of fat

Low-fat margarine	1 teaspoon
Low-fat cream cheese	1 tablespoon
Fat-free salad dressing	1 tablespoon
Some low-fat dressings	1 tablespoon

5 grams of fat

Vegetable oils: olive, canola, sunflower, corn, etc.	1 teaspoon
Soft tub margarine	1 teaspoon
Butter, stick margarine	1 teaspoon
Olives	5 large
Cream cheese	1 tablespoon
Bacon	1 slice
Cream and sour cream	2 tablespoons

8 to 15 grams of fat

Avocado	½ medium
Nuts and seeds	2 tablespoons
Almond or peanut butter	1 tablespoon
Mayonnaise	1 tablespoon
Regular salad dressings	1 tablespoon

EXTRAS

Foods with no fat and few nutrients. Serving sizes are small and provide few calories.

USE IN MODERATION   SERVING SIZES

Diet soft drinks	12-ounce can
Fat-free cream cheese	1 to 2 tablespoons
Fat-free margarine	1 to 2 teaspoons
Fat-free salad dressings, mayonnaise, and sour cream	1 to 2 tablespoons
Jam	½ tablespoon
Ketchup	1 tablespoon
Mustard	1 teaspoon
Sugar, honey	1 teaspoon
Sugar substitutes (Equal)	1 packet
Coffee or tea	1 cup
Spray-on oils (Pam)	to coat pan
Butter substitutes (Molly McButter, Butter Buds)	½ to 1 teaspoon

SUGARS/SWEETS

NO MORE THAN
2 SERVINGS PER DAY   SERVING SIZES

0 to 1 gram of fat

Sugar, honey, syrup	1 tablespoon
**Blackstrap molasses	1 tablespoon
Jelly, jams, preserves	1 tablespoon
Hard candy	2 pieces
Fat-free frozen yogurt or ice cream; sorbet	½ cup
Angel food cake	1 medium slice
Fat-free cookies	2 cookies
Soft drinks	12-ounce can

2 to 5 grams of fat

Graham crackers, vanilla wafers, fig cookies, sugar cookies	2 to 3 cookies
Low-fat ice cream and frozen yogurt	½ cup
Low-fat cakes	1 medium piece
**Pudding, from mix	½ cup
**Sherbet	½ cup

6 to 15 grams of fat

Brownies	1 medium
Chocolate chip cookies	1 to 2
Eclairs	1 small
Most cakes	1 small piece
Fruit pies	1 small piece

>15 grams of fat

**Bread pudding	½ cup
Cheesecake	1 small piece
Fried pies	1

**Source of calcium

ALCOHOL

IF YOU DRINK ALCOHOL,
LIMIT INTAKE TO NO MORE THAN
2 SERVINGS PER DAY   SERVING SIZES

Beer, regular or light	12 ounces
Spirits, straight or mixed in a cocktail	1.25 ounce (or about 1 jigger)
Wine, red or white	4 ounces

Because of the way alcohol is broken down in the body, it may increase the storage of body fat. An occasional drink will not interfere with fitness or weight loss. If you drink on a regular basis, count every serving as 9 grams of fat!

Week 1—Menu Guide

This week, the menu guide is aimed at helping you incorporate all the food groups into your daily diet. It also emphasizes water and an awareness of fat intake. As mentioned earlier, if you do not drink milk or eat yogurt, be sure to choose other high-calcium foods daily.

MEALS

Note: All meals provide a balance of carbohydrate, protein, and fat for optimum energy. If you plan to eat within two hours of exercising, choose the AM snack or a liquid meal.

Morning

Water
Fruit, fresh, canned or dried
100% fruit juice
Grains: cereal and bread
8 ounces low-fat milk or yogurt OR 1 to 2 ounces protein
1 to 2 fat servings
Coffee or tea, if desired; 2 cups maximum

Midday

Water
2 to 3 ounces protein
Any grains
Vegetables
Fruit (optional)
8 ounces low-fat milk or yogurt
1 to 2 fat servings (Okay if other food choices are low fat. Do not add mayonnaise to salami, for example. But, low-fat mayo on water-packed tuna would be okay.)

Evening

Water
2 to 3 ounces protein
Grain or high-carb vegetable
Grain: bread or crackers
Vegetables
Sweet (optional)
1 to 2 fats (within daily fat gram allotment)

SNACKS—DRINK WATER, FOOD IS OPTIONAL

AM

Water
Grain: bread or crackers
Fruit (optional)
4 ounces low-fat milk or yogurt (optional)
1 cup coffee or tea, if desired

Afternoon

Water
Any grain or sweet or fruit
Decaf coffee or tea or caffeine-free diet soda, if desired

Bedtime

Water
Herbal tea, if desired
Grain or fruit, optional and only if hungry

Remember to keep track of what you are eating every day. Use the following two menus to get you started on this week's menu guide. Portion sizes are given only for proteins, milk, fats, and sugars. Let your hunger be your guide for the amounts of other foods to eat. Consult the Power Nutrition Food Groups to get ideas for your own menus.

WEEK 1—SAMPLE MENUS

(BASED ON THE MENU GUIDE)

If the menus, including the snacks, do not contain enough food to satisfy your hunger, eat larger portions of the grains and vegetables.

MENU ONE	FOOD GROUP
Morning Meal	
Large glass of water	
Orange juice	Fruit
Oatmeal with raisins and 1 tablespoon	Grain/Fruit
brown sugar	Sugar
8 ounces skim or low-fat milk	Milk
Toast with ½ tablespoon jam	Grain/Extra
2 slices crisp bacon	Fat
Coffee or tea (with milk, if desired)	Extra
1 teaspoon sugar (or Equal) in coffee, if needed	Extra
AM Snack	
Water	
Saltine crackers	Grain
Banana	Fruit
4 to 6 ounces fruited low-fat yogurt	Milk
Midday Meal	
Large glass of water	
Tuna fish sandwich made with:	
2 ounces water-packed tuna, mixed with	Protein
½ to 1 tablespoon low-fat mayonnaise	Fat
2 slices bread	Grain
lettuce and tomato slices	Vegetable
V-8 juice	Vegetable
8 ounces skim or low-fat milk	Milk
Afternoon Snack	
Water	

	FOOD GROUP
Microwave popcorn, low fat (Newman's Own Light or Orville Redenbacher's Smart Pop, for example)	Grain
Diet soda, caffeine-free	Extra

Evening Meal

Large glass of water	
3 ounces baked chicken breast (Butterball Teriyaki Seasoned Breast Fillets are easy to prepare and delicious)	Protein
Long-grain and wild rice (such as Uncle Ben's; use ½ the fat called for)	Grain
Dinner roll	Grain
Carrots, steamed	Vegetable
Tossed Green Salad* with 1 to 2 tablespoons low-fat salad dressing	Vegetable / Fat
½ cup low-fat ice cream	Sugar

Bedtime

Water	
Celestial Seasonings Sleepy-Time Tea	Extra

MENU TWO	FOOD GROUP

Morning Meal

Large glass of water	
Large smoothie made with:	
banana and frozen unsweetened strawberries	Fruit
apple juice	Fruit
wheat germ	Grain
8 ounces low-fat plain yogurt	Milk
Low-fat granola bar	Grain
Coffee or tea (with milk, if desired)	Extra
1 teaspoon sugar in coffee, if needed	Extra

AM Snack

Water	
Bagel with	Grain
½ tablespoon fat-free cream cheese	Extra

Midday Meal

Large glass of water	
Sandwich made with:	
2 ounces boiled ham and 1 ounce low-fat cheese	Protein
kaiser roll	Grain
mustard	Extra
lettuce and tomato slices	Vegetable
Carrot sticks	Vegetable
8 ounces skim or low-fat milk	Milk
5 olives	Fat

Afternoon Snack

Water	
Apple	Fruit

Evening Meal

Large glass of water	
3 small meatballs in marinara sauce (such as Healthy Choice, or Enrico's brand) over spaghetti noodles	Protein / Vegetable / Grain
French bread, served warm with	Grain
Baked Garlic*	Extra
Large tossed green salad with	Vegetable
1 to 2 tablespoons low-fat salad dressing	Fat
5 ounces red wine (optional)	
2 fig bars	Sweet

Bedtime

Water	
Grapes	Fruit

WEEK 1 IN REVIEW

Answer the following questions to evaluate your progress this week. Congratulate yourself for all your positive steps. Do not dwell on the things you could have done better. Improving your nutritional fitness takes time, remember? Renew your resolve to stick with your plan.

1. List all the things you did well this week with respect to your personal fitness goals. (Use this space to evaluate exercise as well as nutrition.)

2. What, if anything, kept you from doing as well as you would have liked? (time, motivation, illness, etc.)

3. Can you change anything next week to improve your opportunity for success? If so, what, specifically?

4. Reevaluate your goals and revise them if necessary.

My nutritional fitness goals this week are:

_____

_____

_____

_____

_____

_____

_____

*Recipe at end of chapter.

Week 2—Menu Guide

In this week's menu guide, you will notice a decrease in fats from animal sources. The protein sources in the menus are leaner and the milk is either skim or 1% instead of low-fat (2%). That's because animal fat is predominately *saturated* and we need to *keep saturated fats to less than a third of total fat intake*. Also this week, there is more emphasis on whole grains and dietary fiber.

MEALS

Note: All meals provide a balance of carbohydrate, protein, and fat for optimum energy. If you plan to eat within two hours of exercising, choose the AM snack *or* a liquid meal.

Morning

Water

Fruit juice

Fresh or dried fruit

Grains: bran cereal and/or 100% whole-grain bread

8 ounces skim or 1% milk or yogurt OR 1 to 2 ounces protein

1 to 2 fat servings

Coffee or tea, if desired; 2 cups maximum

Midday

Water

2 to 3 ounces lean protein

Any grains, including at least one whole grain

Vegetables

Fruit (optional)

8 ounces skim or 1% milk or yogurt

1 to 2 fat servings (if other food choices are low fat)

Evening

Water

2 to 3 ounces lean protein

Any grains, including at least one whole grain

Vegetables

Sweet

1 to 2 fats (within daily fat gram allotment)

SNACKS—DRINK WATER; FOOD IS OPTIONAL

AM

Water

Grain: bread or whole-grain crackers

Fruit (optional)

4 ounces skim or 1% milk or yogurt (optional)

1 cup coffee or tea, if desired

Afternoon

Water

Any whole grain or sweet or fruit

Decaf coffee or tea or caffeine-free diet soda, if desired

Bedtime

Water

Herbal tea, if desired

Grain or fruit, optional and only if hungry

Remember to keep track of what you are eating every day. Use the following two menus to get you started on this week's menu guide. Portion sizes are given only for proteins, milk, fats, and sugars. Let your hunger be your guide for the amounts of other foods to eat. Consult the Power Nutrition Food Groups to get ideas for your own menus. Tip: In recipes, cut the amount of fat called for in half. This works well in almost everything without affecting texture or flavor. The recipes included in this chapter are already low in fat.

A FEW USEFUL AND DELICIOUS FAT-FREE OR LOW-FAT FOOD PRODUCTS

Promise Ultra nonfat margarine

Low-fat, tub margarine (liquid oil as primary oil source)

Butter Buds

Molly McButter

Nonstick cooking spray (or pump)

Nonfat plain yogurt, drained

Low-fat mayonnaise (Spectrum Naturals brand, preferably)

Snackwell's cookies and crackers

Dole fruit sorbet

Golden Fruit Raisin Biscuits

Evaporated skimmed milk (for coffee or cooking)

Health Valley brand foods

Pritikin brand foods

Healthy Choice brand foods

WEEK 2—SAMPLE MENUS

(BASED ON THE MENU GUIDE)

If the menus, including the snacks, do not contain enough food to satisfy your hunger, eat larger portions of the grains and vegetables.

MENU ONE	FOOD GROUP	MENU TWO	FOOD GROUP
Morning Meal		**Morning Meal**	
Large glass of water		Large glass of water	
Orange juice	Fruit	Grapefruit juice	Fruit
Fresh strawberries, added to	Fruit	Mixed fruit salad	Fruit
Raisin Bran cereal	Grain/Fruit	100% whole-grain toast with	Grain
100% whole-grain toast with	Grain	½ tablespoon jam	Extra
1 to 2 teaspoons low-fat tub margarine	Fat	1 to 2 eggs or egg substitute, scrambled and	Protein
8 ounces skim milk	Milk	cooked with cooking spray	
Coffee or tea (with milk, if desired)	Extra	Coffee or tea (with milk, if desired)	Extra
1 teaspoon sugar (or Equal), if needed	Extra	1 teaspoon sugar (or Equal), if needed	Extra
AM Snack		**AM Snack**	
Water		Water	
Ry-Krisp or Wasa crackers with	Grain	Rice cakes	Grain
fat-free cream cheese	Extra	Raisins, added to	Fruit
Grapes	Fruit	½ cup nonfat plain yogurt	Milk
1 cup coffee or tea, if desired	Extra	Coffee or tea, if desired	Extra
Midday Meal		**Midday Meal**	
Large glass of water		Large glass of water	
2 ounces turkey on	Protein	Salad bar:	
100% whole-grain bread with	Grain	Lettuce and raw vegetables topped with	Vegetable
leaf lettuce, tomato, and sprouts	Vegetable	beans and 2 tablespoons cheese,	Protein
½ tablespoon low-fat mayonnaise	Fat	1 to 2 tablespoons low-fat or fat-free	
Raw broccoli and cauliflower with	Vegetable	salad dressing	Extra
Light Veggie Dip*	Extra	Pasta salad, oil-based dressing	Grain/Fat
8 ounces fruited nonfat yogurt	Milk	Assortment of fresh fruit from salad bar	Fruit
		Crackers, whole-grain, if available	Grain
Afternoon Snack		8 ounces skim or 1% milk	Milk
Water		**Afternoon Snack**	
2 fig bars	Sweet	Water	
Decaf coffee, if desired	Extra	Health Valley Fat Free Granola Bar	Grain
1 teaspoon sugar (or Equal), if needed	Extra	Decaf coffee or tea, if desired	Extra
Evening Meal		**Evening Meal**	
Large glass of water		Large glass of water	
3 ounces **Grilled Tuna Steak***	Protein	3 ounces roasted turkey breast, no skin	Protein
Spinach whole wheat noodles tossed with	Grain	Baked yam with 1 teaspoon low-fat tub	Veg/Fat
1 teaspoon olive oil and 1 tablespoon		margarine	
Parmesan cheese	Fat	Green beans seasoned with 1 tablespoon	
Grilled Zucchini and Mushrooms*	Vegetable	toasted almonds	Veg/Fat
Tossed green salad with	Vegetable	100% whole-grain rolls	Grain
fat-free salad dressing	Extra	Fruit sorbet with 3 vanilla wafer cookies	Sweet
5 ounces white wine (optional)		**Bedtime**	
½ cup low-fat or fat-free pudding	Sweet	Water	
Bedtime		Apple	Fruit
Water			
100% whole-grain toast with	Grain		
½ tablespoon jam	Extra		

*Recipe at end of chapter.

WEEK 2 IN REVIEW

Answer the following questions to evaluate your progress this week. Congratulate yourself for all your positive steps. Do not dwell on the things you could have done better. Improving your nutritional fitness takes time, remember? Renew your resolve to stick with your plan.

1. List all the things you did well this week with respect to your personal fitness goals.

2. In what specific ways did you lower your fat intake and increase whole grains this week?

3. What, if anything, kept you from doing as well as you would have liked? (time, motivation, illness, etc.)

4. Can you change anything next week to improve your opportunity for success? If so, what, specifically?

5. Reevaluate your goals and revise them if necessary.

My nutritional fitness goals this week are:

_____
_____
_____
_____
_____
_____
_____
_____
_____

Week 3—Menu Guide

How about some vegetarian meals? This week the additional focus is on using more vegetable protein and less animal protein. Have at least one vegetarian meal every day. If you are already vegetarian, then this week will be easy.

MEALS

Note: All meals provide a balance of carbohydrate, protein, and fat for optimum energy. If you plan to eat within two hours of exercising, choose the AM snack *or* a liquid meal.

Morning
Water
Fresh or dried fruit
Fruit guice
Grains: bran or whole-grain cereal and/or 100% whole-grain bread
8 ounces skim or 1% milk or yogurt
OR 1 to 2 ounces protein
1 to 2 fat servings
Coffee or tea, if desired; 2 cups maximum

Midday
Water
2 to 3 ounces lean protein
Any grains, including at least one whole grain
Vegetables
Fruit (optional)
8 ounces skim or 1% milk or yogurt
1 to 2 fat servings

Evening
Water
2 to 3 ounces lean protein
Any grains, including at least one whole grain
Vegetables
Sweet
1 to 2 fats (within daily fat gram allotment)

SNACKS—DRINK WATER; FOOD IS OPTIONAL

AM
Water
Grain: bread or whole-grain crackers
Fruit (optional)
4 ounces skim or 1% milk or yogurt (optional)
1 cup coffee or tea, if desired

Afternoon
Water

Any whole grain or sweet or fruit
Decaf coffee or tea or caffeine-free diet soda, if desired

Bedtime
Water
Herbal tea, if desired
Grain or fruit, optional and only if hungry.

Remember to keep track of what you are eating every day. Use the following two menus to get you started on this week's menu guide. Portion sizes are given only for proteins, milk, fat, and sugars. Let your hunger be your guide for the amounts of other foods to eat. Consult the Power Nutrition Food Groups to get ideas for your own menus. You might want to borrow or buy a vegetarian cookbook to get some new ideas for nonmeat meals. Also, visit a health food store or the natural foods section of your grocery store to find convenient vegetarian food products.

WEEK 3—SAMPLE MENUS

(BASED ON THE MENU GUIDE)
If the menus, including the snacks, do not contain enough food to satisfy your hunger, eat larger portions of the grains and vegetables.

MENU ONE	FOOD GROUP
Morning Meal	
Large glass of water	
Orange juice	Fruit
Steel-cut oats cooked with	Grain
raisins and apple chunks	Fruit
1 tablespoon brown sugar, if desired	Sugar
100% whole-grain toast with	Grain
1 to 2 teaspoons low-fat tub margarine	Fat
8 ounces skim or 1% milk (or soy milk)	Milk
Coffee or tea (with milk, if desired)	Extra
1 teaspoon sugar (or Equal), if needed	Extra
AM Snack	
Water	
4 ounces nonfat yogurt with	Milk
Muesli, low-fat granola cereal, or Grape-Nuts	Grain
Midday Meal	
Large glass of water	
Bean Burrito* made with:	
refried beans	Protein
flour tortillas	Grain

	FOOD GROUP
lettuce, tomato, onion	Vegetable
fat-free sour cream, if desired	Extra
Salsa	Extra
Cantaloupe slices	Fruit
Afternoon Snack	
Water	
Low-fat microwave popcorn	Grain
Diet soda, if desired	Extra
Evening Meal	
Large glass of water	
Hamburger made with:	
3-ounce burger made from extra-lean beef	Protein
whole-grain hamburger bun	Grain
piled high with leaf lettuce, tomato, and onions	Vegetable
mustard, ketchup, or low-fat mayonnaise	Extra/Fat
Baked potato topped with chives and	Vegetable
Light Veggie Dip	Extra
12 ounces beer (optional)	
2 peppermint candies	Sweet
Bedtime	
Water	

*Recipe at end of chapter.

MENU TWO	FOOD GROUP
Morning Meal	
Large glass of water	
Grapefruit juice	Fruit
Nutri-Grain waffles topped with	Grain
berries and canned peaches and	Fruit
½ cup nonfat vanilla yogurt	Milk
½ cup skim or 1% milk	Milk
Coffee or tea (with milk, if desired)	Extra
1 teaspoon sugar (or Equal), if needed	Extra
AM Snack	
Water	
Rice cakes with	Grain
1 tablespoon natural peanut or almond butter	Fat
(counts as fat not protein due to small	
serving size)	
Midday Meal	
Large glass of water	
Whole-grain pita pocket bread stuffed with	Grain
Hummus* with	Protein/Fat
lettuce, tomato, and sprouts	Vegetable
Banana	Fruit
8 ounces skim or 1% milk (or soy milk)	Milk
Afternoon Snack	
Water	
Fat-free or low-fat granola bar	Grain

Evening Meal

Large glass of water

Spicy Veggie Stir-Fry* made with:

tofu chunks	Protein
broccoli, carrots, and snow peas	Vegetable
cooked brown rice	Grain
olive and sesame oils	Fat
Cold cucumber slices	Vegetable
Tanya's Frozen Yogurt*	Fruit/Milk

Bedtime

Water	
Herbal tea	Extra

*Recipe at end of chapter.

WEEK 3 IN REVIEW

Answer the following questions to evaluate your progress this week. Congratulate yourself for all your positive steps. Do not dwell on the things you could have done better. Improving your nutritional fitness takes time, remember? Renew your resolve to stick with your plan.

1. List all the things you did well this week with respect to your personal fitness goals.

2. Were you successful in eating less animal protein? Which vegetarian meals did you find satisfying?

3. What, if anything, kept you from doing as well as you would have liked? (time, motivation, illness, etc.)

4. Can you change anything next week to improve your opportunity for success? If so, what, specifically?

5. Reevaluate your goals and revise them if necessary.

My nutritional fitness goals this week are:

_____
_____
_____
_____
_____
_____

Week 4—Menu Guide

It is time to get more creative with vegetables in your diet. Americans simply do not eat enough of them and that may be one of the most significant downfalls of the American diet, with respect to disease prevention. It is also time to become more aware of how much salt you are eating. Up until now, the menu guides and menus have not really mentioned salt at all. This week, you will try some reduced-salt foods and experiment more with spices for seasoning.

MEALS

Note: All meals provide a balance of carbohydrate, protein, and fat for optimum energy. If you plan to eat within two hours of exercising, choose the AM snack *or* a liquid meal.

Morning

Water

Fresh or dried fruit and/or vegetable

Fruit juice

Grains: bran or whole-grain cereal and/or 100% whole-grain bread

8 ounces skim or 1% milk or yogurt

OR 1 to 2 ounces protein

1 to 2 fat servings

Coffee or tea, if desired; 2 cups maximum

Midday

Water

2 to 3 ounces lean protein

Any grains, including at least one whole grain

Vegetables

Fruit (optional)

8 ounces skim or 1% milk or yogurt

1 to 2 fat servings

Evening

Water

2 to 3 ounces lean protein

Any grains including at least one whole grain

Vegetables

Sweet

1 to 2 fats (within daily fat gram allotment)

SNACKS—DRINK WATER; FOOD IS OPTIONAL

AM

Water

Grain: bread or whole-grain crackers

Fruit (optional)

4 ounces skim or 1% milk or yogurt (optional)

1 cup coffee or tea, if desired

Afternoon

Water

Any whole grain or sweet or fruit

Decaf coffee or tea or caffeine-free diet soda, if desired

Bedtime

Water

Herbal tea, if desired

Grain or fruit, optional and only if hungry

Remember to keep track of what you are eating every day. Use the following two menus to get you started on this week's menu guide. Portion sizes are given only for proteins, fats, and sugars. Let your hunger be your guide for the amounts of other foods to eat. Consult the Power Nutrition Food Groups to get ideas for your own menus. Tip: In recipes, reduce the salt called for by one-half. If making casserole dishes or stews, double the amount of vegetables called for. The recipes in this week's menus are already salt reduced.

LOW-SALT PRODUCTS TO TRY

Mrs. Dash spice blends

Papa Dash low-sodium salt

Newman's Own Salsa—lower in sodium than most brands

Worcestershire sauce instead of soy sauce

Health Valley brand soups

Pritikin brand soups

WEEK 4—SAMPLE MENUS

(BASED ON THE MENU GUIDE)

If the menus, including the snacks, do not contain enough food to satisfy your hunger, eat larger portions of the grains and vegetables.

MENU ONE	FOOD GROUP
Morning Meal	
Large glass of water	
Apple juice	Fruit
Fresh grapefruit	Fruit
Spinach Omelette* made with:	
½ cup egg substitute	Protein
2 tablespoons grated low-fat cheese	Protein
spinach and onion	Vegetable
100% whole-grain toast with	Grain
1 to 2 teaspoons fat-free or low-fat tub margarine	Fat

Coffee or tea (with milk, if desired)	Extra
1 teaspoon sugar (or Equal), if needed	Extra
AM Snack	
Water	
(Very likely, you won't be hungry for a snack after the above breakfast.)	
1 cup coffee or tea, if desired	Extra
Midday Meal	
Large glass of water	
Onion or whole-grain bagel with	Grain
fat-free cream cheese	Extra
2 ounces surimi (fake crab)	Protein
Onion and tomato slices	Vegetable
Light 'n Tangy V-8 juice (or low-sodium)	Vegetable
8 ounces nonfat vanilla yogurt	Milk
Afternoon Snack	
Water	
Zucchini Health Muffin*	Grain/Sweet
Decaf coffee or tea, if desired	Extra
Evening Meal	
Large glass of water	
Pasta Primavera* made with:	
fettucini noodles	Grain
2 ounces cubed chicken breast	Protein
broccoli, carrots, pepper, mushrooms, squash	Vegetables
French bread with **Baked Garlic***	Grain
Berries with sorbet	Fruit/Sweet
5 ounces white wine (optional)	
Bedtime	
Water	
Herbal tea	Extra

*Recipe at end of chapter.

MENU TWO**	FOOD GROUP
Morning Meal	
Large glass of water	
Orange juice	Fruit
Grapes	Fruit
Breakfast Beans* made with:	
½ cup pinto beans	Protein
1 egg	Protein
Pico de Gallo*	Vegetable
Flour or corn tortillas	Grain
Coffee or tea (with milk, if desired)	Extra
1 teaspoon sugar (or Equal), if needed	Extra
AM Snack	
Water	
Low-fat or fat-free granola bar	Grain
Coffee or tea, if desired	Extra

Midday Meal

Large glass of water	
Large green salad with variety of raw vegetables	Vegetable
Balsamic or garlic vinegar for dressing	Extra
Fantastic Foods Only A Pinch Lentils and Couscous soup	Prot/Grain
Whole-grain crackers	Grain
8 ounces skim or 1% milk	Milk
Banana	Fruit

Afternoon Snack

Water	
Unsalted jumbo pretzels	Grain
Diet, caffeine-free soda or iced tea	Extra

Evening Meal

Large glass of water	
Wide *no-yolk* egg noodles with	Grain
Onion Béchamel Sauce* (The milk in this recipe is the protein source.)	Veg/Milk
Steamed asparagus	Vegetable
Whole-grain rolls with	Grain
1 to 2 teaspoons low-fat tub margarine	Fat
Bloody Mary made with low-salt tomato juice (optional)	Vegetable
Delicious and Lean Chocolate Cupcake*	Sweet
Decaf coffee or tea, if desired	Extra

Bedtime

Water

*Recipe at end of chapter.
**This menu contains no meat, chicken, or fish and may appear low in protein. But, every *meal* contains complete protein. The menu has a total of 81 grams of protein!

WEEK 4 IN REVIEW

Answer the following questions to evaluate your progress this week. Congratulate yourself for all your positive steps. Do not dwell on the things you could have done better. Improving your nutritional fitness takes time, remember? Renew your resolve to stick with your plan.

1. List all the things you did well this week with respect to your personal fitness goals.

2. Did you meet the recommended intake for vegetables at least five of seven days? If not, how can you, specifically, meet this goal?

3. What, if anything, kept you from doing as well as you would have liked? (time, motivation, illness, etc.)

4. Can you change anything next week to improve your opportunity for success? If so, what, specifically?

5. Reevaluate your goals and revise them if necessary.

My nutritional fitness goals this week are:

_____

_____

_____

_____

Week 5—Menu Guide

This week, pay attention to your sugar/sweet intake. Do you always use sugar or sugar substitute in coffee, tea, or iced tea? Do you always use jam on toast or sweetened yogurt? Do you always eat the sweet serving listed in the menu guide? If so, it is time to wean yourself away from so much sugar. Remember the guideline: No more than two servings per day. Experiment with sugars that provide a little more nutrition than the white stuff, such as blackstrap molasses, pure maple syrup, and all-fruit jams. This week's menus feature fewer sweets and more fruit. Also featured are several nondairy, high-calcium foods (included for those people who do not use dairy products).

MEALS

Note: All meals provide a balance of carbohydrate, protein, and fat for optimum energy. If you plan to eat within two hours of exercising, choose the AM snack *or* a liquid meal.

Morning

Water
Fresh or dried fruit and/or Vegetable
Fruit juice
Grains: bran or whole-grain cereal and/or 100% whole-grain bread
8 ounces skim or 1% milk or yogurt
OR 1 to 2 ounces protein
1 to 2 fat servings
Coffee or tea, if desired; 2 cups maximum

Midday
Water
2 to 3 ounces lean protein
Any grains, including at least one whole grain
Vegetables
Fruit (optional)
8 ounces skim or 1% milk or yogurt
1 to 2 fat servings

Evening
Water
2 to 3 ounces lean protein
Any grains including at least one whole grain
Vegetables
Sweet (optional)
1 to 2 fats (within daily fat gram allotment)

SNACKS—DRINK WATER; FOOD IS OPTIONAL

AM
Water
Grain: bread or whole-grain crackers
Fruit (optional)
4 ounces skim or 1% milk or yogurt (optional)
1 cup coffee or tea, if desired

Afternoon
Water
Any whole grain or fruit
Decaf coffee or tea or caffeine-free diet soda, if desired

Bedtime
Water
Herbal tea, if desired
Grain or fruit, optional and only if hungry

Remember to keep track of what you are eating every day. Use the following two menus to get you started on this week's menu guide. Portion sizes are given only for proteins, fats, and sugars. Let your hunger be your guide for the amounts of other foods to eat. Consult the Power Nutrition Food Groups to get ideas for your own menus. Tip: In recipes, reduce the sugar called for by one-half.

NONDAIRY FOODS HIGH IN CALCIUM
Blackberries
Blackstrap molasses
Broccoli
Corn tortillas
Currants
Figs
Fortified orange juice
Fortified soy milk
Kale
Miso
Salmon, canned with bones
Seaweed
Sweet potatoes
Tofu
Winter squash

WEEK 5—SAMPLE MENUS

(BASED ON THE MENU GUIDE)

If the menus, including the snacks, do not contain enough food to satisfy your hunger, eat larger portions of the grains and vegetables.

MENU ONE	FOOD GROUP
Morning Meal	
Large glass of water	
**Minute Maid calcium-fortified orange juice	Fruit
Shredded wheat with	Grain
skim milk or **soy milk and	Milk
fresh berries (or unsweetened frozen)	Fruit
Whole-grain toast with	Grain
1 ounce low-fat or soy cheese, melted	Protein
Coffee or tea, if desired	Extra
AM Snack	
Water	
Soy smoothie made with:	
½ cup **Fat Free Soy Moo	Milk
frozen, unsweetened peaches	Fruit
apple juice	Fruit
Midday Meal	
Large glass of water	
**Fantastic Foods Cha-Cha Chili	Protein
Baked tortilla chips with salsa (Guiltless Gourmet or Barbara's Amazing Bakes)	Grain
Tossed green salad with vinegar dressing	Vegetable
8 ounces yogurt	Milk
Afternoon Snack	
Water	
Knudsen Fruit Teazer	Fruit
Evening Meal	
Large glass of water	
3-ounce serving of **Salmon Loaf*	Protein
**Baked acorn or other winter squash with	Vegetable
1 teaspoon low-fat tub margarine	Fat
Steamed green beans and baby onions	Vegetable

Whole-grain bread or rolls	Grain
Unsweetened pineapple chunks	Fruit
5 ounces white wine (optional)	

Bedtime

Water	
**Blackstrap Coffee*	Extra

MENU TWO	FOOD GROUP
Morning Meal	
Large glass of water	
**Calcium-fortified orange juice	Fruit
Cranberry Multigrain Cereal*	Grain/Fruit
Whole-grain toast with all-fruit jam	Grain/Extra
(Smucker's Simply Fruit, Polaner All Fruit, for example)	
8 ounces skim milk or **soy milk	Milk
Coffee or tea, if desired	Extra
AM Snack	
Water	
Rice cakes with	Grain
1 tablespoon natural peanut or almond butter	Fat
Midday Meal	
Large glass of water	
Turkey sandwich with:	
2 ounces lean turkey	Protein
whole-grain bread	Grain
½ tablespoon low-fat or fat-free mayonnaise	Fat
piled high with leaf lettuce, tomato, and sprouts	Vegetable
Broccoli/Cauliflower Salad*	Vegetable
Dried apricots and **figs	Fruit
Afternoon Snack	
Pretzels (Try Barbara's or Snyder's of Hanover brand.)	Grain
Flavored seltzer water	Extra
Evening Meal	
Large glass of water	
Black Beans and Rice*	Prot./Grain
Jicama Sticks*	Vegetable
Tossed green salad with salsa or vinegar	Vegetable
French bread, with	Grain
1 teaspoon low-fat tub margarine	Fat
12 ounces light beer (optional)	
**Blackberries, unsweetened, topped with	Fruit
2 tablespoons frozen low-fat yogurt	Extra
Bedtime	
Water	

*Recipe at end of chapter.
**Nondairy food sources of calcium.

WEEK 5 IN REVIEW

Answer the following questions to evaluate your progress this week. Congratulate yourself for all your positive steps. Do not dwell on the things you could have done better. Improving your nutritional fitness takes time, remember? Renew your resolve to stick with your plan.

1. List all the things you did well this week with respect to your personal fitness goals.

2. Did you successfully reduce your sugar intake this week? What foods worked well as sugar replacements?

3. What, if anything, kept you from doing as well as you would have liked? (time, motivation, illness, etc.)

4. Can you change anything next week to improve your opportunity for success? If so, what, specifically?

5. Reevaluate your goals and revise them if necessary.

My nutritional fitness goals this week are:

_____

_____

_____

_____

Week 6—Menu Guide

Well, you have arrived! If you have been following the menu guides for the past five weeks, you are eating well. You have learned to eat balanced meals with your calorie intake spread out evenly over the course of the day. You are now in the habit of drinking more water and eating more whole grains, lots of vegetables and fruits, and low-fat foods. Protein and fat are adequate, but not excessive, in your diet and you get ample calcium. Sodium is less prevalent and you are eating more wholesome foods, providing lots of vitamins and minerals. You have, perhaps, been introduced to some new

FOOD GROUPS AND RECOMMENDED DAILY SERVINGS

Vegetables	At least 3 to 5 servings
Fruits	At least 1 to 2 servings
Grains	6 to 11 servings, using mostly whole grains
Protein	3 to 6 ounces per day, using plant proteins at least three times a week
Milk/Yogurt (cow, soy, or goat)	2 to 3 servings, using skim or 1%
Fats	Use added fat, predominately nonhydrogenated vegetable sources, within daily fat gram allotment
Sugars/Sweets	No more than 1 to 2 servings per day. Choose mostly sweets that contribute nutrients in addition to sugar.

foods and may be shopping more often in the natural foods aisle of your grocery store.

In short, you are now eating a fully *powered* diet and probably no longer need a menu guide. Instead, simply use the recommended intake from each food group as your daily guide to optimum nutrition. The food groups are summarized below, along with some tips for staying on track with Power Nutrition.

TIPS FOR STAYING ON TRACK

- Which food groups do you have the most difficulty getting enough of? Concentrate on eating those foods at breakfast and lunch.
- When it comes to planning your evening meal, determine which food groups you still need for the day. Let the evening meal consist of those foods.
- Always make enough food for leftovers when cooking. That way, you are more likely to have something nutritious on hand when you need a quick meal.
- Plan menus in advance. Planning is the hardest part, especially if you're tired. Getting it out of the way ahead of time saves time and energy.
- Periodically, record a day's food intake or do a twenty-four-hour food recall, such as in Step 2 of this plan (page 50). You can correct any tendencies toward poor eating habits if they are picked up early.

- Use cookbooks and cooking magazines, such as *Eating Well* and *Cooking Light,* to keep menus interesting and tasty.
- Learn to remake some of your old favorite foods into healthier versions rather than give them up completely. After all, eating lean and healthy foods needs to be a way of life, not a temporary *diet* strategy.

WEEK 6—SAMPLE MENU PLANNING GUIDE

Morning Meal	**Food Groups and Servings**
Large glass of water	
8 ounces orange juice	1 Fruit
1½ cups Raisin Bran cereal with	1½ Grain
8 ounces skim milk	1 Milk
1 slice whole-grain toast with	1 Grain
1 teaspoon all-fruit jam	Extra
1 cup instant coffee with skim milk	Extra
AM Snack	
Water	
Blueberry bagel with fat-free cream cheese	1 Grain
Midday Meal	
12-ounce can of Light 'n Tangy V-8	2 Vegetables
Tuna sandwich made with:	
2 slices whole-grain bread	2 Grain
2 ounces water-packed tuna mixed	2 ounces Protein
with fat-free mayo, lots of tomatoes,	
sprouts, leaf lettuce	1 Vegetable
1 large raw carrot	1 Vegetable

Afternoon Snack

_____

Evening Meal

_____
_____
_____
_____
_____

You fill in the blanks based on what is missing from the total recommended servings from each food group. In addition, ask yourself: Are you getting enough water? Are you drinking too much caffeine or alcohol? Are you remembering to replace carbohydrates after a long, tiring workout?

WEEK 6 IN REVIEW
Answer the following questions to evaluate your progress this week. Congratulate yourself for all your positive steps. Do not dwell on the things you could have done better. Improving your nutritional fitness takes time, remember? Renew your resolve to stick with your plan.

1. List all the things you did well this week with respect to your personal fitness goals.

2. What, if anything, kept you from doing as well as you would have liked? (time, motivation, illness, etc.)

3. Can you change anything next week to improve your opportunity for success? If so, what, specifically?

4. Reevaluate your goals and revise them if necessary.

My nutritional fitness goals this week are:

_____
_____
_____
_____
_____
_____

Putting Power Nutrition into Your Life

TROUBLESHOOTING GUIDE
Are you having trouble meeting your fitness goals or following the Power Nutrition Plan? Below are solutions to some of the most common problems encountered when trying to become nutritionally fit.

Problem: I'm not used to eating breakfast.
Solution: Sure, breakfast is important, but you may not be hungry enough to eat it first thing in the morning. In that case, eat your _breakfast_ meal during your midmorning coffee break. Or perhaps you are hungry by the time you leave for work, but there is no time to eat. Pack breakfast with you and eat it on the way to work. Smoothies and sandwiches are easy to handle in the car or on the bus.

Problem: I get too sleepy after eating a big lunch.
Solution: Perhaps you are simply overeating in order to eat everything on the menu guide. Remember, eat only until comfortably satisfied, not stuffed.

Or you may be affected by too many carbohydrates at lunch. Try cutting down or eliminating fruit, grains, and starchy vegetables at lunch. Eat a bigger portion of protein (about 4 to 5 ounces) and a salad. A high-protein, low-carbohydrate lunch will keep you more alert in the afternoon. You can eat more carbs and less protein at your evening meal.

Problem: Work requires eating out a lot, making it difficult to follow the menu guide.
Solution: Get a copy of _The Restaurant Companion_ by Hope Warshaw (Surrey Books, 1990). This handy reference will teach you how to eat low-fat foods in a variety of restaurants. Also, learn to become assertive when ordering in a restaurant. Ask how foods are prepared and request more vegetables. Order salad dressing and sauces _on the side._ You can always order fresh fruit even if it isn't listed on the menu. Look for menu items labeled as _heart healthy._ Try the vegetarian entrees; they can be a healthier choice.

If you end up eating with an important client who wants to go to his or her favorite high-fat restaurant, don't worry about it. Just try to work within your daily fat gram allotment. Sometimes friends or business associates try to insist you eat certain (usually high-fat) foods with them. This is so *they* feel better about what they want to eat. Learn to decline tactfully if you would rather make a healthier choice. You could say, "You go ahead. My stomach can't tolerate sausage (or whatever) anymore." Or, "That sounds great. What I'm really hungry for, though, is turkey on whole wheat."

Problem: I hate to cook! I need recipes that are easy and fast.

Solution: Explore your grocery store for convenient, healthy products, such as Healthy Choice frozen dinners, Fantastic Foods soups, and Lundberg Family Farms One-Step Rice & Lentil dishes. In the following section, "Planning Tips," there is a list of foods to keep on hand that are quick and nutritious. The natural foods section is a good place to find healthy, convenient foods.

Check out the following cookbooks for healthy meals you can prepare quickly.

Healthy Cooking for Two, by Brenda and Angela
  Shriver, The Summit Group, 1994.
Microwave Gourmet Healthstyle Cookbook, by Barbara Kafka, William Morrow and Co., 1989.
Quick and Healthy, by Brenda Ponichtera, R.D.,
  ScaleDown, The Dalles, Oregon, 1991.
*Simply Colorado: Nutritious Recipes for Busy
  People,* Colorado Dietetic Association,
  (303) 830–1980.

Problem: My hectic schedule keeps me from eating regularly. I miss lunch a lot and dinner is often eaten after 8 P.M.

Solution: You need to have an emergency nutrition kit available. This means stocking your desk drawer or your car with healthy snacks that, when necessary, can be a meal. Skipping meals will only zap your energy level and may lead to overeating later in the day or evening. If your schedule forces you to rely on several minimeals throughout the day, so be it. Simply prepare yourself with healthy choices instead of relying on vending machines.

Try meal replacement bars, such as PowerBars, XTRNR bars, Bear Valley MealPack, and Great Cakes. These are much better than a candy bar and just as quick. Other helpful items you can stash easily include Healthy Valley Fat Free Granola Bars, small pop-top cans of tuna, low-fat crackers, bagels, assorted dried fruits, and small cans of fruit juice or V-8 juice.

Problem: The menu guides have too much food at each meal. I can't possibly eat all that!

Solution: The menu guides may *appear* to have a lot of food because each meal is itemized with foods from all the different food groups. Let's assume you normally go to the local deli for lunch and may have a corned beef sandwich, chips, and soda for lunch. Your meal consists of grain (bread), protein (corned beef), perhaps vegetables (lettuce, tomato, kraut), fat (chips, fatty meat), and sweet (soda). Your total intake is approximately 610 calories and 22 fat grams. If, at the same deli, you chose a salad meal, such as the one described in Week 2, Menu 2, you would eat 626 calories and 17 fat grams. So, for about the same amount of calories (energy), you get *a lot more nutrition* and less fat with a Power Nutrition meal.

Whole grains, fresh vegetables, and fruits are bulky and take longer to eat than fatty, processed foods. It looks like you have more food on your plate. What you really have is more nutrition on your plate for less fat and calories. A Power Nutrition meal translates into more energy and feeling better.

Problem: If I eat breakfast, I'm hungrier at lunch. I end up eating too much and can't lose weight.

Solution: Well, let's not forget it is normal to eat several times a day. That includes eating breakfast *and* lunch, dinner, and probably one or more snacks. You may have been skipping breakfast and eating a light lunch to make up for overeating in the late afternoon and evening. But this pattern doesn't work; it only insures you will, again, be ravenous in the latter part of the day. It's time to break this cycle if you really want to lose body fat and achieve nutritional fitness.

If eating breakfast makes you hungrier all day, perhaps you aren't eating enough. A slice of toast or glass of juice won't sustain you for long. Eating a larger, more balanced breakfast that includes some protein will usually carry you through to lunch quite nicely. And you will be more productive and alert all morning. If you haven't been eating breakfast, it will take some time to get your body used to it again. Give yourself at least two weeks of eating a Power Nutrition breakfast before you decide it isn't working.

Problem: I don't have time for all this planning and recording. I usually lose weight with Slim-Fast. Is there anything wrong with using it or something similar?

Solution: Perhaps you are struggling with the commitment that permanent change requires. Perhaps you simply want quick results with little effort on your part. That's what diets promise and can't deliver! Any of the hundreds of diets available will allow you to lose weight, for as long as you follow the diet. The problem with diets is they simply do not work for 95 percent of the people who use them. Sure, you may lose weight initially, but it doesn't stay off. That's because most diets are impossible, if not unhealthy, to follow for extended periods of time. Another reason, diets do not teach you how to eat; they teach you how to go hungry!

The Power Nutrition Plan is absolutely doable! And it teaches you how to sustain nutritional fitness for a lifetime. The planning and recording seem burdensome in the beginning, but they really take very little time. Follow the planning tips and other suggestions for making this as easy as possible. The record keeping takes only a few minutes, if done as you go. Another ten to fifteen minutes in the evening to evaluate your daily progress is not much to ask, considering the results you will get.

The short-term success achieved with dieting is not *real* success; it is fantasy. The weight is quickly regained, accompanied with disappointment and frustration. Eventually, you give up, feeling like a complete failure. I urge you to *get out of the dieting trap*. Be patient with yourself and continue to tackle your nutritional goals, one at a time. The results, perhaps a little longer in coming, will be much more rewarding than any temporary weight loss a diet can give you.

Problem: I *want* to follow the plan, but can't seem to stick with it more than a day or two.

Solution: Stop getting in your own way! This happens to most of us at some point when trying to change something as ingrained as eating habits. Examine your *self-talk*. What kind of things are you saying to yourself about the plan and your ability to follow it? Is it mostly negative? Do you try to use guilt to motivate yourself? These are common, usually unconscious, self-defeating tactics used by *dieters*. The Power Nutrition Plan is not about dieting or being perfect. Use positive language to reinforce progress and forgive yourself for slipups.

Are your goals realistic? Are you trying to change something that doesn't need to change? For example, are you trying to lose body fat when you don't need to? Perhaps you are trying to change too many things at once. Reevaluate the goals you have identified and try to simplify them. Insure success by taking *baby steps* on your road to fitness.

You may benefit from working with a registered dietitian, experienced in the areas you need help with. Look in the yellow pages or call your local hospital for names of professionals in your area. You can also contact the American Dietetic Association's nationwide nutrition network at (800) 366–1655. The network helps you determine what type of nutrition counseling you need and can make an appropriate referral in your location.

PLANNING TIPS

Healthy meals don't just happen unless you think *nutrition* when you think about food. Planning menus ahead is an invaluable tool in helping you stay on track with the Power Nutrition Plan. You may shy away from planning because of the time involved, but I spend less than one hour a week planning menus. That hour saves me time later in trying to figure out what to cook. Also, if I am tired at the end of the day and haven't pre-planned dinner, I am more likely to opt for a quick dinner out or a frozen pizza. Here are some simple strategies for planning and preparing healthy menus:

- Look through cookbooks to select recipes/dishes. Select four or five dinner meals for the week.
- Shop according to the recipes so that you have everything you need on hand.

QUICK BREAKFAST FOODS TO KEEP ON HAND	CONVENIENT PACKABLES FOR LUNCH AND SNACKS	EASY-TO-PREPARE FOODS TO KEEP ON HAND
A variety of dry cereals—shredded wheat, bran flakes, low-fat granola, muesli, Grape-Nuts, etc.	Light 'n Tangy V-8 juice	Bean Cuisine Creative Dishes
Skim or 1% milk	Sparkling fruit juice and water—Sundance, EverFresh, Fruit Teazer	Butterball seasoned, skinless chicken breasts
Nonfat or low-fat yogurt, plain and fruited	Instant bean and lentil soups—Nile Spice or Fantastic Foods	Lundberg Family Farms One-Step Gourmet Rice & Lentils
Frozen, unsweetened fruit	Fat-free bean dip—Bearitos or Guiltless Gourmet	Fantastic Foods Tabouli Salad Mix (use ½ the oil)
Bagels	Fat-free tortilla chips—Amazing Bakes, Guiltless Gourmet, Slim Chips, etc.	Prewashed spinach
Cottage cheese		Frozen vegetables, plain
Fat-free cream cheese	Nonfat or low-fat cheese	Canned beans—black, garbanzo, etc.
Health Valley Fat Free Granola Bars	Peanut butter, the natural kind	Refried beans—fat-free or vegetarian refried
Health Valley Fruit Bakes (not the fat-free ones, they are too dry)	Whole-grain crackers—Kavli, Wasa, Ryvita	Tortillas (serve with beans)
Health Valley Fat Free Muffins	Low fat crackers—saltines, Snackwell's, Health Valley	Fresh veggies that store well—carrots, onions, potatoes
Fresh fruit	Pretzels, preferably low-salt	Chinese noodles (cook in three minutes)
Frozen juices	Rice cakes	Variety of noodles/pasta
Weight Watchers Breakfast On-The-Go English Muffin Sandwich	Carrots, prewashed	Couscous
Small cans or boxes of 100% fruit juice, such as Minute Maid	Pocket bread (fill with veggies, hummus, etc.)	Marinara pasta sauce—Healthy Choice, Enrico's, Ragú Today's Recipe, or any other low-fat version
Frozen egg substitute (thaws quickly in microwave)	FiBar	Uncle Ben's Country Inn Recipes
Eggo Nutri-Grain Waffles	Meal replacement bars—PowerBar, XTRNR, Great Cakes, Bear Valley MealPack	Uncle Ben's Long Grain & Wild Rice mix
Pancake mix, such as Aunt Jemima Complete Pancake & Waffle Mix	Pineapple, snack-sized, canned in juice, with pop-top	Low-fat frozen meals—Healthy Choice, Lean Cuisine, Tyson, etc.
Pure maple or low-sugar syrup	Tuna, small pop-top cans	Popcorn, microwave—Orville Redenbacher's Smart Pop, Jolly Time Light
Raisins and other dried fruits		
Whole-grain bread		

- Prepare extra amounts of foods that are called for in more than one dish. For example, you could have baked chicken with rice and then use the leftovers to make a vegetable/chicken stir-fry.
- Always cook enough for leftovers. Use these for the next day's lunch whenever possible. Freeze the rest for an easy meal later. You can even make your own *TV dinners* by freezing individual meals on divided plates.
- Keep plenty of quick breakfast and lunch items on hand to fill in when there are no leftovers. Some suggestions are listed above.

SURVIVING THE GROCERY STORE

I actually *enjoy* going to the grocery store, checking out the new products, and selecting healthy, delicious foods. But I know a lot of people lose their imagination when it comes to food. Grocery shopping becomes a tedious chore they try to get through as quickly as possible. They buy the same foods over and over only to find themselves bored with the task of putting food on the table. It doesn't have to be that way!

The next time you go grocery shopping:

- Go when you are not already exhausted.
- Always have a shopping list to ease the trauma of decision making. This is especially helpful if you do end up at the store feeling tired.
- Allow yourself plenty of time. Read a few food labels and get acquainted with new products. Comparison shop on the basis of ingredients and fat grams in addition to price. For example, if you are looking for a granola bar, choose one that lists a real food as the first ingredient—fruit or whole grain—as opposed to a sugar. Then check the fat grams before deciding which brand to buy.
- Plan to purchase one new food each week—a new vegetable or low-fat item, for example. The *natural foods* aisle is a great place to explore. You will find unusual grains, as well as some healthy convenience foods.
- Leave the kids at home, unless they are old enough to be helpful.
- Don't go with a ravenous appetite or an overly full

belly. If you arrive at the store hungry, take the time to get a snack before you start shopping.

THINGS TO CONSIDER ON A FOOD LABEL

Recent changes in food labeling laws make it easier to understand the nutritional value of foods. Here are some basics to know:

Ingredients Are Listed in Descending Order by Weight. The item listed first is present in the largest amount, based on weight, not volume or calories. The further down the list, the less there is of that item.

The Bold Print Is Marketing. Even though health claims are regulated by law, food companies take as much liberty as possible in promoting their products. Read the nutritional information before deciding if the product meets your standards.

Pay Attention to Serving Size. It is the amount of food that corresponds to the nutrition facts presented. Under the new regulations, serving sizes are now standardized for similar products, making it easier to compare brands.

Nutrition Information. Now called Nutrition Facts on food labels, nutrition information has been updated to provide data more pertinent to health issues today. Calories from fat are given in addition to total calories. Also new is the requirement to list grams of sugar and dietary fiber, along with the total amount of carbohydrate present.

Since deficiency of B vitamins is no longer a major health concern in the United States, B vitamins are no longer listed. Now only vitamins A and C, calcium, and iron are required. Of course, sodium, protein, saturated fat, cholesterol, and total fat grams are still listed.

% Daily Value. This refers to the amount of nutrients present compared to the amounts recommended in a 2,000-calorie diet. The 2,000-calorie reference diet is based on average needs for women, children, and men over age fifty.

Daily Values Footnote. This lists the daily values (not percentage) for fat, saturated fat, cholesterol, sodium, carbohydrate, and dietary fiber in the 2,000-calorie reference diet. Some labels will also give daily values for a 2,500-calorie diet, an average amount needed by teenage boys, men under fifty, and very active people.

When the Bold Print Says "93% Fat Free, 7% Fat." If you see this, it usually refers to fat by weight, not by calories. You will often see this on meat products. The fat by calories could be way over 30 percent. Check the fat grams and calories per serving to decide if it is a low-fat product.

Easy Guideline. Any food with 3 or fewer fat grams per 100 calories is a low-fat food. You don't have to eat low-fat foods exclusively; it is your total fat intake that counts. But it is helpful to compare the fat content of different brands of the same food.

Fat-Free Foods. There are literally hundreds on the market now. Some are useful and others are just fat-free junk foods. Be aware that many low-fat products have traded sugar and additives for the fat. Just because a food is fat-free doesn't make it healthy.

COOKING TIPS THAT REALLY WORK!

- Always read a recipe entirely before beginning to prepare it. Get out all the necessary ingredients before you begin; this will save time later on.
- Invest in some good nonstick cookware and the utensils that won't scratch them.
- Canned products are usually cheaper than the same product in jars.
- Use nonfat yogurt or blended cottage cheese instead of sour cream.
- Reduce the fat in most recipes by half without affecting flavor or quality.
- Sauté or stir-fry vegetables in water or broth instead of oil. Or if using a nonstick skillet, coat it with a cooking spray or pump, such as Pam, first. Then you can get by with using only 1 teaspoon of oil for cooking.
- Use 2 egg whites in place of 1 whole egg to cut fat

and cholesterol. Separating the eggs yourself is less expensive than buying egg substitutes.
- To substitute liquid oil for solid fats, use one-quarter less oil than the recipe calls for. Example, use 3 tablespoons oil instead of 4 tablespoons shortening. You will have to experiment with this method in baked goods to get the right consistency.
- Cut the sugar by one-third to one-half in baked goods and desserts. Add extra spice or flavoring, such as orange peel, to enhance the impression of sweetness.
- Substitute nonfat dry milk for part of the sugar in cookies and loaf breads to increase calcium and protein.
- You can safely cut the salt by half in most recipes without altering flavor.
- Experiment with herbs and spices to replace both salt and added fat in recipes. Dry fresh herbs in the microwave for ten to fifteen seconds, on low.
- Increase the fiber in baked goods by using whole-grain flour for half of the total flour called for. If you choose to use all whole-grain flour, use 2 tablespoons *less* per cup.
- Add oat bran or wheat germ when cooking hot cereals to increase fiber and nutrients.
- Add more fruit or vegetables than called for in casseroles or other recipes.
- Add grated carrots or zucchini to meat loaf.
- Cook with a mixture of fat-free cheese and low-fat cheese instead of regular cheese. This works well in casseroles, on pizza, or other dishes with baked cheese.
- Omit the oil and salt in the cooking water for rice or pasta. They aren't necessary. Rinse cooked pasta with cool water immediately after cooking to keep it from being sticky.
- To enhance the flavor of beans without fat, use chilies, coriander, cumin, tumeric, oregano, thyme, or savory.
- To reduce gas formation from beans, boil the beans in water for three minutes and let them soak for eight hours or so. Add one or two strips of kombu seaweed (found in the natural foods department) during cooking. You can remove the

seaweed before serving, if desired; it does not flavor the beans.

- Do not soak fresh produce to clean it. This leaches out water-soluble nutrients.
- Fresh vegetables are superior in nutrition to canned and frozen ones only if they are handled properly. Cook them with as little water as possible, cover while cooking, and cook only until tender. Use steaming, stir-frying, or pressure cookers instead of boiling. Do not overtrim or overchop vegetables, as this causes more nutrients to be lost.
- Use glass containers in the microwave whenever possible. Chemical compounds in plastic containers can migrate into fatty foods (another good reason to cut the fat!).

WHEN IN RESTAURANTS

- Initially, choose restaurants that you are familiar with. Before you get there, plan what you will order. (Save room during the day for a little extra fat from the restaurant meal.) Then look at the menu to confirm it is a good choice by evaluating how it is prepared.
- Request sauces be brought on the side or eliminated. *Be assertive; after all, you are the paying customer!*
- Ask questions about how foods are prepared: "Are the vegetables seasoned with butter or some other source of fat?"
- Don't be shy about making special requests: "Please substitute a baked potato for the french fries and bring the sour cream on the side." Some waiters will act as though it can't be done or be miffed that you are making their job more difficult. *Too bad!* They are there to serve you. You are paying them to do it and it is your right to get what you want if at all possible. You may have to gently, but firmly, remind your waiter of that.
- Choose items that are *steamed, poached, grilled, or barbecued* instead of *fried, deep-fried, topped with cheese, or in cream sauce.*
- Look for items that are marked as *heart healthy* or *low fat.* Many restaurants now offer such items.

- It is entirely possible to follow the Power Nutrition Plan while eating out. Remember, there are no forbidden foods. By knowing your daily fat gram allotment, you can eat whatever you want and still stay within your fat budget.
- Instead of viewing restaurant meals as opportunities to splurge, focus on the benefits of eating out: not having to cook or clean up, being waited on, pleasant atmosphere, etc.
- If you eat out frequently, pick up a copy of *The Restaurant Companion,* by Hope Warshaw, Surrey Books, 1990.

DO YOU NEED NUTRITIONAL SUPPLEMENTS?

There is a virtual plethora of products available for fitness enthusiasts and people concerned either with losing or gaining weight. Some supplements probably have potential benefits, others are safe, but ineffective, and still others are utterly ridiculous. Unfortunately, there isn't room in this book to explain the differences. Nutritional science has only recently begun to explore the benefits of nutritional supplements for fitness. We have a lot to learn. Unfortunately, the supplement industry is not well regulated. It is easier to make a product based on theory than to actually determine its effectiveness in well-controlled scientific studies. Consult a qualified health professional knowledgeable about supplements to evaluate your personal needs. My best advice? *Caveat emptor:* Buyer beware.

In my experience as a nutrition counselor, if most people put as much time and money into their food intake as they do searching for a miracle pill, they would be further ahead in the fitness game. So, first, focus on following the Menu Guides presented in the Power Nutrition Plan. If you want the added *insurance* of a vitamin/mineral supplement, take a multiple vitamin that contains around 100 percent of the U.S. RDA for each nutrient. (These products will not likely contain 100 percent of the recommended calcium intake due to the bulky nature of calcium. If you can't meet your calcium needs with food, you will have to take a calcium supplement.)

TIPS FOR WEIGHT LOSS

The Power Nutrition Plan is designed to help those who need to lose weight. Here are some additional strategies for maintaining a healthy body weight.

1. Eat when you are hungry and stop when you are satisfied. If you aren't hungry, save the food for later.

2. Set a realistic weight goal and plan to lose slowly, no more than one-half to two pounds a week. In addition to eating a low-fat diet, cut your calorie intake by no more than 200 to 500 calories a day.

3. Weigh yourself only once a week, at most! Better yet, rely on how you feel and how your clothes fit to determine if you are making progress.

4. Don't deprive yourself of foods you really want. Eat them in reasonable portions and when you are hungry. Remember, there are no forbidden foods.

5. Drink plenty of water, eight or more glasses a day.

6. Utilize the Week in Review sheets in the Power Nutrition Plan. Remember to keep a daily record of food intake and fat grams.

7. Do not expect yourself to be perfect. Forgive yourself when you overeat or underexercise. A setback does not have to spell disaster unless you let it.

8. Celebrate your successes! Reward yourself for healthy behaviors—eating healthy and exercising—not for losing weight. It is these behaviors that must be firmly established in order to maintain weight losses. Do not, however, use food as the reward!

9. Wear clothes that fit and look nice on you now. Get rid of your fat clothes, along with any skinny clothes you purchased after your last starvation diet. If you cannot realistically maintain that skinny body, having clothes around that don't fit will just make you feel bad.

10. Live today as though you had already reached your goal weight. The things in life that make it wonderful can be had at any weight. Everyone wants to be attractive. But life is about more than being thin. If you learn to enjoy yourself now, losing weight and keeping it off will be much easier.

TIPS FOR WEIGHT GAIN

Gaining muscle weight takes time, especially if you come from a family of naturally thin people. The important thing is to be patient and diligent about your weight-gain endeavors. Trying to bulk up too fast will only result in your getting fat! There are many overweight men who fondly remember those days in their teens and early twenties when they had to force-feed themselves to gain weight. The following guidelines will help you build muscle weight, not fat weight.

1. Expect to gain about one-half to one pound per week. Gaining faster than that may well mean you are putting on fat weight. (It is a good idea to have your percentage of body fat measured before beginning your weight gain diet; see page 50.)

2. DO NOT SKIP MEALS! You will need at least three meals per day. Eat larger portions of the high-carbohydrate foods, such as grains, breads, cereals, starchy vegetables, and fruits. Don't pile on the fat, but don't skip it either. Use the form "How Much Fat Can I Eat?" on page 41. Figure your daily fat gram allotment at 30 percent of total calories.

3. Eat snacks as often as you are hungry. Snacks need to consist of healthy foods and not be so large that they curb your appetite for meals.

4. Drink high-calorie liquids such as fruit juice and milk instead of iced tea or coffee with meals. You do need to drink some plain water also, but at least half your liquids should contain calories.

5. Surprisingly, your need for increased protein while gaining weight can easily be met through food. You do not need to purchase expensive protein supplements. In fact, getting too much protein is not healthy. If you believe you cannot eat enough protein in your diet, talk with a sports nutritionist before spending money on a

product that may be unnecessary and even detrimental.

6. A high-calorie weight-gain supplement may come in handy if you have a hard time eating enough food to meet your increased calorie needs.

7. Learn to choose the higher-calorie foods within each food group. Some examples are listed below.

8. Of course, weight training is critical to your ability to gain muscle instead of fat. If you do not already lift weights, seek out a trainer who is experienced in this area of fitness.

LOWER CALORIE	HIGHER CALORIE
Orange juice	Grape juice
Grapefruit juice	Apple juice
Applesauce	Dried fruit
Rice Krispies	Granola
Cheerios	Grape-Nuts
Vegetable soup	Split pea soup
Green beans	Corn
Summer squash	Winter squash

SUMMING IT UP

Feeding your body well offers numerous benefits. You will be more energetic, feel better, and perhaps prevent or delay illness. Good nutrition cannot guarantee that you will develop the shape you desire, but it goes a long way in helping you meet your full potential for a healthy, fit body. Eating to support exercise will give your body an extra push when it is most needed. Eating to support life will pay off in all your endeavors. *Bon appétit!*

Power Nutrition Recipes

Nutrition analysis was performed by the author, using manufacturer's data and the Nutritionist IV program, version 2.0, from N-Squared Computing, Salem, Oregon.

WEEK 1 RECIPES

TOSSED GREEN SALAD

This salad is not meant to be iceberg lettuce with dressing. No nutritional value there! Instead, create a nutritious salad by using a variety of leaf lettuces, spinach, escarole, other greens, and radicchio. Some grocery stores now sell a mix of these salad greens, prewashed and ready to use.

Make salads easy by washing and drying all of the greens right after purchase. Store them in large resealable bags. Then they are ready to throw together whenever you need a salad.

Use seasoned vinegar, such as balsamic or garlic, as a fat-free, low-sodium dressing. Low-fat cottage cheese, salsa, or the Light Veggie Dip (Week 2 recipe) can also be used as dressings. Of course, there are a multitude of low-fat and fat-free salad dressings available in any grocery store.

BAKED GARLIC

Makes 4 to 6 servings

1 head fresh garlic
1 teaspoon olive oil

Preheat oven to 325°. Remove outer paperlike coating from garlic, but do not peel or separate cloves. Place garlic on a piece of foil. Drizzle the oil over garlic. Tightly seal the edges of the foil, leaving some space around the garlic. Bake 1 hour. (Special cookware for baking garlic is now available in kitchen stores and catalogues.) Garlic can be baked ahead of time and reheated. It keeps a few days in the fridge.

Separate cloves. Squeeze cooked garlic out of its shell and spread on bread in lieu of butter. Delicious!

Nutritional information per one-quarter head of garlic: 33 calories, 0.6 gm protein, 5 gm carbohydrate, 1 gm fat (31 percent fat calories), 0 sodium, 47 mg potassium, 0 calcium, 0 dietary fiber. Count as an *extra* food.

WEEK 2 RECIPES

LIGHT VEGGIE DIP

Makes 11 servings, 2 tablespoons each

1 cup nonfat or 1% cottage cheese

¼ cup plain, nonfat yogurt

2 tablespoons nonfat sour cream (Naturally Yours Real Dairy No Fat Sour Cream is best)

½ teaspoon Dijon mustard

Pinch of sugar

¾ teaspoon Mrs. Dash Garlic & Herb Seasoning

Place all ingredients in a blender. Mix until smooth. Serve with raw vegetables or over baked potatoes.

Nutritional information per serving: 21 calories, 3 gm protein, 1 gm carbohydrate, <½ gm fat (11 percent fat calories), 101 mg sodium, 33 mg potassium, 26 mg calcium, 0 dietary fiber. Count as an *extra* food.

GRILLED TUNA STEAK

Makes 5 servings, 3.3 ounce each

This recipe was adapted from one by the National Fish and Seafood Council. I reduced the sodium content by using Worcestershire instead of soy sauce and omitting the salt.

1 lb. fresh tuna, cut into five steaks

Marinade:

1 tablespoon lemon juice

2 tablespoons Worcestershire sauce

2 tablespoons orange juice

1 tablespoon tomato paste, no salt added

½ teaspoon minced garlic

½ teaspoon oregano

1 tablespoon parsley, fresh or dried

Pepper to taste

Mix all ingredients for marinade. Add tuna, turning to coat well. Let tuna stand at least 20 minutes in marinade. Grill fish for 5 minutes on each side, periodically basting with marinade. Do not overcook or fish will be dry and tough. Note: Place fish on a perforated pan on the grill to keep it from breaking apart when turning.

Nutritional information per serving: 179 calories, 27.5 gm protein, 3 gm carbohydrate, 6 gm fat (30 percent fat calories), 108 mg sodium, 396 mg potassium, 20 mg calcium, 0 gm dietary fiber. Count each serving as 3 ounces of protein.

GRILLED ZUCCHINI AND MUSHROOMS

Makes 4 servings, 1 mushroom and ½ zucchini each

This recipe was adapted from "Grilled Garlic Squash," Simply Colorado, *published by the Colorado Dietetic Association, 1990.*

1 teaspoon minced garlic

1 teaspoon olive oil

1 teaspoon cooking sherry

1 teaspoon water

½ teaspoon lemon juice

½ teaspoon summer savory

Pinch or two of salt

4 large mushrooms, stems cut even with cap or removed

2 medium zucchini, cut in half lengthwise

Mix first seven ingredients together and set aside. Prepare vegetables. Brush sauce on bottom of mushrooms and cut side of zucchini. Grill or broil (with cut side toward heat) 4 minutes. Brush remainder of sauce on vegetables and continue cooking 4 minutes more.

Nutritional information per serving: 35 calories, 2 gm protein, 4 gm carbohydrate, 2 gm fat (38 percent fat calories), 58 mg sodium, 353 mg potassium, 21 mg calcium, 1.5 gm dietary fiber. Count as 1 vegetable serving. Although this recipe is 38 percent fat calories, when eaten with the other menu items, total fat calories for this meal are less than 30 percent.

WEEK 3 RECIPES

BEAN BURRITO

Makes 4 servings, 1 burrito each

Pam or other nonstick cooking spray or pump
2 green onions, chopped
¼ teaspoon minced garlic (You can use preminced garlic or substitute garlic powder, to taste)
1 16-ounce can fat-free or vegetarian refried beans (I like Rosarita brand)
2 cups leaf lettuce, torn into small pieces
1 tomato, chopped or thinly sliced
4 large flour tortillas
4 tablespoons fat-free sour cream (Real Dairy No Fat Sour Cream brand tastes best, or substitute nonfat plain yogurt)
4 tablespoons salsa

Coat a nonstick skillet with cooking spray. Briefly sauté onion and garlic. Mix in beans. Heat, covered, over very low heat. Stir occasionally. Meanwhile, prepare lettuce and tomato. Heat tortillas. You can put them between two damp paper towels and heat in a microwave for 60 to 90 seconds. Another method is to heat them individually on the bottom of a dry, very hot iron skillet, turning frequently until soft and warm.

When tortillas are ready, fill each one with one-quarter of the bean mixture. Top with lettuce, tomato, and 1 tablespoon each of sour cream and salsa. Roll up and enjoy! If you plan to take the burrito in a sack lunch, put the beans in the tortilla and roll. Reheat in a microwave and then top with the rest of the ingredients. Also, any leftover beans make a great bean dip with fat-free tortilla chips!

Nutritional information per burrito: 303 calories, 13.5 gm protein, 55 gm carbohydrate, 6 gm fat (16 percent fat calories), 811 mg sodium, 223 mg potassium, 111 mg calcium, 2½ gm dietary fiber. Count each burrito as 1 grain, 2 ounces of protein, and 1 vegetable.

HUMMUS

Makes 7 servings, ¼ cup each

Adapted from a recipe for chickpea dip found in The New York Times New Natural Foods Cookbook *by Jean Hewitt, Avon Publishing, 1971.*

1 can (15.5 ounces) chickpeas (garbanzo beans)
4 tablespoons sesame tahini (available in the natural foods section of the grocery store)
½ tablespoon olive oil
⅓ cup lemon juice
1 tablespoon minced garlic

Combine all ingredients in a blender. Mix until smooth. Put in a pita pocket bread with fresh cucumber slices, tomato, and sprouts. Leftovers keep several days in the fridge.

Nutritional information per serving: 213 calories, 8 gm protein, 19 gm carbohydrate, 12 gm fat (50 percent fat calories), 226 mg sodium, 195 mg potassium, 77 mg calcium, 4 gm dietary fiber. Count as 1 ounce of protein and 2 fat servings. Although this dish is 50 percent fat calories, when combined with the rest of the menu items, this meal is less than 30 percent fat calories.

SPICY VEGGIE STIR-FRY

Makes 5 servings, 1 cup each

This recipe was inspired, in part, by Jane Brody's "Simple Tofu Stir-Fry," in Jane Brody's Good Food Book, *Bantam Books, 1985.*

Sauce:
¼ cup chicken or vegetable broth
1 tablespoon Worcestershire sauce
1 teaspoon lemon juice
1 tablespoon Mirin or dry sherry

Stir-Fry:
Pam or other nonstick cooking spray
1 teaspoon olive oil
1 teaspoon sesame oil (Use chili oil if you like it really hot!)
1 tablespoon minced garlic
1 tablespoon sesame seeds, preferably unhulled
½ teaspoon crushed red pepper

½ pound firm tofu, cut into small cubes
2 carrots, sliced thin, on the diagonal
2 cups broccoli florets (from 1 medium stalk)
6-ounce package frozen Chinese pea pods

Mix together all sauce ingredients and set aside.

Coat a large nonstick skillet with cooking spray. Heat olive and sesame oils over medium heat. Add garlic, sesame seeds, and red pepper. Sauté briefly and then add tofu cubes. Toss tofu with seeds and garlic to coat. Continue stirring while tofu browns for about 2 minutes. Remove tofu from skillet and set aside.

Add carrots and 2 tablespoons water to skillet. Reduce heat to low, cover, and cook until carrots begin to soften, stirring occasionally. Remove lid, add broccoli and cook, uncovered, 2 minutes more. Then add pea pods, toss, and cook for 1 minute. Add tofu and sauce. Toss all ingredients well. Cover and cook until heated thoroughly, about 3 minutes. Serve over rice.

Nutritional information per serving: 148 calories, 10.5 gm protein, 13 gm carbohydrate, 7 gm fat (40 percent fat calories), 103 mg sodium, 163 mg calcium, 516 mg potassium, 4 gm dietary fiber. Count as 1½ ounces of protein and 2 vegetable servings. Although the stir-fry alone is 40 percent fat calories, when served over rice, the percentage fat calories drops to below 30 percent.

TANYA'S FROZEN YOGURT

Makes 3½ servings, ½ cup each

My good friend Tanya Evtuhov shared this wonderful treat with me.

1 cup frozen, unsweetened blueberries (or any
    other unsweetened, frozen fruit)
1 cup nonfat, vanilla yogurt

Using a blender, thoroughly mix the fruit and yogurt. Eat right away or store in airtight container in the refrigerator. Absolutely wonderful!

Nutritional information per serving: 74 calories, 3.5 gm protein, 15.5 gm carbohydrate, 0.3 gm fat (3 percent fat calories), 40 mg sodium, 167 mg potassium, 118 mg calcium, 1 gm dietary fiber. Count each serving as a partial fruit and milk/yogurt serving.

WEEK 4 RECIPES

SPINACH OMELETTE

Makes 1 serving

Nonstick cooking spray
  1 green onion, chopped (optional)
1½ cups fresh spinach, torn into small pieces
  ½ cup Egg Beaters or other fat-free egg substitute
    (You can use 1 whole egg and 2 egg whites; this
    adds 5 grams of fat)
Pinch of salt, pepper to taste
  2 tablespoons low-fat shredded cheese, any flavor

Coat a small, nonstick skillet with cooking spray. Over medium-low heat, cook onion and spinach, covered, until spinach is partially wilted, about 3 minutes. Pour egg substitute over and around the spinach, covering the bottom of the skillet. Add pepper to taste and a pinch of salt. Cook on low until almost done. Sprinkle cheese on top and continue to cook until egg is set. To *finish* the omelette, either fold it in half and press lightly to be sure all egg is cooked or cook under a broiler for a few minutes. Note: If you cook egg with the lid on, it cooks fast and needs no *finish* step. However, the egg has a steamed flavor.

Nutritional information: 117 calories, 16.5 gm protein, 6 gm carbohydrate, 3.5 gm fat (27 percent fat calories), 400 mg sodium, 747 mg potassium, 252 mg calcium, 2 gm dietary fiber. Count as 2 ounces of protein and 1 vegetable serving.

ZUCCHINI HEALTH MUFFINS

Makes 8 large muffins or 16 small,
1 large or 2 small per serving

Nonstick cooking spray
2¼ cups whole wheat flour
 ¼ cup sugar
 ¼ cup nonfat milk powder
 1 teaspoon cinnamon
 ¼ teaspoon salt
 1 teaspoon baking soda
 ½ teaspoon baking powder
 ½ teaspoon ginger
1½ medium zucchini, shredded
 8 ounces plain nonfat yogurt
 ¼ cup pure maple syrup
 ¼ cup unsweetened applesauce
 ½ cup nonfat egg substitute (such as Egg Beaters)
 1 cup seedless raisins
 1 teaspoon vanilla extract

Preheat oven to 350°. Spray eight large or sixteen small muffin cups with nonstick cooking spray.

In a medium bowl, combine the dry ingredients. Stir thoroughly.

In a large bowl, combine the remaining ingredients. Mix thoroughly with a wire whisk.

Add flour mixture to the zucchini mixture, using spoon to mix just until the flour is moistened.

Spoon batter into cups. Bake for 30 minutes (less if you're making small muffins) or until a toothpick inserted in center of each muffin comes out clean. Cool muffins thoroughly on a wire rack before removing them from the muffin pans. Eat plain or slice and heat under a broiler and serve with applesauce or all-fruit jam. These muffins are flavorful, almost fat free, and not as sweet as traditional zucchini muffins. To make them sweeter, use nonfat vanilla yogurt instead of plain or use additional sugar instead of the nonfat milk powder.

Nutritional information per large muffin: 254 calories, 9 gm protein, 57 gm carbohydrate, 0.8 gm fat (3 percent fat calories), 228 mg sodium, 502 mg potassium, 128 mg calcium, 5.7 gm dietary fiber. Count each large muffin as 1 grain and 1 sweet serving.

PASTA PRIMAVERA

Makes 4 large servings

Adapted from "Perfect Pasta Primavera" in Jane Brody's Good Food Book, *Bantam Books, 1985. You can use any fresh or frozen vegetables in this recipe, equal to about 4 cups chopped or sliced, total. The ones used here give this dish a lot of color as well as flavor.*

 2 carrots, cut on the diagonal
 1 cup chopped broccoli (can use stems)
 ½ green pepper, chopped
 3 large mushrooms, sliced
 1 yellow squash, sliced ¼ inch thick
Nonstick cooking spray
 1 teaspoon olive oil
 1 to 2 cloves minced garlic
 2 skinless, boneless chicken breasts, cut into bite-sized pieces
12 ounces fettucini noodles

Sauce:
 2 teaspoons margarine (or 4 teaspoons low-fat margarine)
 2 tablespoons flour (dissolved in water)
 1 cup skim milk
 ½ cup chicken broth
 ¼ cup grated Parmesan cheese
 1 teaspoon dried basil

Begin heating water for noodles. Meanwhile, steam all vegetables until crisp-tender, about 5 to 7 minutes for the carrots and broccoli. The others will take less time. As vegetables are steaming, coat a nonstick skillet with cooking spray. Heat the olive oil over medium heat. Add garlic and sauté for 1 minute. Add chicken, tossing to coat with the garlic. After chicken is browned, reduce heat to low and cover. Cook until chicken is tender and no longer pink. Mix chicken with vegetables and keep warm in a low-temperature oven.

Add noodles to rapidly boiling water. While noodles are cooking, prepare the sauce. Melt margarine over medium-low heat in a small saucepan. Add half of the dissolved flour, mixing with a wire whisk.

Gradually stir in milk and chicken broth. Add rest of dissolved flour, stirring with the whisk to prevent lumps. Cook until sauce begins to thicken. Add Parmesan cheese and basil. Continue to stir until cheese melts and sauce thickens a little more. Pour sauce over vegetable/chicken mixture, tossing gently to coat. Serve over cooked noodles. This dish cools off quickly, so serve immediately.

Nutritional information: 563 calories, 29.5 gm protein, 85 gm carbohydrate, 12 gm fat (19 percent fat calories), 310 mg sodium, 743 mg potassium, 231 mg calcium, 4 gm dietary fiber. Count as 2 ounces of protein, 2 vegetable, and 3 grain servings.

BREAKFAST BEANS

Makes 4 servings

1 can plain black beans
4 whole eggs

Pour can of beans, including juice, into a nonstick skillet over medium heat. When beans are slightly warm, carefully break eggs over the top of the beans. Cover and cook on medium-low heat until eggs are poached. Carefully scoop out a portion of beans with one egg on top. Serve with warm tortillas and salsa or Pico de Gallo (see below).

Nutritional information per serving: 219 calories, 16 gm protein, 27 gm carbohydrate, 5.5 gm fat (23 percent fat calories), 140 mg sodium, 450 mg potassium, 55 mg calcium, 4.6 gm dietary fiber. Count as 2 ounces of protein.

PICO DE GALLO

Makes 32 servings, 2 tablespoons each

At my house, this condiment goes quickly, so I always make a big batch. You may prefer to cut it in half. If this turns out too hot, dilute it with more tomato.

15 fresh jalapeño peppers
 1 medium white onion
 5 Roma tomatoes
 4 tablespoons fresh cilantro (or to taste)
Pinch or two of salt

Wearing rubber gloves, carefully remove stems and seeds from peppers. (Depending on the peppers, this can be very hot and the seeds will only make it hotter. If you don't wear the gloves, you will soon regret it!) Finely chop the peppers, onion, tomatoes, and cilantro. An onion chopper or food processor is helpful, especially for the onions and peppers. However, the tomatoes can easily be too juicy, so chop them by hand. Gently mix together all ingredients. Stir in salt. This dish should have very little juice; it isn't salsa. It is a wonderful condiment for eggs, fish, chicken, chili, and beans. You can use it in cooking or as a dip with fat-free tortilla chips.

Nutritional information per serving: 12 calories, 0.6 gm protein, 3 gm carbohydrate, 0.1 gm fat (6 percent fat calories), 10 mg sodium, 108 mg potassium, 5 mg calcium, 0.7 gm dietary fiber. Count as ½ vegetable serving.

ONION BÉCHAMEL SAUCE

Makes 8 servings, ½ cup each

This recipe was adapted from one shared by a fellow onion and garlic lover, Mark Burrows. It is chock full of both! You can make this with soy milk, such as Health Valley Fat Free Soy Moo; it will be slightly sweeter than with cow's milk.

2 tablespoons olive oil
3 large onions, quartered and sliced
6 large cloves of garlic, sliced thick
4 tablespoons whole wheat flour
2 cups skim milk
Pinch of nutmeg
¼ to ½ teaspoon salt, or to taste
½ teaspoon white pepper

Heat olive oil in a large, nonstick skillet until hot. (If a drop of water pops when placed in the oil, it's hot enough.) Sauté onion and garlic over medium heat until translucent, about 10 minutes.

Meanwhile put flour and ½ cup of the milk in a glass jar. Shake until flour is dissolved. Set aside. Into onions, stir in the nutmeg and the remaining 1½ cups of milk; heat until bubbling. Then slowly add the flour mixture, salt, and pepper, stirring continuously. Turn heat low and simmer, covered, for 2 to 3 minutes. Serve over noodles.

Nutrient analysis per serving of sauce: 113 calories, 17 gm carbohydrate, 4 gm protein, 3.7 gm fat (29 percent fat calories), 169 mg sodium, 314 mg potassium, 106 mg calcium, 2.5 gm dietary fiber. Count as 1 vegetable and a partial milk serving.

DELICIOUS AND LEAN CHOCOLATE CUPCAKES

Makes 1 dozen, 1 cupcake per serving

A modified version of the "Double Chocolate Cupcakes" recipe from Light & Easy, Oxmoor House, 1990.

1½ cups all-purpose flour
½ cup plus 1½ tablespoons sugar
¼ cup unsweetened cocoa powder
1 teaspoon baking powder
½ teaspoon salt
½ cup orange juice
⅓ cup water
2 tablespoons canola oil
½ tablespoon apple cider vinegar
1 teaspoon vanilla extract
⅓ cup *mini* semisweet chocolate chips
1 teaspoon powdered sugar for dusting

Preheat oven to 375°. Put paper liners in a muffin pan. Combine the dry ingredients in a medium-sized bowl, mixing thoroughly. In a separate bowl, mix together the liquid ingredients. Make a well in the center of the flour mixture. Pour in the wet ingredients and mix the two until just moistened. Gently fold in the chocolate chips. Fill each muffin two-thirds full. Bake 12 minutes or until a toothpick, inserted in middle, comes out clean. (At high altitude, it takes about 20 minutes to cook.) Cool cupcakes on a wire rack. Dust the tops with the powdered sugar.

Nutritional information per serving: 150 calories, 2 gm protein, 27 gm carbohydrate, 4 gm fat (25 percent fat calories), 160 mg sodium, 105 mg potassium, 7 mg calcium, ½ gm dietary fiber. Count as 1 sweet.

WEEK 5 RECIPES

SALMON LOAF

Makes 6 servings

This recipe was adapted from one by the Canned Salmon Institute.

Nonstick cooking spray
1 can (14¾ ounces) pink salmon
1½ cups cooked brown rice
1 small can (8½ ounces) cream-style corn
½ green pepper, chopped
2 green onions, chopped
¾ cup grated low-fat cheese, Monterey Jack/Colby blend
2 egg whites, beaten
¼ teaspoon Mrs. Dash seasoning
¼ teaspoon sesame chili oil (or use 3 drops Tabasco sauce)

Preheat oven to 350°. Coat an 8-inch square glass pan with cooking spray. In a medium bowl, flake apart the salmon with the liquid. Add all remaining ingredients, combining thoroughly. Turn into the glass pan. Bake for 1 hour. Let stand at room temperature for 5 minutes before serving. This dish is good cold too.

Nutritional information per serving: 233 calories, 21 gm protein, 21 gm carbohydrate, 7.5 gm fat (29 percent fat calories), 630 mg sodium, 373 mg potassium, 283 mg calcium, 1.7 gm dietary fiber. Count as 2½ ounces of protein and a partial grain and vegetable serving.

BLACKSTRAP COFFEE

Makes 1 serving

Mix 1 teaspoon blackstrap molasses with 1 cup hot water. Add milk, if desired.

Nutritional information per cup (without milk): 15 calories, 0 protein, 6 gm carbohydrate, 0 fat, 13 mg sodium, 196 mg potassium, 51 mg calcium, 0 fiber. Count as an *extra* food.

CRANBERRY MULTIGRAIN CEREAL

Makes 2 large servings

I always have plenty of grains on hand to make this cereal. If you prefer, you can use a premixed multi-grain cereal, such as Quaker Multi-Grain Cereal.

¾ cup water
¾ cup apple juice
⅓ cup dried, sweetened cranberries (can substitute raisins)
3 tablespoons Zoom or other whole wheat hot cereal
2 tablespoons oat bran
3 tablespoons Cream of Rye cereal
3 tablespoons quick oats
Pinch of salt

Combine water, apple juice, and cranberries in a small saucepan. Heat to boiling. Meanwhile, combine the cereals and salt. When liquid is boiling, gradually stir in cereal mixture. Reduce heat to low and cook about 2 minutes, stirring occasionally. Turn off heat, cover, and let stand 1 minute. Serve with milk, if desired; needs no additional sugar.

Nutritional information per serving (without milk): 225 calories, 5 gm protein, 54 gm carbohydrate, 1.5 gm fat (5 percent fat calories), 211 mg sodium, 404 mg potassium, 34 mg calcium, 4 gm dietary fiber. Count as 2 grain and 1½ fruit servings.

BROCCOLI/CAULIFLOWER SALAD

Makes 4 servings, 1 cup each

2 cups broccoli florets (from 1 medium stalk; save the stalk and use it in stir-fry or salad.)
½ head of cauliflower, florets divided
1 green onion

Dressing:
¼ cup plain, nonfat yogurt (pour off liquid)
1 tablespoon low-fat mayonnaise
Pinch of celery seed
Pinch of dill weed
¼ teaspoon basil
Pinch of salt

Have a large pot of water boiling. Blanch broccoli and cauliflower in boiling water for 1 to 2 minutes, no longer. (I use a pan big enough to hold a colander, put the vegetables in the colander, and then insert it into the boiling water.) Cool the vegetables immediately in the refrigerator or a sink of cold water. Meanwhile, chop the green onion and set aside.

For the dressing, mix together all ingredients. When the vegetables are cooled, cut them into bite-sized pieces. Add the onion and dressing. Toss thoroughly. Chill before serving. Tastes best when fresh.

Nutritional information per serving: 49 calories, 4.5 gm protein, 7 gm carbohydrate, 1.5 gm fat (23 percent fat calories), 79 mg sodium, 511 mg potassium, 73 mg calcium, 4 gm dietary fiber. Count as 1 vegetable serving.

BLACK BEANS AND RICE

Makes 6 servings, 1 cup beans and 1 cup rice per serving

This recipe was adapted from a recipe in New Recipes from Moosewood Restaurant.

2 cups brown rice (yields 6 cups cooked)
Nonstick cooking spray
1 tablespoon olive oil
1 medium onion, chopped
3 cloves garlic, minced
1 medium carrot, chopped
½ green bell pepper, chopped
½ teaspoon cumin
½ teaspoon coriander
Salt and pepper to taste
1 tablespoon dried parsley
1 can (14.5 ounces) stewed tomatoes with juice
2 cans (15 ounces each) black beans, drained

Begin cooking rice. Meanwhile, coat a large non-stick skillet with cooking spray. Add olive oil and sauté the onion and garlic for 3 minutes. Add carrot and continue cooking for 3 minutes. Add green pepper and sauté 5 minutes more. Add spices and tomatoes with juice. Simmer until all vegetables are tender. Add drained beans. Simmer 10 minutes more. Serve over brown rice with fat-free sour cream or yogurt.

Nutritional information per serving: 376 calories, 13 grams protein, 72 grams carbohydrate, 4.6 grams fat (11 percent fat calories), 120 mg sodium, 704 mg potassium, 77 mg calcium, 8 grams dietary fiber. Count as 2 ounces of protein and 2 grain servings.

JICAMA STICKS

Makes 8 servings

This recipe, slightly modified, was discovered in Cuisine of the American Southwest *by Anne Lindsay Greer, Cuisinart Cooking Club, Inc., Harper & Row, 1983.*

1 small to medium jicama
Several fresh limes
½ teaspoon chili powder (or paprika)
1 to 2 tablespoons fresh, chopped cilantro

Peel the jicama with a sharp knife, also removing the fibrous, inner layer. Slice the white flesh of the jicama into strips. Squeeze lime juice over the jicama strips. Then sprinkle with chili powder and cilantro and toss.

Nutritional information is not available for this vegetable. This is a low-fat dish as all vegetables are low in fat (except avocado) and no fat is added in the recipe. Count as 1 vegetable serving.

CHAPTER SIX

The Lower Back

BY BRYON HOLMES, M.S.

You are in a privileged and small minority if you don't suffer from lower back pain. Lower back pain will cause 80 percent of all Americans to miss at least one week of work during their lifetime. It is the most expensive health care cost in America. Eighty billion dollars a year can be directly attributed to the treatment of lower back problems.

The Unguarded Moment

An isolated human spine from a fresh cadaver can only withstand about five pounds of pressure before it buckles or collapses. This underscores the importance of soft tissues (muscle, ligaments, and tendons) that surround the spine and allow it to perform the normal physiological functions for which it is designed. All injuries occur when some external load or force exceeds an individual's structural capacity. Ninety percent of all lower back pain may be attributed to soft-tissue damage. Most lower back injuries occur during an "unguarded moment." This moment happens when an individual has to suddenly react to his or her environment. It also occurs when one turns, twists, stoops, or bends in an unusual manner.

Acute and Chronic Pain

Back pain can be categorized as two phases: acute pain and chronic pain. Back pain is considered acute during the first six weeks. Most lower back pain (80 percent) will disappear within six weeks, regardless of any intervention. This explains why the most common medical advice given during the acute phase is to take it easy and let the body heal itself. The use of passive modalities such as ice, heat, ultrasound, massage, acupuncture, acupressure, rolfing, and chiropractic can make you feel better while your body recovers, but provides no proven physiological benefit to accelerate the healing process.

When back pain continues beyond six weeks it is considered chronic. An individual who is suffering from chronic lower back pain will develop new muscle recruitment patterns that compensate and substitute for a weak and painful lower back. This is a primitive neuromotor survival strategy that allowed our ancestors to escape danger in the event of injury. This phenomenon is apparent to anyone who has observed a wounded animal continue to be mobile despite its injuries. The natural reaction to back pain is to block or guard any movements that require the back to work. This will temporarily prevent the back musculature from being exposed to external forces. Doing this relieves short-term pain, but the long-term effects can be devastating. Pain leads to disuse; disuse leads to muscular atrophy; atrophy leads to weakness. Weakness predisposes an individual to recurrent injury because of the inability to withstand normal usage. This continuous cycle is referred to as the *chronic deconditioning syndrome*. Chronic disuse atrophy, or the deconditioning syndrome, can be compared with an individual who has an arm in a cast for six to eight weeks. After removal of the cast, an obvious weakness in muscle strength is apparent. The human body physiologically adapts to the demands placed upon it. The muscle group in question has essentially adapted to no stimulation by allowing unused muscle to atrophy and weaken.

Prevention

Strength of the trunk extensors is reduced in the patient with chronic back pain. Adequate strength of the trunk muscles is necessary for a return to full function. It is necessary to increase the functional and structural integrity of the lower back by increasing the efficacy of the soft tissues. Most lower back pain is pre-

ventable and can be treated and managed successfully. You can increase a muscle's contractile ability (strength) by exposing it to regular overload stimulation (strength training). In other words, by isolating and strengthening the muscles, you can treat and prevent back pain. Increasing your levels of strength increases your structural integrity and your ability to withstand the unguarded moment. Specific exercise is the only effective way to prevent lower back problems. It is also the only effective way to rehabilitate and control the recurrence of chronic lower back pain once it has developed.

When we examine the normal movement of the trunk we see approximately 182 degrees of movement. Approximately 110 degrees occur from the contraction of the buttocks and hamstrings as they rotate the pelvis around the head of the femur. Another 72 degrees of movement occur through the lumbar spine. It is the muscles of the lumbar spine used for this movement that atrophy and become inhibited in the presence of pain. Unfortunately, this also leads to the degradation of tendons, ligaments, and intervertebral disks. The normal poor blood supply to a disk does not allow the metabolic waste products to be removed. Disk nutrients are delivered by means of diffusion, which requires disks to be loaded and unloaded much like a sponge. This is done with the help of the movement of the surrounding muscles. If the lower back muscles are not working properly, this normal process does not occur and pain persists due to a disk's inability to repair itself. Normal and healthy lower back muscles are also important for the tendons, ligaments, and fascia (sheath surrounding muscles), which are in various states of repair and need this muscle movement to encourage proper alignment of new cellular tissue. Movement will also facilitate the production of synovial fluid in the facet joints. This fluid is the body's natural lubricating substance that allows joints to move smoothly.

In chronic pain patients, the lumbar spine must be isolated during exercise to get stronger. During trunk extension, the hip flexors are the primary movers and the lumbar extensors are the secondary movers. If the lumbar extensors are to get strong, they must be isolated so that they can be exposed to greater workloads than usual; then they become stronger and prepared to withstand the unguarded moment. At the present time, there is only one device on the market that has a restraining mechanism to prevent pelvic rotation as the trunk extends—the MedX lower back machine.

Lower Back, Legs, and Buttocks

The legs and buttocks play an important and intricate role in the prevention and rehabilitation of lower back pain. The muscles of the buttocks and hips support and assist the back in most movements. Just as a chain is only as strong as its weakest link, we are only as strong as our weakest body part involved in a movement. With strong legs and buttocks it is possible to perform more lifts, work longer, and move freely in our environment with good posture. If we have weak legs and buttocks, then the back is exposed to greater loads as our lifting posture declines and greater demands are placed on the lower back. This is a scenario ripe for injury as one muscle group is required to substitute for the other.

Abdominals

Weak abdominal musculature allows the abdomen to sag, creating a greater load on the lower back, forcing it to hold up the mass in front of it. Strengthening the abdominals creates greater intraabdominal pressure; increased pressure forces a more upright positioning of the spine. The net result is a decreased load on the lumbar disks. Poor posture contributes to lower back pain. Increasing the strength of the lumbar extensors and the abdominals will help improve posture and decrease the incidence of back pain. Strong lower back muscles and strong abdominals work together in maintaining a pain-free healthy back.

Upper Back and Chest

As stated earlier, good posture is essential to lower back wellness. It is common for there to be an imbalance between the chest and back. Because we tend to do everything in front of us, the chest and shoulders tend to be stronger than the back, causing the upper torso to roll forward and shifting the torso into a forward posture. To alleviate this and to align the spine correctly, it is important to exercise the upper back as much as the chest. This will balance and center the torso, thereby improving posture.

Hamstring Flexibility

Flexibility in the hamstrings (backside of thigh) is important to the lower back because the hamstrings attach into the pelvis. The erector spinae in the lower back also attaches into the pelvis. A tight hamstring will prohibit the range of motion of the erector spinae when one bends over (trunk flexion), thereby limiting its mobility and ability to gain strength in a full range of motion. One must maintain flexibility in the hamstrings to avoid this. A good exercise for this is the hamstring stretch (see page 101). Generally, range of motion is limited due to soft tissue damage; this may be intramuscular adhesions (an abnormal joining together of separate tissues, caused by inflammation), contractures in tendons (a permanent shortening of a tendon), or scar tissue. If you perform hamstring strengthening exercises through your full range of motion you will receive strengthening benefits about 18 degrees beyond where you stop. As your strength improves, you will have the ability to overcome the resistance caused by the soft tissue and your range of motion will return to normal.

Lower back pain is usually caused by a combination of factors. If you have chronic lower back problems, it is important that you work with a qualified professional to treat the problem holistically.

The Exercises and Program

The following exercises will help strengthen the muscles of your lower back. They are listed in order of difficulty, from least difficult to most difficult. Choose an exercise that fits your fitness level and incorporate it into your legs and buttocks routine. Do your lower back exercise at the end of your routine; this allows the back to remain strong and fresh while performing your other exercises.

BASIC GUIDELINES FOR BACK STRENGTHENING

Always work within a range of motion in which you feel no pain. If it is painful to reach certain positions, stop short of them during exercise. *Exercises designed to increase strength will increase strength 15 degrees beyond the end point of the movement.* Therefore, stopping movement just prior to a position of discomfort will provide significant strengthening benefits beyond that range of motion. Never use a sudden movement when performing a strength exercise even though it is harder to do a slow, controlled movement. Sudden movements use momentum. By performing a slow, controlled movement, you will not be able to handle as much resistance, but muscular fatigue (overload) is still accomplished, and the risk of injury is greatly reduced.

LOWER BACK EXERCISES

Opposite Arm and Leg, on Knees: Start on all fours, resting on your hands and knees. You should look straight down, neither tucked or looking up. From this position, simultaneously raise and straighten your right arm and left leg until they are parallel to the ground (or as close to parallel as you can) without going past the parallel position. Hold for two seconds and

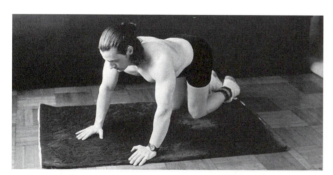

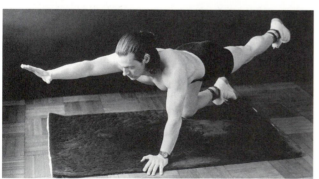

come back slowly to the starting position. Repeat with left arm and right leg. Start with ten repetitions on each side and build up to twenty repetitions. (Note: Never use momentum to complete your exercise; when you get tired, rest, then continue on.)

Opposite Arm and Leg on Stomach, Face Down: Lie face down on the floor, arms extended overhead, palms on the floor. From this position, simultaneously raise your right arm and left leg as high as you comfortably can. Hold for two seconds and come back to the floor slowly. Repeat with left arm and right leg. Build up until you can complete twenty repetitions on each side.

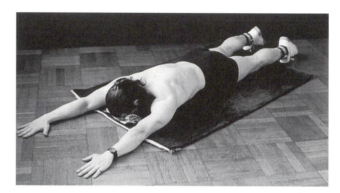

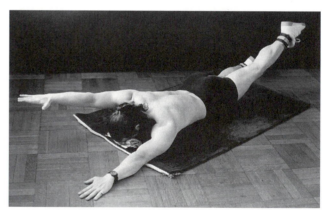

Basic Trunk Extension: Lie face down flat on the floor, leaving your arms at your side. Slowly raise your chest off the floor as high as you comfortably can. Hold for two seconds and come back to the floor slowly. Gradually increase until you can do twenty repetitions easily. If your feet come off the ground on either this or the intermediate trunk extension, you need to support your feet: either by placing them under something such as a couch, or by having a partner hold them down.

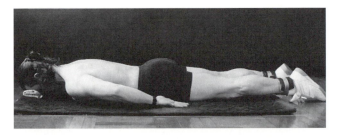

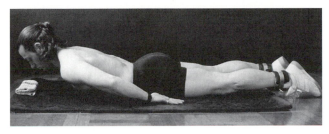

Intermediate Trunk Extension: Lie face down with a firm pillow under your pelvis; place your heels under a couch, leaving your arms to your side. Slowly, raise your chest off the floor as high as you comfortably can. Hold for two seconds and come back to the floor slowly. When you can do twenty repetitions easily, place another pillow under your pelvis. This will increase the difficulty and range of motion of the exercise.

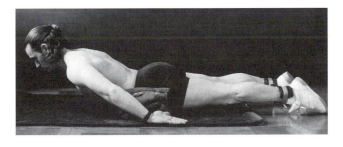

Advanced Trunk Extension: Lie face down on a bed, table, exercise bench, or Roman chair. Have someone hold your ankles as you slide forward until your pelvis is on the edge of the table and your trunk is hanging off. Slowly, raise up as high as you can, hold for two seconds, and then return to starting position. When you can accomplish twenty repetitions, start holding weighted objects in your hands as you do the exercise.

FOR THOSE WITH LOWER BACK PROBLEMS

If you have lower back problems, you face special challenges when working out. It is important for you to start slowly and build gradually. You may feel that you can do more during the early phases, but remember it is quality, not quantity, that is important. If you skip to higher levels, you may not establish the strength base necessary to prevent injury. So start with the first level and progress according to recommendations. Your lower back problems didn't develop overnight and restoration of function won't either.

If you have lower back problems, it is imperative that you check with a doctor before beginning an exercise program. When exercising, it is also important that you learn how to distinguish between good and bad pain as discussed on pages 24–25. You should *not* exercise through spasm, lingering pain, or shooting, peripheral pain.

Each exercise has a lower back rating. Check it before choosing exercises. *Low risk* does not mean the exercise is guaranteed to be safe for your back. It means you are at lower risk of injury. You should also never jerk or perform sudden, extreme movements. Once you have developed a solid base of strength, you will be able to move to more advanced exercises. Just remember to go slowly and work with a doctor, physical therapist, or fitness trainer when in doubt.

The important thing to remember is, if you have lower back pain, part of the problem is lower back weakness. You have to strengthen the weak area. Proper stretching and specific lower back exercises will help strengthen and prevent recurring back pain. If you take care of your back, it will last a lifetime, but strength and movement are the keys. As we say in rehabilitation, "If it's not moving, it's probably dead."

Complete Wellness

DEBORAH M. HOLMES, M.S.

In this chapter we will look at the physiological pathway of the body that exercise affects. By understanding these pathways we can see how exercise can affect the body in many different ways. Oftentimes it is not understood how a simple exercise session can influence all the other systems of the body—for example, how exercise affects digestion, sleep patterns, hormones, etc.

We will also discuss the amount of exercise it takes to achieve these benefits—how much is enough versus how much is too much. Understanding this gives everyone a baseline to design their own comprehensive program and to achieve the goals they want.

We will look at overall wellness goals for a better life, describe how fitness and health fit into the overall realm of wellness, and show the importance of exercise as it relates to the physical aspect of wellness.

Last, there is a routine designed to show how an individual can incorporate these exercises into a normal, healthy exercise regimen.

The Benefits of a Little Exercise

The problem in today's exercise world is the constant insistence that more is better: "Train harder, run faster; no pain, no gain." It's no wonder greater than 70 percent of the American population give up on exercise every year. Why do things need to be hard in order to be beneficial? They don't. Slowly, research is beginning to show that sometimes less is better.

It's important to understand both extremes of an exercise program in order to know what you should be doing in an exercise session, these two extremes being "too much" and "too little" exercise. A well-composed exercise program will put you somewhere in the middle of these extremes. We need to challenge our bodies just beyond our present exercise abilities without doing "too much." It's not beneficial to the body as a whole to fail at an exercise program. This is why we should consider the opposing extreme, looking to see just how little it takes to achieve the results we are after, testing even the slightest muscle stimulation for benefits.

Let's look at what an exercise does to the body, examining how little it takes to stimulate your entire body to achieve some of the results you want. You must remember that there are hundreds of benefits achieved through exercise. Not only will you look better, but you will achieve benefits that include: sleeping better, decreased stress, better digestion, clearer thought processes, improved coordination, higher energy levels, higher metabolism, more regularity of body functions and systems, to name a few. Just how does this all work? Let's start with the body-mind connection.

When we begin with a single contraction of any muscle, we have more than just a muscle moving. Every movement is a small part of a larger, complete process. We know that in order for that muscle to move, more must happen within the body. A single muscle movement creates microscopic movements of muscle fibers deep within the muscle itself. Active muscle proteins called actin and myosin play a big part in allowing the myofilaments of the muscle to slide back and forth, allowing each muscle fiber the opportunity to connect with another so that shortening of a muscle occurs, therefore allowing the muscle to contract.

For a skeletal muscle to contract there must be a stimulus. These stimuli are normally transmitted by the nerve cells, or neurons from the brain. These motor neurons connect to the muscle fibers at locations called neuromuscular junctions in the muscles themselves. When the impulse reaches the muscle fiber a chemical is released called acetylcholine (ACh). ACh leads to muscle excitation. Once the muscle has been triggered to contract, the neuromuscular impulse travels back up to the brain in order to create more stimu-lation impulses or to relax—depending on what the muscular body is requiring at the time.

Now with the stimulation having traveled back to the brain, further excitation of other neuromuscular junctions can occur. ACh also excites other neuroglandular junctions (areas between motor neurons and glands of the body) and causes some firing between certain brain and spinal cord cells. The different glands of the body secrete many substances; two types are exocrine glands (secreting their products into ducts that empty at the surface, examples being mucus, perspiration, oil, wax, and digestive juices), and endocrine glands (secreting their products into the blood, examples being pituitary, thyroid, and adrenal glands). Endocrine glands always secrete hormones, which are chemicals that regulate various physiological activities. Exercise affects the different hormonal and other systems of the body through common connections triggered by the motorneurons that originated in the brain itself.

Forcing a muscle contraction causes various stimulations to occur within the body by placing a demand on the brain to respond with its motorneuron-body connections. Following the physiological path of stimulation shows how the "whole" body benefits from muscle stimulation and/or by exercise as a whole. By understanding how this body-mind connection works, we can see that exercise affects our bodies more than by just making us look good.

We often hear about the different effects that hormones have on the body but rarely have the opportunity to know what specific ones actually do. Below are just a few examples of some of the hormones stimulated and their results, through exercise. *Examples of hormonal stimulation include:*

- Norepinephrine: regulates sleeping, dreaming, and mood.
- Dopamine: affects emotions and subconscious movements of skeletal muscles.
- Serotonin: induces sleep, sensory perception, and regulates temperature.
- Peptides (a chain of amino acids that occur naturally in the brain): form the building blocks of protein.

- Endorphins: suppress pain; linked to memory and learning, sexual activity, control of body temperature; regulate hormones that affect the onset of puberty, sexual drive, and reproduction.
- Angiotensin: helps regulate blood pressure.
- Cholecystokinin: causes pancreas to release digestive juices and gallbladder to release bile; there is also some indication that it may be related to the control of appetite.
- Neurotensin: regulates blood glucose levels and possible pain pathways.

How much exercise does it take to get these kinds of benefits for the body? Not a lot. For a nonactive person, often it only takes a stretching routine to stimulate these muscle fibers. Any amount of movement that stimulates increased muscle contractions (not necessarily heavy contractions) and increased blood flow into and out of the muscles themselves can have increased effects on the brain and body. This is beneficial to know when you are beginning an exercise program, because even minor increases neuromuscularly will increase your hormonal excretions; these increases lead to feeling better about yourself. When you feel better about yourself, you will be encouraged even further into a healthy lifestyle. This will aid you in achieving the goals that you set for yourself within an exercise program.

How much is enough? Science says that the minimal amount of exercise to achieve basic health benefits is: aerobic conditioning (swimming, jogging, walking, cycling) for twenty minutes at least three times a week; strength conditioning (one exercise for each body part, one set of fifteen repetitions) for two or three sessions a week; flexibility conditioning (for each body part) about ten minutes at least three times a week.

Is this enough for you? Yes, if your personal goal is to achieve basic fitness and health goals. However, if you are after something more (examples: weight loss, competition training, rehabilitation) you will need either to do more of the specific exercise or to modify your training in order to achieve the goals you desire. If you are unsure of what you need to do to modify your workout routine in order to achieve your fitness goals, consult an exercise specialist in your area. A good exercise specialist will be able to guide you toward reaching these goals.

Why Spot Training Is Unhealthy

With a book like this, the questions of "spot reducing" or "spot training" always arise. After all, this book only discusses training for the butt and thighs. Does training only one part of the body do any good? Can it be harmful?

Research proves time and time again that there is no such thing as spot reducing. In order to reduce any part of your body you need to follow a complete wellness package that includes proper diet, proper exercises, and proper motivations all geared toward reducing your body composition. With a wellness package that includes your body as a whole, you will find that those unwanted "spots" will reduce and you will create a much more beautiful body as a whole.

The exercises in this book are geared toward one particular part of the body. So does this mean that we are promoting spot training? No. What we mean by *spot training* is working only one part of your body, or one muscle group continuously, without any attention given to other muscle groups. Common examples of this kind of training are concentration on abdominals, inner thighs, calves, biceps, and chest. These tend to be aesthetic areas where both men and women want to achieve "the look."

When you begin designing a strength training package you need to consider what your personal goals are. It is good to have goals in mind such as "I want to tone up my entire body," "I want to reduce the size of my thighs," "I want to see my triceps muscle when I extend my arm." Yes, many of these goals are for "the look," and there is nothing wrong with this. What's important is how you achieve your goals. Your personal goal is always the beginning of any exercise program design.

Spot training is an unhealthy way to train. Every muscle has another muscle that opposes it bimechanically—for example, the triceps versus the biceps; these must equally maintain or increase strength in order to maintain balance within the skeletal structure. If you were to train only your triceps and neglect all other muscle parts, you would be spot training. If you keep a balanced training routine, you will be able to avoid unnecessary joint and structure problems. Any good exercise specialist will guide you away from this kind of exercise program.

Spot training can eventually lead to a number of physical problems. Problems associated with spot training or overtraining a particular muscle group begin with muscle strength imbalances. These imbalances will continue to cause more problems by creating structure imbalances that eventually will cause joint and ligament problems. You see this problem often where a training goal is to develop incredible thighs (quadriceps muscles); a person with this goal works his or her quads overtime and this often results in knee injuries. The problem begins because of the lack of attention given to muscle balance in training by not including exercises for the hamstring muscles. If the quadriceps muscles become stronger without the hamstrings becoming equally strong, eventually the quadriceps will begin to pull the patella (kneecap) out of alignment and from there cause further complications with the knee joint itself.

What this shows is that no matter how much or how little you exercise, your routine needs to include balance between opposing muscle groups, and the routine should include exercises for all muscles of the body. If you have a training routine that incorporates this strategy, then what you can do is put special emphasis or "extra spot training" attention on those parts of your body that are more of a concern to you. That is how we want you to use this book.

Concentrating on the butt and thighs is important to you. Make sure to add it to your comprehensive workout. Never neglect the other parts of your body completely. Simply add additional exercises to those areas of concern. There are many examples of this kind of training with many world-class athletes. For example, a speed skater must have thighs of steel, but he or she also incorporates a program with upper body strength training. A speed skater would train every body part but emphasize extra spot training for the thighs.

Remember to always look at your exercise program as a whole, from the fingertips to the tips of your toes and every single cell in between. If you do, you will be happy with the overall results achieved through your exercise program.

The Building Blocks of Wellness

The mind and body are directly related to everything that affects our lives today. Wellness is a state of being where the mind and body are able to productively live and work together as one complete unit.

That is why when you are reading and studying the benefits of strength training in a book like this, you need to know what else affects your overall wellness profile. After all, your wellness profile will be affected by the addition of, and the changes to, your exercise program. You need to assure yourself that when you begin this new exercise program all dimensions within your wellness profile will support your total personal profile. For example, will you be able to fit this exercise program into your work schedule, will you be able to financially afford this exercise program, will you have a social support system, will you believe in yourself and what you can do, will you emotionally dedicate yourself to this program, will you continue to learn more about your exercise program, and then continue with dedication in order to achieve the results that you want to achieve?

These are all building blocks of your personal wellness profile. These building blocks consist of six major dimensions of wellness that affect each of us: physical, emotional, spiritual, intellectual, vocational, and social. Each dimension is directly related to another. The approach you use in developing these dimensions will reflect in the type of lifestyle you have chosen to lead and allow you to make appropriate activity changes in your daily life. Every dimension treated as an equal can bring about a fulfilling "wellness profile."

Keep in mind that all six building blocks are smaller parts of the whole picture. It would be like looking at a whole pie, cut into six pieces, each piece being its own size depending on how much that wellness aspect affects your individual life.

At the beginning of this chapter we took a look at what exercise does physiologically to the body. Let's end this portion of the chapter by seeing how exercise affects the six dimensions of wellness. Here (see page 96) is a chart

WELLNESS DIMENSIONS	EXERCISE BENEFITS
PHYSICAL	Makes you look and feel better. Fights many aspects of disease processes. Increases stimulation to all body systems. Improves sleep. Improves skills and body function.
EMOTIONAL	Decreases stress reactions. Increases self-confidence. Balances hormonal extremes (affecting mood swings). Improves thought processes. Improves self-image.
SPIRITUAL	Encourages self-care. Promotes self-healing. Encourages more involvement with groups and organizations. Has positive effect on belief system.
INTELLECTUAL	Stimulates thought processes. Increases blood flow to brain. Allows for intellectual stimulation. Helps with focus. Stimulates mind during sluggish times of day or evening.
VOCATIONAL	Improves general health therefore improving output. Results in less sick days. Increases tolerence levels. Improves mental stamina. Burns stress from workday.
SOCIAL	Is fun to do with others. Creates common bond with others. Improves patience skills. Increases positive feelings about self. Reflects positive image on others. Gives good excuse to avoid unsupportive or unhealthy social situations.

that shows some of the benefits your wellness profile will receive when you participate in an exercise program.

Creating stronger muscles is extremely important and affects your physical wellness profile. However, having a strong butt and thighs will not put you in a state of optimal health; it is only one stepping-stone toward improving your personal profile. This is why we have taken the time in this chapter to discuss "wellness." The all-encompassing world of living involves strengthening all the dimensions that directly affect your lifestyle. After all, wellness *is* the lifestyle you have chosen to live.

The Four Components of Exercise

Exercise is the one portion of the wellness profile that directly affects all other components of wellness. Therefore, we need to take a look at exercise and learn how to put together an exercise program.

The four components of physical exercise are cardiovascular fitness, muscular strengthening, muscular endurance, and flexibility. To have a well-rounded physical wellness profile you need to include each of these four components in your exercise program.

CARDIOVASCULAR FITNESS

Cardiovascular fitness is achieved by performing activities that tax the heart, lungs, and circulatory systems. When cardiovascular exercise is performed, the body puts a demand on the oxygen exchange systems of our bodies. Needed oxygen is taken in from the lungs into the circulatory system, then distributed to the muscles that are being used during exercise. The oxygen then helps break down the stored fats into energy for use by the working muscle. This entire exchange system forces the lungs and heart to become extremely efficient, so that the working muscles can continue their activities.

The American College of Sports Medicine states that thirty minutes of cardiovascular exercise at least three times a week is a substantial way to receive health benefits. A cardiovascular program consists of activities that allow you to reach 65 to 85 percent of your maximum heart rate for a duration of no less than twenty minutes. The kinds of exercises that we are discussing are walking, jogging, swimming, bicycling, and aerobic dancing. Maintaining these kinds of exercises longer than twenty minutes may provide additional benefits if performed correctly.

Finding Your Target Heart Rate: The following formula will determine your target heart rate for doing cardiovascular work. The following example is for someone who is thirty years old.

At birth your maximum heart rate is 220 beats per minute. Each year you age, your maximum heart rate decreases by one beat. So to determine your maximum heart rate, you subtract your age from 220.

For training purposes, you want to achieve between 65 and 85 percent of your maximum heart rate, so to figure out what your ten-second pulse rate should be, multiply your maximum heart rate (220 minus your age) by .65 and .85, and then divide those figures by 6 (because there are six ten-second periods in every minute). The two resulting figures are the low and high ends for your ten-second pulse during training. When working out, you want to keep your heart rate between these parameters. So for a thirty-year-old:

$220 - 30 = 190$ beats per minute
    (*Maximum heart rate*)
$190 \times .65 = 124$ beats per minute
    (*Lower end of target*)
$190 \times .85 = 162$ beats per minute
    (*Upper end of target*)
$124 \div 6 = 21$
    (*Lower end of target ten-second pulse*)
$162 \div 6 = 27$
    (*Upper end of target ten-second pulse*)

In the middle of your exercise session, count your number of heartbeats in ten seconds by checking your pulse at your wrist or on your neck. It should be somewhere between the upper and lower ends of your target pace. So in the example above, a thirty-year-old would want to be between twenty-one and twenty-seven beats in the ten-second count.

Cardiovascular Exercise Routine: The following are general guidelines for a progressive cardiovascular program.

Weeks 1 and 2:	5 minutes easy pace
	5 minutes target pace
	5 minutes easy pace
	Total time: 15 minutes

Weeks 3 and 4:	5 minutes easy pace
	5 minutes target pace
	2 minutes easy pace
	5 minutes target pace
	5 minutes easy pace
	Total time: 22 minutes

Weeks 5 and 6:	5 minutes easy pace
	10 minutes target pace
	2 minutes easy pace
	10 minutes target pace
	5 minutes easy pace
	Total time: 32 minutes

Weeks 7 and 8:	5 minutes easy pace
	15 minutes target pace
	2 minutes easy pace
	15 minutes target pace
	5 minutes easy pace
	Total time: 42 minutes

Maintenance (after eight weeks):	5 minutes easy pace
	10 to 30 minutes target pace
	5 minutes easy pace

STRENGTH TRAINING AND ENDURANCE

Strength training provides both increased strength gains and increased endurance to the muscles, joints, bones, and ligaments of the body. The kind of benefits that you can achieve with strength training include developing a stronger posture and structural features, stronger bones, increased strength for daily activities, greater muscle tone and flexibility, and strength in joints.

Strength training should include exercises designed for all major muscle groups of the body, and should be performed at least two to three times per week. Strength training can be done a variety of ways by using free weights, strength machines, or through other resistive kinds of training methods. There are a variety of strength training programs that will help you to achieve the benefits that you are after.

Your strength training program needs to include exercises for all parts of your body. You should strength train using larger muscle groups first, followed by your smaller muscles near the end of your workout.

If you are unfamiliar with these exercises it is important that you are trained properly. Do not begin any strength program without proper instruction from someone educated in the field of strength training. Learning proper form and concepts from the beginning will allow for a safe and effective exercise program.

EXERCISES TO CHOOSE FROM

Back
Pullovers
Upright rows
Bent-over rows
Single-arm rows
Lat pulldown (*behind the neck*)
Lat pulldown (*to the chest*)
Rear flys
Low back extensions

Legs
Leg extension (quadriceps)
Leg curls (hamstrings)
Squat
Lunge
Abduction exercises
Adduction exercises
Calf raises

Chest
Bench press
Flat bench flys
Incline bench press
Incline flys
Pullovers
Wide arm push-ups

Triceps
Triceps extensions
Overhead extensions
Triceps kickbacks
Close grip bench press
Dips
Close grip push-ups

Shoulders
Lateral raises
Overhead press

Front raises
Rear flys

Biceps
Straight curls
Individual curls
Concentration curls
Hammer curls

Extras to Add
Side bends
Neck exercises
Forearm strength training
Abdominals (from *The Complete Book of Abs*)

When beginning your program be sure to choose an exercise weight that will allow you to reach a point of fatigue within a reasonable number of repetitions. Reaching fatigue means achieving the maximum number of lifts where you cannot lift the weight another time during the set. It's important that you do not get "hung up" on *numbers*—that is, worrying about how many you need to do. Don't get stuck on sets of ten, sixteen, or twenty. You need to determine the set number each time you exercise, write down the number of repetitions that you physically have done after each exercise, then on the next day that you exercise attempt to do more repetitions. When you are comfortably lifting between twelve and sixteen repetitions, increase the amount of training weight during your next exercise session.

Strength Training Routine: The following are general guidelines for a progressive strength training routine.

Weeks 1 and 2: Perform one set of each.	1 exercise for your back
	1 exercise for your chest
	1 exercise for your shoulders
	1 exercise for your biceps
	1 exercise for your triceps
	1 exercise for your quadriceps
	1 exercise for your hamstrings
	1 stomach exercise

Weeks 3 and 4: Perform one set of each.	2 exercises for your back 2 exercises for your chest 1 exercise for your shoulders 1 exercise for your biceps 1 exercise for your triceps 1 exercise for your quadriceps 1 exercise for your hamstrings 1 exercise for your calves 1 stomach exercise
Weeks 5 and 6: Perform one set of each.	3 exercises for your back 2 exercises for your chest 2 exercises for your shoulders 1 exercise for your biceps 1 exercise for your triceps 1 exercise for your quadriceps 1 exercise for your hamstrings 1 exercise for your total legs/gluteals 1 exercise for your calves 1 stomach exercise
Weeks 7 and 8:	Begin two sets of each exercise. Continue adding variety into your program.
Maintenance (after eight weeks):	Continue at two to three sets of each exercise. Mix up your workout, allowing for variety. Continue to increase weight when needed.

STRETCHING

Flexibility is extremely important in the comprehensive program of physical fitness, and is the easiest type of exercise to maintain, because it can be done just about anywhere. Flexibility also works the muscles, ligaments, and joints. It is important for maintaining posture, joint mobility, range of motion, and helps keeps the ligaments and tendons from tightening. Flexibility needs to be done at least three times a week, and should provide stretches for all major muscle groups and joints. Flexibility is most effective when performed at the end of your exercise routine.

Neck Stretch: Each movement should be done once. Then move on to the next movement without resting. Drop head forward, chin to chest. Hold for ten seconds. Looking straight ahead, lower your right ear to your right shoulder. Hold for ten seconds. Lower your left ear to your left shoulder. Hold for ten seconds.

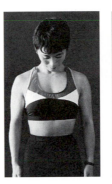 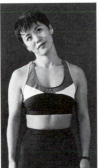 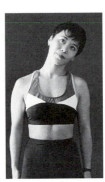

Shoulder Roll: Standing, raise your shoulders high on your neck and roll them backward. Perform five reps. Then repeat the movement, but roll your shoulders forward. Perform five reps. Then bring your shoulders up toward your ears and hold for a count of five and release.

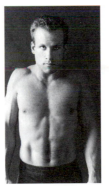 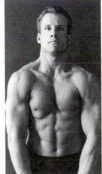 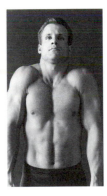

Shoulders Stretch: Grasp hands in front of your body and turn palms forward while fingers remain interlocked; stretch shoulders forward, as you reach out as far as possible, rounding your back. Hold for fifteen seconds and perform two reps. Maintain hand position, stretch up, straight overhead. Hold for fifteen seconds and perform two reps.

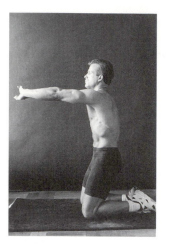
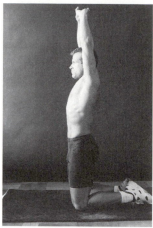

Side Bend: Stand with your feet together, arms fully extended over your head, hands touching. Bend at your waist over your right side. Hold position for ten seconds. Then bend at your waist over your left side. Hold this position for ten seconds.

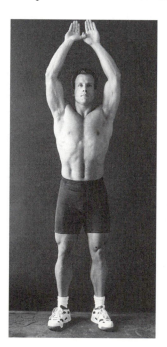
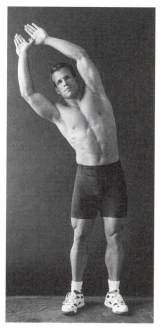

Side Bend Two: Spread legs wide, letting one hand slide down the leg while the other hand goes easily over your head. Slowly come up and perform the movement on the other side.

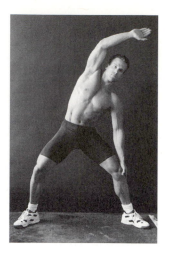

Knees-to-Chest Hug: Lie flat on your back; bring both knees to your chest. From this position, wrap your arms around your legs and hug your knees to chest. At the same time, bring your chin to your chest. Hold for fifteen seconds.

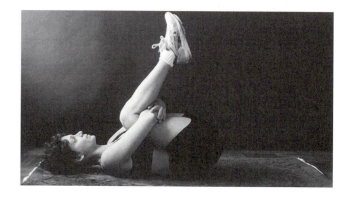

Knees to Side: Lie flat on your back, knees bent, feet flat on the floor. Let both legs fall to one side. Hold for ten seconds. Then let the legs fall to the other side. Hold for ten seconds.

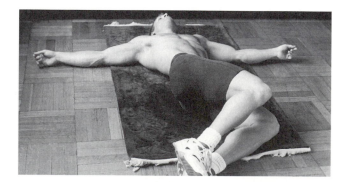

Elongation Stretch: Lie flat on your back, arms fully extended over your head, legs fully extended on the floor. Extend from your fingertips to your toes, lengthening your body in both directions. Hold for fifteen seconds.

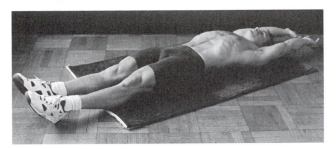

Hamstring Stretch: Lie on your back, legs bent, feet flat on the floor. Grab one leg behind the knee, straighten the leg, and gently pull it toward your head (chin to chest). Hold for fifteen seconds. Repeat with the other leg.

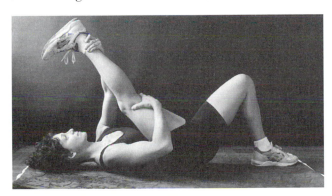

Quadriceps Stretch: Turn on one side and lie comfortably with shoulder under ear. Reach behind your back for your top ankle and gently pull it back. Then switch sides. Hold on each side for fifteen seconds.

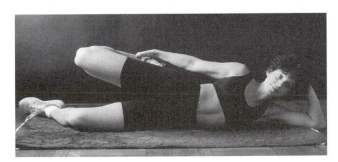

Back and Stomach Stretch: Lie on your stomach, hands under your chest (palms down). Slowly pressing up with your arms, straighten them as much as you can and arch your back. Relax lower body. Look up, attempting to get your chin as high as possible. Hold for fifteen seconds.

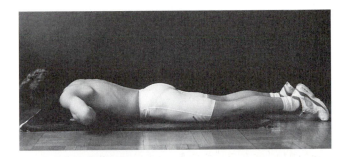

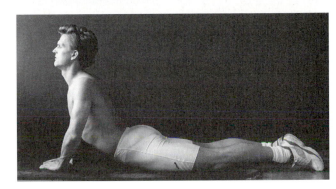

Back Arch: Come up on your hands and knees (all fours). Place hands under your shoulders and hunch your back up like a cat and lower your head. Hold for fifteen seconds and perform two reps. Then arch your back in the opposite direction. Hold for fifteen seconds.

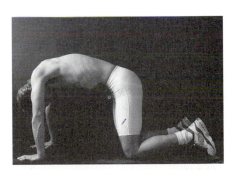

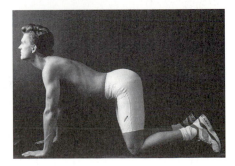

Chest Stretch: Kneeling erect, clasp your hands behind your lower back and slowly try to extend your hands up and back. Hold for fifteen seconds.

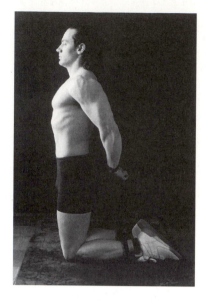

Single Leg Stretch: Sit on floor with one leg extended out in front, other leg bent toward your body, with the sole of your foot touching the thigh of your other leg. Reach with both hands toward toes. Hold for fifteen seconds. Repeat on other side.

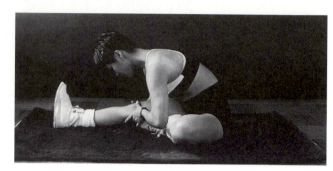

ADVANCED STRETCHING

As you continue to get stronger with your exercise program it would be beneficial to increase your stretching program to include more specific stretching techniques. Stretching at the end of a hard workout is a very good way to alleviate tightness, cool down the muscles, and help avoid unnecessary soreness the following day.

When beginning your stretching program, please consult an exercise instructor so that you will know proper form and procedures for stretching.

The following advanced stretches can be added to your program for added emphasis on lower body flexibility.

Hips Stretch: Lying on your back, extend left leg out straight on the floor. Bring right thigh perpendicular to body. Gently pull right leg across your body with left hand

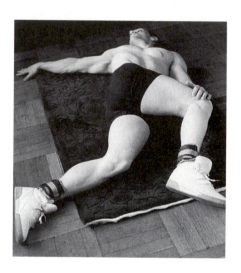

keeping both shoulders on the floor. Look in the opposite direction of the twist. Hold for fifteen seconds. Repeat on other side.

Groin Stretch: Sitting upright on the floor bring the bottoms of your feet together as you bring the feet in as close to the body as possible. Gently add pressure to the inner thighs with elbows pushing

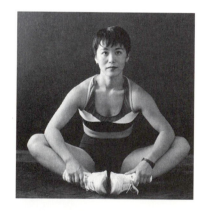

down for greater stretch. Hold for fifteen seconds.

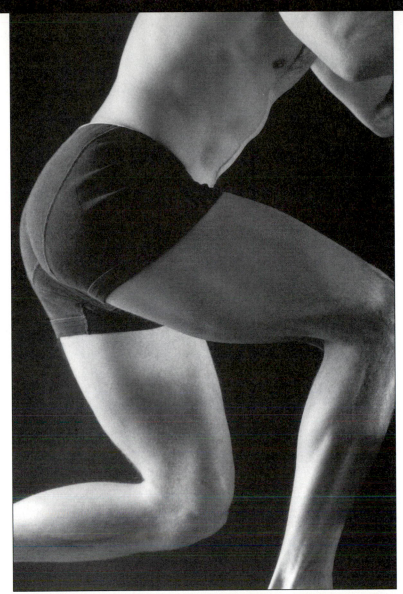

PART THREE

The Exercises

Introduction to the Exercises

There are hundreds of exercises and variations that work your butt and legs. You will find that most exercise books or videos will give you between ten and twenty to choose from. Over the next seven chapters you will learn over one hundred. The reason you are given such an extensive selection is to offer you a wide variety from which to choose; this both allows you to discover what works for you, and also to create change, which equals growth. These factors help to motivate you, which in turn leads to a better performance in your workout. The result: You are much less likely to quit—and that means success.

As you read through the exercises in the following chapters keep in mind what you read in this chapter and apply it to each exercise. When starting a routine refer back to this chapter and review all of the guide-lines set up for you for each exercise that you will be performing.

A Key to the Exercises

Each exercise is presented in a format designed to help you make intelligent exercise choices. This section explains the different parts of the format.

DIFFICULTY LEVELS
The exercises are ranked from 1 to 3: 1 being the easiest; 2, intermediate; and 3, advanced. Choose exercises that correspond to your fitness level and exercise experience. These, of course, are general categories. Depending on your individual strengths and weaknesses, you will find particular exercises more or less

difficult than the next person. Remember, increasing difficulty is a way to increase intensity, which causes muscle adaptation. So as a general guideline, start with the easiest exercises, build strength, and move to more difficult movements.

It is important to note that Combination exercises (exercises that work two or more areas—i.e., front and back) tend to be rated in the advanced category because of the numerous muscle groups involved and their more difficult demands on muscle coordination. These exercises are very effective and specific to many aspects of sports and everyday life. Because of this it is essential to start with some Combination lifts. Since you should build up in intensity when exercising, it is important to start with the least difficult Combination exercises and move on to the most difficult.

LOWER BACK

Because everybody's lower back is different, we rank each lower back exercise according to its "risk" factor. The purpose of ranking the exercises this way is not to discourage you from doing certain exercises or to encourage you to do those that will prove too strenuous. The ranking system is a warning: Proceed carefully. If you have a history of lower back problems, you need to exercise with extra care. You should also consult a doctor to discuss exercise in relation to any specific problem. Again, these rankings are general guidelines to help you find the appropriate exercises that fit your needs and experience.

The three lower back rankings are: Low Risk, Moderate Risk, and High Risk. These rankings are based on a combination of the following criteria:

1. *The range of motion involved in the movement.* Smaller, isolated movements such as Seated Adductions are safer than Squats.
2. *Single or compound movement.* A single movement would involve one of the areas (i.e., front or back) working alone, as in a Seated Adduction or Leg Extension. A compound movement involves two or more areas working together, as in a lunge. Single-area movements are generally safer.
3. *External support.* The more external support the

lower back has, the safer the movement will be. So any movement where you keep your lower back pressed against the floor, wall, or a seat back is generally safer than movement without such support. It is important to discuss the use of weight belts to support the lower back. Weight belts are a useful tool to support the lower back while exercising. However, they are often overused. When performing exercises on the lower body, you need to consciously stabilize the lower back throughout the exercise. This helps to strengthen the lower back. If you use a weight belt, you minimize the opportunity to strengthen the lower back. It is therefore necessary to develop a logical strategy of when to utilize a weight belt. Generally speaking, it is a good strategy to avoid using a weight belt when performing high-volume, low-weight exercises, and to use it when performing low-volume, high-weight exercises. This, of course, is an individual decision and should be based on your particular needs.

4. *Length of the lever involved in the movement.* The longer the lever is (torso or legs) and the farther away it moves away from your center in its range of motion, the more torque (stress) on the lower back. Therefore, straight-leg movements (Standing Kickbacks) tend to be more stressful than bent-leg movements (Bent-Leg Kickbacks). Also, the upper body flexion is influenced by how far the weight is from the center—a Stiff-Leg Dead Lift (weight closer to center at point of flexion) is less stressful than a Good Morning (weight further from center at point of flexion).
5. *Single or compound plane of movement.* A single plane of movement is safer than a compound movement. For example, a Back Extension takes place on a single plane as opposed to a Back Extension with a Twist, which takes place on two planes: up and down, and rotation.
6. *Motor skill rating of the exercise.* An exercise that is more difficult to coordinate is also potentially more difficult to stabilize. Thus many multi-segment lifts such as the Squat have the potential to be stressful.

7. *Speed of movement.* Explosive or hard-to-control movements such as Box Lunges have the potential to be stressful to the lower back.

In addition to the above, it is also important to note that an increase in the intensity (weight) of any exercise can create stress on the lower back. As always, improper technique can create stress on the lower back as well. But knowing the general principles that are involved with potential lower back strain gives you the tools to modify certain exercises to fit your lower back needs.

AREA

The exercises are grouped into areas of emphasis: front (front portion of the lower body—i.e., quadriceps); back (back portion of the lower body—i.e., butt or hamstrings); inside (inner portion of the lower body—i.e., adductors); outside (outer portion of the lower body—i.e., abductors); Combination exercises (exercises that incorporate two or more of the above-mentioned areas). Being able to correctly visualize which muscles you are working is essential to understanding the exercise.

Similar exercises are grouped together when possible. For example, all squats, lunges, abduction, and adduction exercises are put into one group. Such groupings make it easier to see variations in the exercise.

INSTRUCTION

This is the exercise itself: the starting position, movement, and proper exercise technique.

TRAINER'S TIPS

For each exercise, you can make use of the trainer's tips section like a personal trainer. Some of the tips are specific to the exercise, others are reminders that are true for every exercise. You need to hear these tips over and over until they become second nature. The following tips are essential for working the butt and legs:

- Keep speed of movement controlled through the entire range of motion so you can feel constant tension.

- Feel your muscles work (focus your mind on the correct area) and try to maintain tension through all ranges of motion.
- Use caution if you have lower back problems. Overkicking or jerky motions can make the exercise potentially dangerous.
- Maintain a stable upper body when performing an exercise.
- Try not to completely lock out the knee in any exercise. Always decelerate just short of locking knees out.
- Always use proper breathing techniques (see page 23).
- Always keep neck and back in alignment. Don't look up or down.
- Don't squeeze bar or machine with hands during exercise.

Speed of Movement

It is important to be aware of your speed of movement when you do the exercises. There are two basic types or classifications:

1. *Concentric or Positive Phase*—Move with authority or explosiveness (one to two seconds).
2. *Eccentric or Negative Phase*—Move under control (three to four seconds).

How explosive you are on the concentric phase depends on: (1) what your current strength base is; you should have at least four weeks of strength training before really emphasizing explosiveness; (2) what you are training for; explosiveness is specific to many sports; (3) variety in training.

Controlling the eccentric phase (e.g., lowering the weight back to the stack on a Leg Extension) is very important to get the maximum training effect in a workout and also to prevent injury. If you force the muscle to work through the eccentric phase rather than relying on gravity or momentum, you will receive the maximum benefit throughout the full range of motion. Also, it is common to hurt oneself on the eccentric phase by letting gravity take the weight down; using gravity puts the joint and muscle under undue stress because of the potential bouncing at the end of the motion and because when the muscle relaxes (loses control), it then has to suddenly regain control.

Remember that following these guidelines on speed is very important for getting the most out of your workout and for guaranteeing that you will have a safe workout.

Eccentric Emphasis Training

For a variety of reasons you may at some point wish to perform eccentric emphasis training. This means that you will emphasize the eccentric or negative phase of the exercise. Generally, it is best to emphasize the eccentric phase after concentric failure occurs, which means that you have reached your maximum point at the concentric half of the exercise, and cannot continue. At this point, some exercisers have a partner "spot" them (i.e., lift the weights) for the concentric phase so that they may perform the eccentric phase of the exercise, thus reaching a maximum point for both phases of that exercise. In such cases, you may take as long as five to ten seconds on the eccentric phase or you may add weight to the eccentric phase. In either case you are attempting to overload the eccentric phase by increasing the intensity through this range of motion.

Pulsing

Pulsing is holding a movement at the top of its range of motion, then moving back and forth, about one to two inches, keeping constant tension on the muscle being exercised. This tiny movement pumps the muscle. An example would be taking the Leg Extension up almost to a lockout and then bending and straightening within a range of one to two inches.

Exercise Variety

As mentioned, where possible we have grouped similar exercises together in series. These exercises have similar movements with different variations added: for example, the lunge series. In each exercise many of the mechanics are the same with slight variations in the movements, changing the emphasis of the exercise. In one case, the leg may be pulling, in another pushing. You may step forward on one exercise and back on another. The differences allow you to work the leg from different angles and in different modes. This shocks the muscle, causing adaptation or growth. Also, the more angles you hit the leg from, the more completely it is trained, and the more options you have for specificity in training the leg. Using different types of lunges is an example of how you can achieve one of the most important training principles—variety. Without variety you will get bored, the muscle will grow complacent, instead of being shocked into growth periods, and the muscle won't achieve its best overall development.

Controversial Exercises

There are exercises in this part that may be considered by many to be dangerous because of the potential for injury if done incorrectly. In particular, the Squat is a victim of this mind-set. For the most part, the negative bias about the Squat and its variations is the result of people performing the Squat incorrectly. The myth that the Squat is bad for the knees does not hold water if the Squat is performed using the correct technique. In fact, the Squat is a very effective and important exercise. It improves running, jumping, and throwing abilities. It also promotes joint integrity for the knee (just the opposite of a common misconception).

There is, however, truth to some of the concerns about squatting. The most important is the possibility of injuring the back while squatting. If not performed correctly the lower back can be at risk, possibly more so on the Squat than on other exercises. It is therefore advisable that someone with a history of lower back problems should proceed with caution when performing this exercise (use perfect technique and lower weights), and in many cases should not perform it. Instead this person should look for alternative exercises. A person with no back problems should be able to perform the Squat without any problem.

If you have a history of knee problems you should also proceed with caution and consult a specialist before starting a squatting regimen.

Bar Positions

The position of the bar when performing certain exercises is very important. Changing its location will change the center of gravity, thus changing the emphasis from one muscle group to another. There are two main bar positions that are primarily used when performing the Squat or the Lunge. Always remember, when loading the bar you always walk forward into a squat or power rack, and back out with the bar once it has been secured.

FRONT POSITION

There are two ways to "rack" the bar in the front position. The first way is to grip the bar like you normally would with both hands about shoulder width apart, or slightly wider if more comfortable. Walk in toward the bar until it is tight against your throat and resting on top of the front of both shoulders. Your elbows should be raised as high as they can be throughout the lift with your hands lightly gripping the bar.

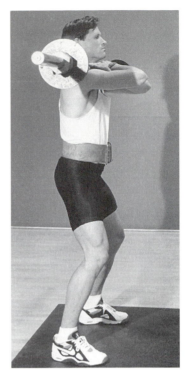

The second way to rack the bar is to cross grip it. Approach the bar the same as before setting the bar tight against your throat and resting on the front of your shoulders. Reach through with both hands and arms until the bar is as tight to your throat as possible, then bend your right arm at the elbow and grip the bar just inside your left shoulder. Do the same with your left arm, gripping just inside the right shoulder, so your arms are crossed, left over right. Keep both elbows elevated as high as possible throughout the lift.

BACK POSITION

To rack the bar in back, first center yourself on the bar by gripping with both hands about shoulder width apart, or wider if more comfortable. Walk under the bar, placing the bar just below your neck on upper back. If you place it too high and it rests on the C7 vertebra of your neck it will be very uncomfortable and could lead to injury. Grip loosely with both hands.

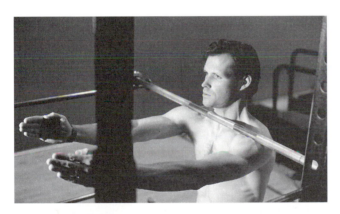

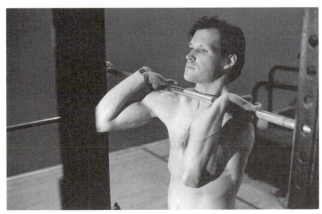

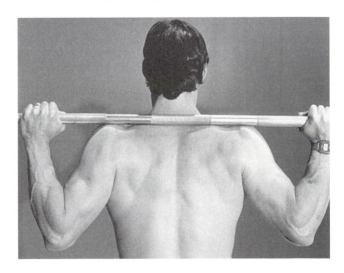

Dumbbell Positions

Correctly positioning dumbbells when performing a lift guarantees safety and maximum results. Once again, changing the position affects the center of gravity of the lift, thereby offering variety and changing the way an exercise feels. There are four main dumbbell positions used primarily when squatting or lunging.

DUMBBELLS AT SIDE

Place the dumbbells at your side. The key is to not allow the extra weight to affect your posture. Maintain an upright upper torso with your shoulders square and back, your chest out, and your head and neck aligned with your back. Look straight ahead.

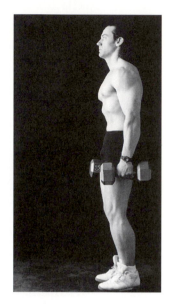

DUMBBELLS RACKED

Position the dumbbells as if they were a bar and you had them racked for a front squat. You may rotate your hands in and flair your elbows out and up if you wish. This will allow you to rest the handle part of the dumbbell on the top of your shoulders. Once again, it is important to maintain good posture.

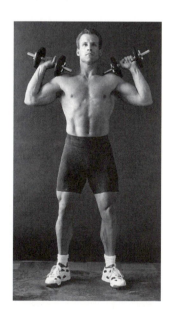

Variation 1: Single dumbbell can also be placed below the neck, like racking the bar in back (page 109).

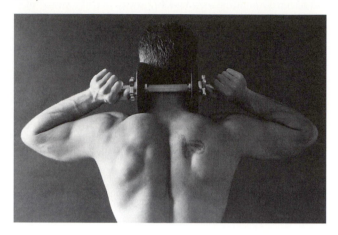

Variation 2: Dumbbells can rest on each shoulder. Balance the handle of the dumbbell on the shoulder while weight rests on the outside (front and back) of your shoulders.

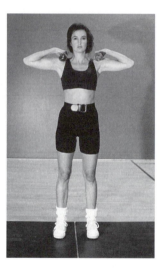

DUMBBELLS OVERHEAD (OR BAR OVERHEAD)

Extend both dumbbells directly overhead, just as if you were performing a standing dumbbell shoulder press. Maintain good posture throughout exercise. Avoid arching your lower back while in this position. Obviously this position prohibits exercising with as much weight as you would in the other positions, but it will increase you heart rate more rapidly and thus is a good position for an aerobic workout. This position can also be utilized with a bar. (See Overhead Squat, page 166.)

Rubber Bands and Ankle Weights

Practically all of the exercises performed with a cable and weight stack for resistance can also be performed using either a rubber band or ankle weights for resistance.

Foot Positions

There are various foot positions that can be incorporated in different exercises to change the angle of the working muscle. It is important to realize that the foot position is not changed for the sole purpose of creating a new angle for the foot, but rather to rotate the leg in or out thus changing the angle from which the quads, hips, butt, hamstrings, and calves work. When you change your foot position, it is important that you keep your knee aligned with your foot. There are five main foot positions that are used when exercising the lower body.

Neutral: This position is when the foot is pointed straight ahead. The entire leg is also in alignment with the foot.

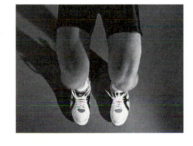

Inversion: This position is when the foot is angled (rotated) in. The entire leg is rotated at this angle, thus the leg is rotated in, starting from the hip.

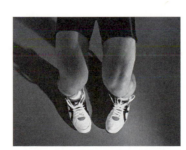

Eversion: This position is when the foot is angled (rotated) out. The entire leg is rotated out with the angle, thus the leg is rotated out, starting from the hip.

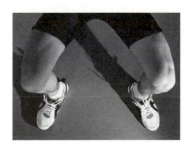

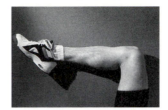

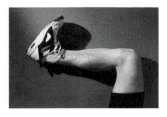

Plantar Flexion (Pointed): This position is when the toes are pointed straight and away from the head (often referred to as pointed down). Plantar (pointed) can be applied when the foot is straight, inverted, or everted.

Dorsi Flexion (Flexed): This position is when the toes are pointed straight and back toward the head (often referred to as flexed back). Dorsi flexion (flexed) can be applied when the foot is straight, inverted, or everted.

Foot Positioning and Movement

Four movements in particular, and calf work in general, can use a variety of the above foot positions. These four movements are adduction, abduction, extension, and flexion. Below are the desired foot positions for the four main types of movement and for calf work.

ADDUCTION

An everted (rotated out) position is best when performing adduction movements. This allows the leg to rotate out, which then focuses the work on the inside. The eversion can be applied with the foot in a plantar or dorsi flexion, with dorsi flexion probably better. Common exercises would be those listed in chapter eleven.

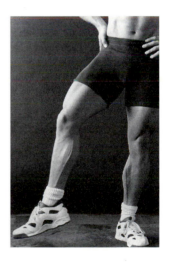

ABDUCTION

An inverted (rotated in) position is best when performing abduction movements. This allows the leg to rotate in, which then focuses the work on the outside. The inversion can be applied with the foot in a plantar or dorsi flexion. Common exercises would be those listed in chapter twelve.

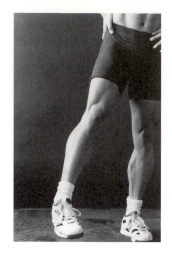

EXTENSION

All five foot positions (neutral, inversion, eversion, and plantar and dorsi flexion) can be used for extension movements. This allows you to hit the muscles from a variety of angles. Just remember that the leg rotates with the foot. A common extension exercise that this could be applied to would be Leg Extensions.

FLEXION

All five foot positions can be used for flexion movements. Changing foot positions will enable you to focus on the muscles from a variety of angles. Again, remember that the leg rotates with the foot. A common flexion exercise that this could be applied to would be Leg Curls.

CALF WORK

All three angled positions (neutral, inversion, and eversion) can be used to hit the muscles from a variety of angles. Just remember that the leg rotates with the foot. Two common calf work exercises that this could be applied to would be any Toe Raise and any Heel Raise.

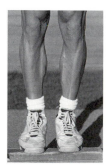 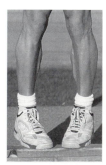 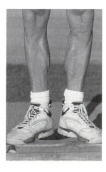

Important Body Positioning

It is important to position yourself correctly during any exercise that you perform. The following are guidelines to follow when performing exercises in these particular situations.

TORSO POSTURE FOR SQUATTING AND LUNGING

In setting up the upper body follow these guidelines. The chest should be out, shoulders back, lower back straight, and eyes looking straight ahead (head and neck should be aligned with spine). This position keeps the upper body stable and protects the lower back.

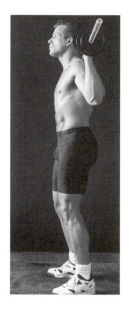

KNEE POSITION FOR SQUATTING, LUNGING, AND PRESSING

When performing any of these exercises it is important to keep the knee in a good position. This is especially important for women because of a wider pelvic girth, which makes knee alignment

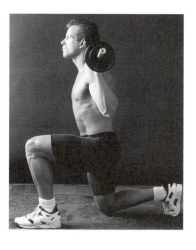

that much more essential. It is key to have proper alignment from the very start. In any starting position knees are slightly bent and aligned with toes. The desired position is to bend to a 90-degree angle or slightly past with the shin perpendicular to the ground on any Squat or Lunge. When performing any pressing action do not allow the knee to come forward past the toes. This position keeps the knee in alignment with the calf and foot, thus allowing the stress to be displaced through the lower leg. Do not allow the knee to go out over the toe because most of the stress of the movement will go right through the knee.

POSITION FOR CABLE CROSS OR PULLEY WORK

When performing cable work it is important to observe two things: distance and posture. When performing standing cable work you will want to hang on to the apparatus with the hand nearest to it. You should position yourself an arm's length away from the apparatus so that there is room to take an exercise through a full range of motion. Your posture should be straight up and down with your head, neck, and back in alignment. Stay square throughout the exercise. Don't allow the cable to twist you. When seated or lying, position yourself so that the attached leg is at least two to three feet from the weight stack.

POSITION ON ALL FOURS

This position is common in cable work and floor exercises. You assume a position on your hands and knees. In this position you should keep your head aligned with your spine (your head should not be tilted back, nor should your chin be tucked in toward the chest) and your back should remain flat, not hunched or rounded.

On all cable work make sure you are far enough away from the weight stack to keep constant tension on the working muscles. This means the weights can't hit the stack before you've completed the movement.

CHAPTER NINE

The Back

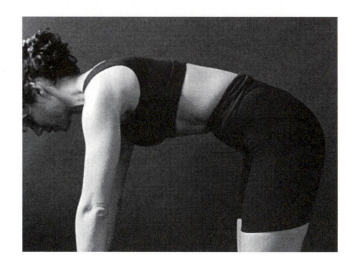

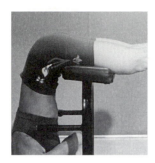

Exercise: Back Extension

DIFFICULTY: 2
LOWER BACK: HIGH RISK
AREA: BACK (GLUTES, HAMSTRINGS)

STARTING POSITION: Lie face down on a Roman chair or off the end of a bench with someone holding your legs. Your torso should be far enough out on the Roman chair or the bench to allow your upper body to bend down to a 90-degree angle. To start the exercise you will be extended and parallel to the ground. You may place your hands on your ears or across your chest.

MOVEMENT: Lower your torso in controlled motion toward the floor until you reach a 90-degree bend (or until you feel tightness in your lower back or hamstrings). Return to starting position by raising your torso until it's parallel to the floor.

TRAINER'S TIPS:
- Avoid raising above parallel on the extension phase.
- Control downward phase; don't let gravity take you down.
- Focus your mind on your butt and lower back as you extend up.
- Squeeze your butt together as you raise torso.
- This exercise can be performed holding weights behind the head or across the chest.

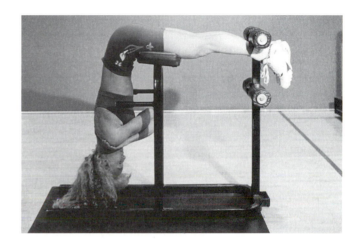

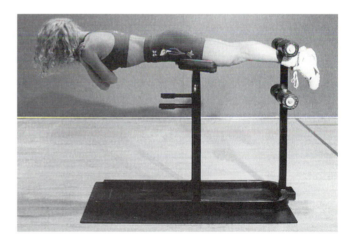

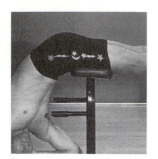

Exercise: Back Extension with a Twist

DIFFICULTY: 2
LOWER BACK: MODERATE RISK
AREA: BACK (GLUTES, HAMSTRINGS)

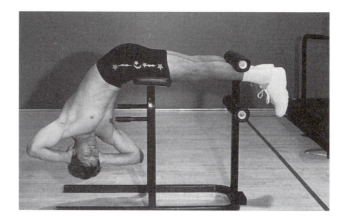

STARTING POSITION: Lie face down on a Roman chair or off the end of a bench with someone holding your feet. You should be far enough forward on the pad or off the bench to allow your torso to bend at a 90-degree angle. Twist your upper body so one shoulder rotates toward the ceiling and you are looking to the side. You may place your hands on your ears, across your chest, behind your back, or you may hold a stick or bar behind your head.

MOVEMENT: Lower your torso in a controlled motion toward the floor. Maintaining your twist, raise your torso parallel to the floor. Return to starting position maintaining twist. Perform all reps on one side and then on the other.

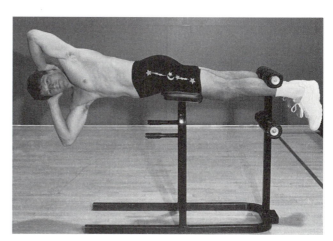

TRAINER'S TIPS:
- Avoid overtwisting; turn only as far as comfortable, not beyond.
- Concentrate on your glutes and lower back as you raise.
- This exercise can be performed holding weights behind the head or across the chest.
- Focus your mind on the working muscle.

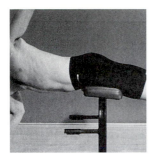

Exercise: Extended Back Rotations

DIFFICULTY: 2
LOWER BACK: MODERATE RISK
AREA: BACK (GLUTES, HAMSTRINGS)

STARTING POSITION: Lie face down on a Roman chair or off the end of a bench with someone holding your feet. Your pelvis should be on the pad or bench, allowing you to maintain a parallel position to the ground. Your entire body is parallel to the floor. You may place your hands on your ears or across your chest, or you may hold a pole behind your head.

MOVEMENT: Twist your upper torso to the right as far as comfortable while remaining parallel to the ground. Twist to tightness and return to starting position. Perform the same movement to the left.

TRAINER'S TIPS:
- Avoid overtwisting; turn only to tightness, not beyond.
- Maintain parallel position throughout the exercise.
- Focus your mind on your butt and lower back as you twist.
- This exercise can be performed holding weights behind the head or across the chest.

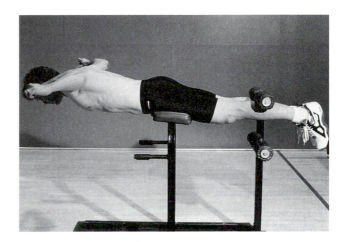

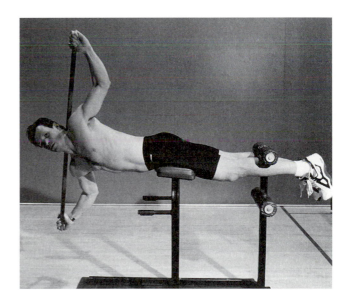

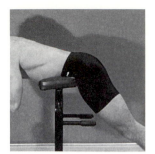

Exercise: Prone Double-Leg Raises

DIFFICULTY: 1
LOWER BACK: HIGH RISK
AREA: BACK (GLUTES, HAMSTRINGS)

STARTING POSITION: Lie on your stomach on a Roman chair so your legs are hanging off, with knees slightly bent. Hang on to the front of the chair for support, head straight and in alignment with your spine.

MOVEMENT: Lower your legs until they are an inch from the floor. Raise them back to starting position. Do not move them past parallel.

Variation: This exercise can be done one leg at a time.

TRAINER'S TIPS:
- Avoid raising above parallel on the extension phase. Raising too far will arch the back and cause undue stress on the lower back.
- Control downward phase; don't let gravity control the movement.
- Focus your mind on your butt and lower back as you extend. Contract your butt.
- This exercise can be performed with a rubber band, ankle weights, or body weight for resistance.

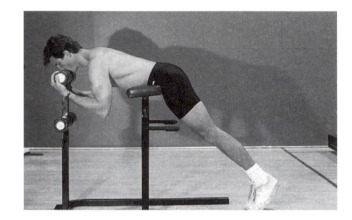

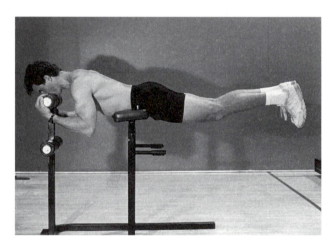

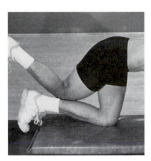

Exercise: Bent-Kick Crosses

DIFFICULTY: 2
LOWER BACK: MODERATE RISK
AREA: BACK (GLUTES, HAMSTRINGS), OUTSIDE (ABDUCTORS)

STARTING POSITION: Get down on all fours on the floor, back flat.

MOVEMENT: Keeping your exercising leg bent at a 90-degree angle throughout the exercise, push the leg back and up until you feel tightness in the butt, and then return to the starting position. Repeat with other leg.

TRAINER'S TIPS:
- On the backward motion of this movement move your foot toward the ceiling.
- Do not overpush. Your thigh should be parallel to the ground at the top of the motion.
- Keep motion controlled so you can feel constant tension in the butt.
- Feel your butt tighten as you raise and try to maintain tension through both ranges (back and forward) of motion.
- You can also perform this exercise with a rubber band, ankle weights, cable attachment, or body weight for resistance.

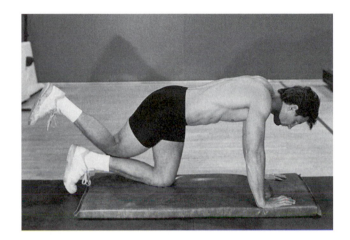

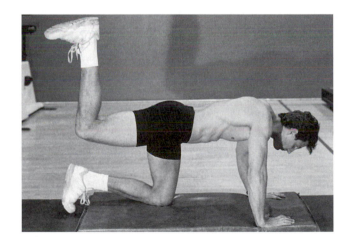

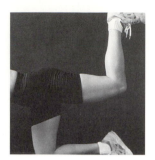

Exercise: Bent-Leg Kickbacks

DIFFICULTY: 2
LOWER BACK: MODERATE RISK
AREA: BACK (GLUTES, HAMSTRINGS)

STARTING POSITION: Get on all fours on the floor, back flat.

MOVEMENT: Keeping your exercising leg bent at a 90-degree angle throughout the exercise, raise the leg back and up until you feel tightness in the butt (you should feel as though you are raising the sole of your foot toward the ceiling). Return to even or slightly in front of the nonworking leg. Repeat with other leg.

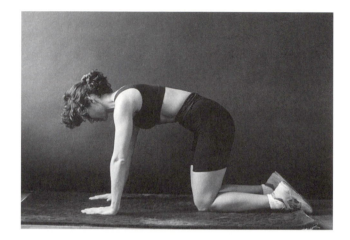

TRAINER'S TIPS:
- Do not overpush. Your thigh should be parallel to the ground at the top of the motion. Do not raise the leg higher, as this will cause the lower back to arch.
- Keep motion controlled so you can feel constant tension in the butt.
- Feel your butt tighten as you raise, trying to maintain tension through both ranges (back and forward) of motion.
- Overkicking or jerky motions can make the exercise potentially dangerous for the lower back.
- You can also perform this exercise with a rubber band, ankle weights, cable attachment, or body weight for resistance.
- Focus your mind on the working muscles.

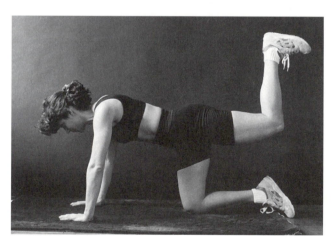

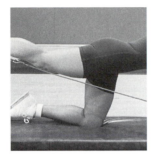

Exercise: Bent-Leg to Straight Kickbacks

DIFFICULTY: 2
LOWER BACK: MODERATE RISK
AREA: BACK (GLUTES, HAMSTRINGS), FRONT (QUADRICEPS)

STARTING POSITION: Get on all fours facing the weight stack, back flat. Attach working leg to the ankle cable attachment.

MOVEMENT: Simultaneously raise and extend the leg (keep a slight bend in the knee) so thigh is parallel to the floor. Bend lower leg back to 90-degree angle and return to even or slightly in front of the unattached leg. Repeat with other leg.

TRAINER'S TIPS:
- Keep motion controlled so you can feel constant tension in the butt.
- Feel your butt tighten as you raise and try to maintain tension through both ranges (back and forward) of motion.
- Overextending or jerky motions can make the exercise potentially dangerous for the lower back.
- You can also perform this exercise with a rubber band, ankle weights, or body weight for resistance.

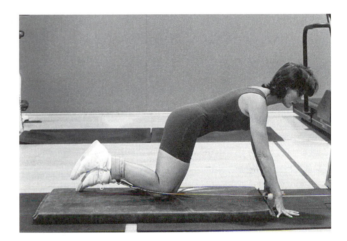

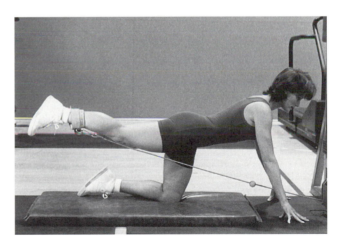

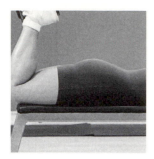

Exercise: Flat Dumbbell Leg Curls

DIFFICULTY: 2
LOWER BACK: MODERATE RISK
AREA: BACK (HAMSTRINGS)

STARTING POSITION: Lie on your stomach (on a bench or on the floor) with both legs straight. If on a bench your knees should be just off the edge. Hold the dumbbell between both feet with your toes pointed (as pictured). Arms are placed comfortably at your sides or underneath your forehead.

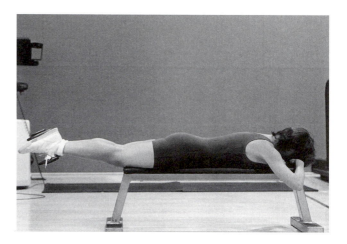

MOVEMENT: Raise your heels toward your butt to a 90-degree angle. Hold for a count and return to starting position under control. Maintain tension by not quite touching the bench or floor on your return to the starting position.

TRAINER'S TIPS:
- Avoid raising your pelvis during the movement.
- Feel your hamstrings tighten as you raise and try to maintain tension through both ranges (back and forward) of motion.
- Keep toes pointed throughout motion.
- Avoid jerky movements.

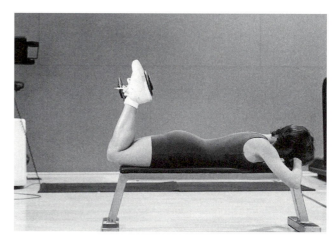

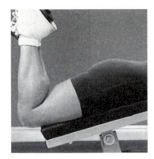

Exercise: Incline Dumbbell Leg Curls

DIFFICULTY: 2
LOWER BACK: MODERATE RISK
AREA: BACK (HAMSTRINGS)

STARTING POSITION: Lie on your stomach, with both legs straight, on a bench elevated at one end. The angle of the bench should be between 30 and 45 degrees. Hold on to top of bench with both hands, securing the dumbbell between feet with your toes pointed.

MOVEMENT: Keeping your pelvis flat, raise your heels toward your butt to a 90-degree angle or past. Hold for a one count and return to starting position. Maintain tension by not quite touching the bench on your return.

TRAINER'S TIPS:
- Maintain tension on your hamstrings throughout the entire range of motion, both the raising and the lowering phase.
- Keep toes pointed throughout motion.
- Avoid jerky motions.
- Focus your mind on your hamstrings throughout the movement.

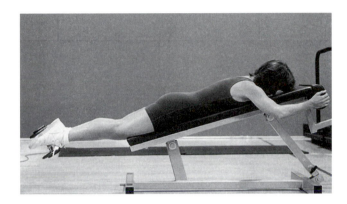

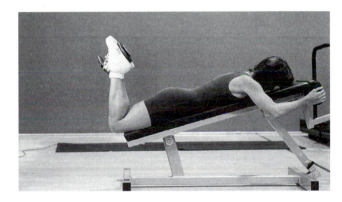

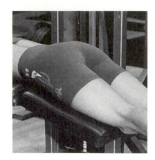

Exercise: Leg Curls

DIFFICULTY: 1
LOWER BACK: MODERATE RISK
AREA: BACK (HAMSTRINGS)

STARTING POSITION: Lie on your stomach on a leg curl machine with the lifting pad located just above the ankles. Knees should be just off the bench.

MOVEMENT: Keeping your pelvis flat, raise your heels toward your butt to a 90-degree angle or past. Hold for a one count and return to starting position. Maintain tension on your hamstring by not allowing plates to touch weight stack at the bottom of the movement.

Variations: Foot position can affect the angle in which you work the hamstrings, emphasizing a particular area. Feet flexed or pointed with toes angled out will emphasize the outer area, while feet flexed or pointed with toes angled in will emphasize the inner area. This exercise can also be performed by raising two legs up, and then one leg down to emphasize the eccentric phase.

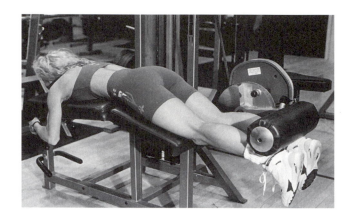

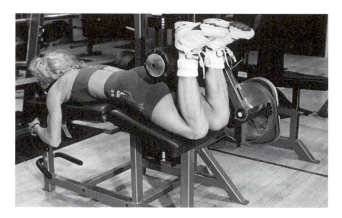

TRAINER'S TIPS:
- Avoid raising your pelvis as you raise your heels.
- Most leg curl machines now have adjustable lifting arms (pads). If you have this variable you should set the lifting arm at the lowest setting without hyperextending your knee.
- Keep knees just off the bench. If your knee is on the bench it can be easily hyperextended.
- Feel your hamstrings tighten as you raise, and try to maintain tension through both motions.
- You can also perform this exercise one leg at a time either by alternating legs or by completing a full set with one leg and then a full set with the other leg.

- This exercise can be performed using ankle weights or a rubber band.
- The newer leg curl machines have an angle built into the bench to relieve pressure on the lower back. If your bench is flat, place a pillow under your pelvis to relieve pressure.
- Avoid jerky motions.

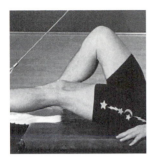

Exercise: Lying Straight-Leg Kickdowns

DIFFICULTY: 1
LOWER BACK: MODERATE RISK
AREA: BACK (GLUTES, HAMSTRINGS)

STARTING POSITION: Lie on your back, head toward weight stack, and hook working leg to ankle cable attachment (which is attached to the high cable pulley). To start, your working leg (slightly bent at the knee) is at a 90-degree angle to the body.

MOVEMENT: Keeping your knee slightly bent throughout the exercise, drive your heel to the ground. Return to starting position under control. Repeat with other leg.

TRAINER'S TIPS:
- On the down motion of this exercise squeeze your butt.
- Getting into the starting position can be somewhat awkward. Therefore it is recommended that you use a light weight.
- Keep motion controlled so you can feel constant tension in the butt.
- Use caution if you have lower back problems. Lack of control on the up motion or jerky motions can make the exercise potentially dangerous.
- Keep lower back pressed against the floor at all times.

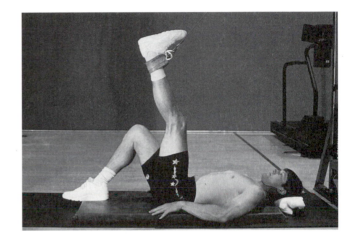

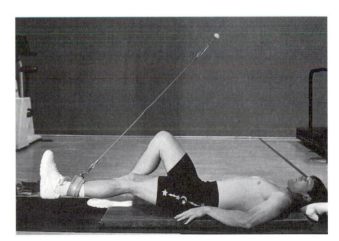

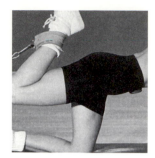

Exercise: Mountain Climber Leg Curls

DIFFICULTY: 2
LOWER BACK: MODERATE RISK
AREA: BACK (HAMSTRINGS, GLUTES)

STARTING POSITION: Get down on all fours, butt toward the weight stack, and hook leg to ankle cable attachment. Your working leg should be extended back and straight out, off the floor and parallel to the ground with other knee resting on the floor. Keep the back flat.

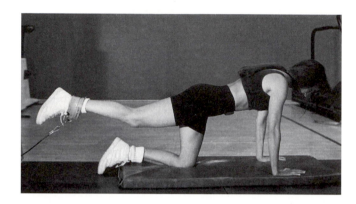

MOVEMENT: Bring your heel as close to your butt as you can without raising or lowering your thigh. Return to starting position. Repeat with other leg when finished.

TRAINER'S TIPS:
- Don't move your upper body, or arch or round your back.
- Keep motion controlled so you can feel constant tension in the butt and hamstrings.
- Focus your mind on your hamstrings throughout the exercise.
- This exercise can be performed with a rubber band, ankle weights, or body weight for resistance.

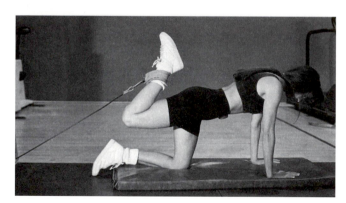

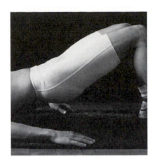

Exercise: Pelvic Lifts

DIFFICULTY: 1
LOWER BACK: LOW RISK
AREA: BACK (GLUTES, HAMSTRINGS)

STARTING POSITION: Lie on your back, knees bent, feet flat, hands at your side, palms down.

MOVEMENT: Lift your pelvis straight up toward the ceiling, squeezing your butt together until your back is straight; do not lift so high your back is arched.

Variation: This exercise can be performed with weights, i.e., Pelvic Lifts (Weighted), by placing a weight on your hips, and moving through the range of motion.

TRAINER'S TIPS:
- Keep motion controlled so you can feel constant tension in the butt.
- Pause at the top of the motion and squeeze the butt together.
- Focus your mind on your butt.

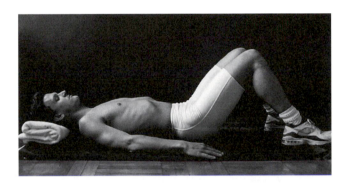

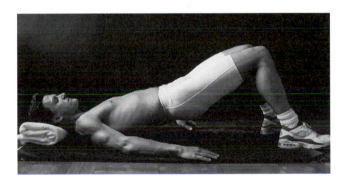

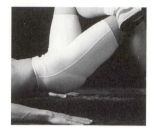

Exercise: Single-Leg Pelvic Lifts

DIFFICULTY: 2
LOWER BACK: LOW RISK
AREA: BACK (GLUTES)

STARTING POSITION: Lie on your back with one knee bent, foot flat on the floor. Your other leg is crossed, ankle resting just above the knee of other leg. Your hands should be at your sides.

Variations: Lie on your back with one leg bent, foot flat on the floor, your leg extended, knee slightly bent. This extended leg can have a variety of foot positions (straight, pointed out, or pointed in).

MOVEMENT: Lift your pelvis straight up toward the ceiling, squeezing your butt together as you lift. Raise your pelvis to a straight back, not beyond.

TRAINER'S TIPS:
- Roll your spine up and down through the motion.
- Control the motion keeping constant tension in the butt.
- Feel your butt squeeze together as you raise. Pause at the top and squeeze the butt together hard.

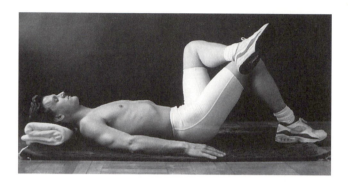

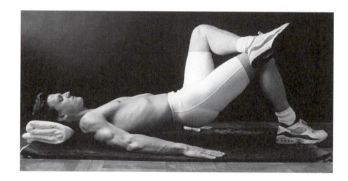

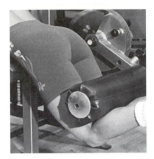

Exercise: Backward Leg Raises

DIFFICULTY: 2
LOWER BACK: MODERATE RISK
AREA: BACK (GLUTES, HAMSTRINGS)

STARTING POSITION: Lie on your stomach on a leg curl machine with the lifting bar located on the back side of your knees. Raise your feet so your lower legs are at a 90-degree angle to your thighs.

MOVEMENT: Keeping your legs bent at a 90-degree angle throughout the exercise, raise your legs until you feel tightness in the butt. Return to starting position without letting the weight plates touch the stack.

TRAINER'S TIPS:
- On the lifting motion of this exercise raise the soles of your feet toward the ceiling.
- Your thighs should be parallel to the ground or below at the top of the motion. Do not lift higher as this will cause the lower back to arch.
- Most leg curl machines now have adjustable lifting arms (pads). If you have this variable you should set the lifting arm at the lowest setting.
- Keep motion controlled so you can feel constant tension in the butt.
- Feel your butt tighten as you raise and try to maintain tension through both ranges (back and forward) of motion.
- Use caution if you have lower back problems. Overlifting or jerky motions can make the exercise potentially dangerous.
- You can also perform this exercise one leg at a time either by alternating legs or by completing a full set with one leg and then a full set with the other leg.
- Make sure to start out using very light weights.
- Focus your mind on the working muscles.

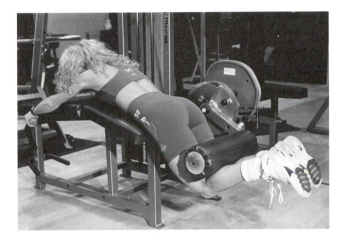

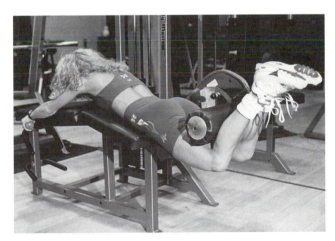

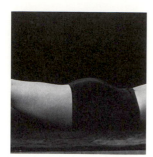

Exercise: Prone Single-Leg Raises

DIFFICULTY: 1
LOWER BACK: MODERATE RISK
AREA: BACK (GLUTES, HAMSTRINGS)

STARTING POSITION: Lie on your stomach with your legs extended, arms overhead, and your forehead flat to the ground.

Variations: (1) Place hands palms up under hips, or (2) fold hands in front and rest forehead on hands.

MOVEMENT: Raise working leg (keeping slightly bent at the knee) until you feel tightness in your butt. Return to starting position. Your leg should remain extended throughout the exercise. Repeat with other leg.

TRAINER'S TIPS:
- Do not raise leg so high that you feel pain in the lower back.
- Keep motion controlled so you can feel constant tension in the butt.
- Squeeze the butt as you raise the leg. Pause at the top and contract for a one count.
- Maintain a stationary position with your upper body throughout the exercise.

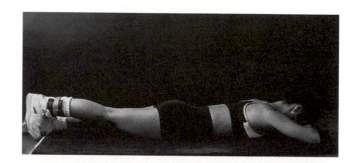

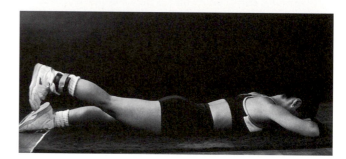

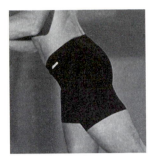

Exercise: Standing Kickbacks

DIFFICULTY: 1
LOWER BACK: MODERATE RISK
AREA: BACK (GLUTES, HAMSTRINGS)

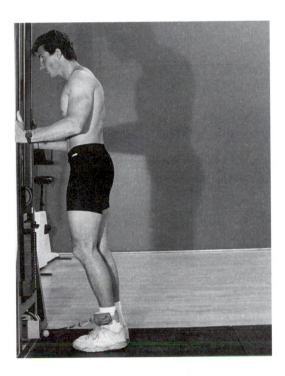

STARTING POSITION: Stand facing weight stack using your hands to hang on for balance (keep your hands away from moving weights). You should be leaning slightly forward with your entire body in alignment (straight). Attach your working leg to the ankle cable attachment.

MOVEMENT: Move your working leg back, keeping the knee slightly bent throughout the motion. Move leg until you feel tightness in butt. Do not overextend the movement and arch your back. The leg should then return even with your stationary leg. Repeat with other leg.

TRAINER'S TIPS:

- Control the movement through both ranges of the motion, squeezing your butt as you move leg back and maintaining tension in your butt as your leg comes forward.
- Focus your mind on the working muscles.
- Maintain the same bend in the knee throughout the entire movement. If you bend and straighten the leg during the exercise, other muscle groups will come into play and make the exercise less effective.
- Kicking or jerky motions make the exercise potentially dangerous for the lower back.
- You can also perform this exercise with a rubber band, ankle weights, or body weight for resistance.

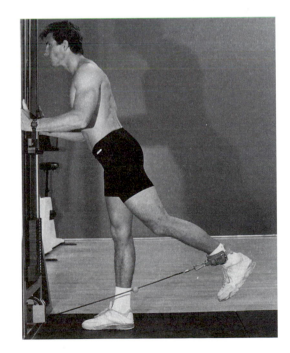

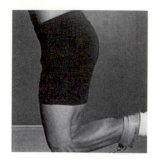

Exercise: Standing Leg Curls

DIFFICULTY: 2
LOWER BACK: LOW RISK
AREA: BACK (HAMSTRINGS)

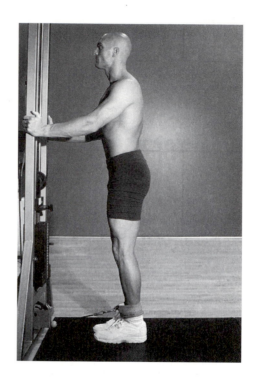

STARTING POSITION: Stand facing the weight stack and attach your leg to the ankle cable attachment. Both knees are slightly bent and the foot is flexed on the working leg. Maintain proper body alignment.

MOVEMENT: Keeping your torso and thigh stationary, raise your heel toward your butt, bending your knee to 90 degrees or more. Hold for a one count and return to starting position, keeping tension on the muscle, not allowing plates to touch weight stack at the bottom of the movement. Repeat with other leg.

TRAINER'S TIPS:

- Avoid jerking or moving your torso. Keep upper body stationary throughout exercise and avoid arching your back.
- Feel your hamstrings tighten as you raise heels, maintaining tension through lowering and raising phases of motion.
- Keep knee of working leg next to stationary leg. Do not let knee move forward or backward.
- Use caution if you have lower back problems. Strict technique will prevent the likelihood of injury.
- There are standing leg curl machines; the technique is the same. This exercise can also be performed with ankle weights, a rubber band, or body weight for resistance.

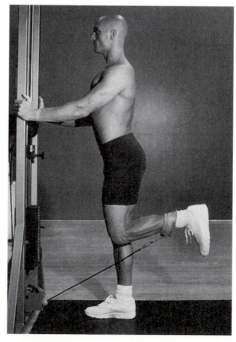

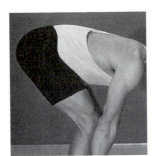

Exercise: Stiff-Leg Dead Lift

DIFFICULTY: 3
LOWER BACK: HIGH RISK
AREA: BACK (GLUTES, HAMSTRINGS)

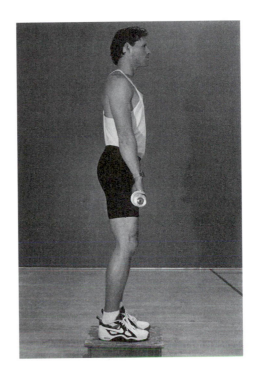

STARTING POSITION: Stand with feet slightly apart and pointed straight ahead (you may stand on a box or bench to allow for a greater range of motion). Your knees should be slightly bent. Hold dumbbells or bar in front.

MOVEMENT: Keeping the dumbbells or bar as close to the body as possible, bend forward at the hip maintaining your flat back and bent knees. Lower resistance until you feel tightness in the hamstrings. Extend back up to starting position.

TRAINER'S TIPS:
- Keep your back straight throughout the exercise.
- Support the movement by contracting your abs.
- Keep knees slightly bent throughout the movement. Whatever bend in your knees that you start with maintain throughout.
- Keep motion controlled and focus on your hamstrings and butt, especially as you extend back up to your starting position.
- Return all the way back to the starting position making sure that your shoulders are slightly rolled back and your chest is out at the top of the motion.
- Feel your butt squeeze together as you raise.
- Do not bounce down; control downward phase of the motion.
- This exercise may be performed without weights.
- If you have a lower back problem approach with extreme care and start out with no weights. Increase your range of motion slowly.

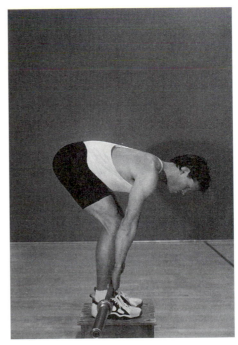

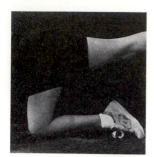

Exercise: Straight-Leg Rotations

DIFFICULTY: 1
LOWER BACK: MODERATE RISK
AREA: BACK (GLUTES), OUTSIDE (ABDUCTORS), INSIDE (ADDUCTORS)

STARTING POSITION: Get on all fours and extend working leg back and parallel to the ground. Your head and neck should be aligned with the spine, head looking straight down.

MOVEMENT: Keeping your working leg straight, make a small circular clockwise motion. Repeat the same number of repetitions counterclockwise. Repeat with other leg.

TRAINER'S TIPS:
- Avoid making too big a circle, keeping circle small to avoid stress on the lower back.
- Keep the rest of your body stationary throughout the exercise.
- Focus on your butt as you circle the leg.
- This exercise can be performed using ankle weights.

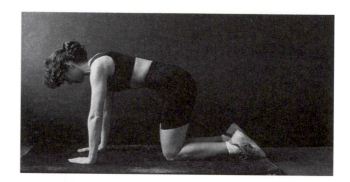

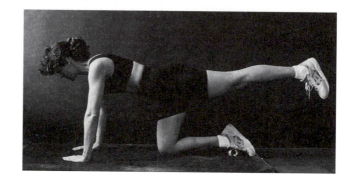

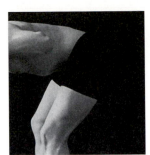

Exercise: Good Mornings

DIFFICULTY: 3
LOWER BACK: HIGH RISK
AREA: BACK (GLUTES, HAMSTRINGS)

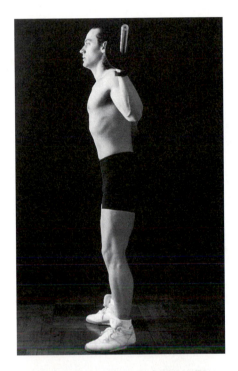

STARTING POSITION: Stand with your feet slightly wider than shoulder width apart, toes slightly turned out. Your knees should be slightly bent, your shoulders back, and your chest out. Hold bar behind neck or place hands behind ears.

MOVEMENT: Bend forward at the hip, keeping your back flat and your knees slightly bent throughout the movement. Bend until your torso is parallel to the ground, maintaining a straight line with your torso, neck, and head (don't allow your chin to drop forward or your shoulders to hunch). Raise torso back up to starting position.

TRAINER'S TIPS:
- Support the movement by contracting your abs throughout the entire range of motion.
- Keep knees slightly bent throughout the exercise. Whatever bend in the knees that you start with maintain throughout.
- Keep motion controlled and focus your mind on your hamstrings and butt, especially as you extend back up to the starting position.
- Return all the way back to the starting position, making sure that your shoulders are slightly rolled back at the top of the motion.
- Squeeze your butt on the way up.
- Do not bounce down or perform the downward phase of the motion out of control.
- This exercise may be performed without weights.

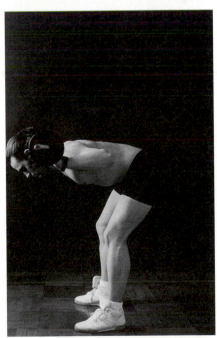

CHAPTER TEN

The Front

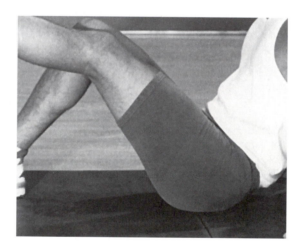

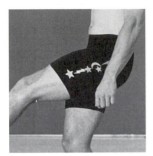

Exercise: Front Kicks

DIFFICULTY: 1
LOWER BACK: LOW RISK
AREA: FRONT (HIP FLEXORS, QUADRICEPS)

STARTING POSITION: Stand with back to weight stack and your working leg attached to an ankle cable strap. Both legs should be slightly flexed at the knee. If support is available in front of you, use your hands to balance; otherwise balance free form.

MOVEMENT: Move the attached leg forward to about a 45-degree angle and return under control to the starting position. Do not allow weights to touch stack. Repeat with other leg when finished.

TRAINER'S TIPS:
- Maintain stationary position with your torso.
- Focus your mind on your thighs and hip flexors, contracting on the forward movement and maintaining the contraction as you return to the starting position.
- Avoid jerky motions.
- Keep working leg slightly bent throughout the movement.
- This exercise can also be performed with a rubber band, ankle weights, or body weight for resistance.

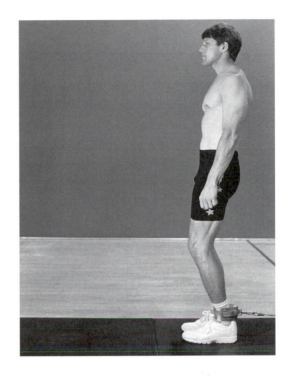

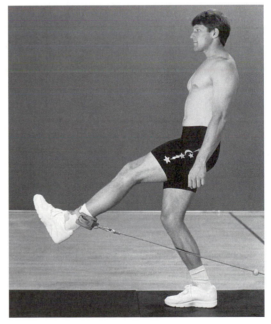

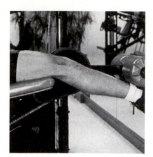

Exercise: Leg Extension

DIFFICULTY: 1
LOWER BACK: LOW RISK
AREA: FRONT (QUADRICEPS)

STARTING POSITION: Sit with ankles behind lifting arm, hands supporting at your sides.

MOVEMENT: With your legs bent at 90 degrees or more, extend both legs up, keeping a slight bend at the top of the movement. Hold for a count and bend back down to the starting position. Do not let the weights touch the stack, keeping constant tension on the muscles.

Variations: Foot positions will affect the angle of the lift, emphasizing the inner or outer area of the thigh. If the foot is flexed back or pointed down, and the hip is rotated out (toes angled out), the emphasis will be on the inner area. If the foot is flexed back or pointed down, and the hip rotated in (toes angled in), the emphasis will be on the outer area. You can also perform this exercise one leg at a time either by alternating legs or by completing a full set with one leg and then a full set with the other leg. An eccentric overload can be accomplished by lifting with two legs and lowering with one.

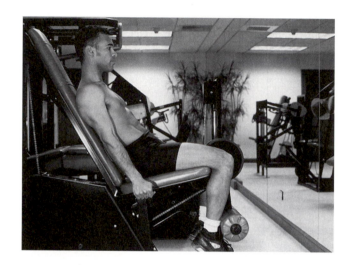

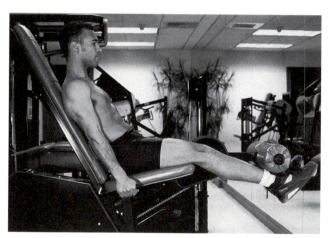

TRAINER'S TIPS:
- Maintain stable position with your torso throughout lift.
- This lift can also be performed off a chair with ankle weights, a rubber band, or body weight for resistance.
- Focus your mind on the working muscles.

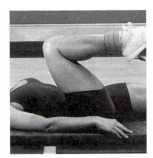

Exercise: Lying Kneebacks

DIFFICULTY: 1
LOWER BACK: LOW RISK
AREA: FRONT (HIP FLEXORS, QUADRICEPS)

STARTING POSITION: Lie on your back with feet toward the weight stack; unattached leg is bent with foot flat on the floor. Working leg is straight and hooked to ankle cable attachment. Hands are at your sides.

MOVEMENT: Bring knee of working leg back toward chest (the knee should come as close to the chest as possible while keeping your lower back pressed against the floor). Return to starting position under control. Repeat with other leg when finished.

TRAINER'S TIPS:
- Maintain stationary position with your torso, never allowing your lower back to lose contact with the ground.
- Focus your mind on your thigh and hip flexors as you bring the knee back toward the chest.
- Maintain the contraction as you return to the starting position.
- Avoid jerky motions.
- This exercise can also be performed with a rubber band, ankle weights, or body weight for resistance.

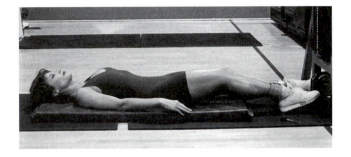

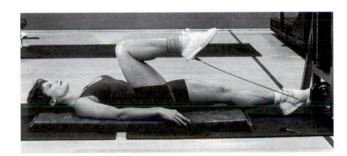

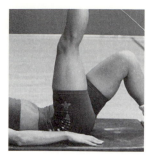

Exercise: Lying Leg Raises

DIFFICULTY: 1
LOWER BACK: LOW RISK
AREA: FRONT (HIP FLEXORS, QUADRICEPS)

STARTING POSITION: Lie on your back on the floor with feet toward weight stack. Unattached leg should be bent with foot flat on the floor. The working leg should be slightly bent at the knee and hooked to ankle cable attachment. Hands are at your sides.

MOVEMENT: Lift the working leg up and back, keeping the knee slightly bent throughout the entire exercise. Lift as high and as far back as possible without allowing the lower back to lose contact with the ground. Return to starting position under control. Repeat with other leg when finished.

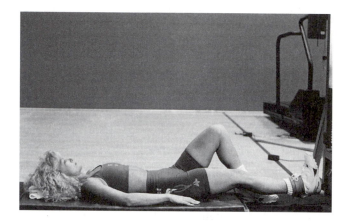

TRAINER'S TIPS:

- Maintain stationary position with your torso.
- Focus your mind on your thighs and hip flexors, contracting as you lift your leg, and try to maintain the contraction as you return to the starting position.
- Avoid jerky motions.
- Keep knee of working leg slightly bent throughout the motion.
- Maintain contact to the ground with your lower back throughout the exercise.
- This exercise can also be performed with a rubber band, ankle weights, or body weight for resistance.

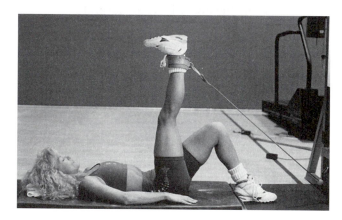

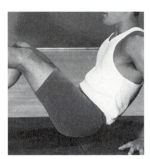

Exercise: Seated Leg Raises

DIFFICULTY: 1
LOWER BACK: MODERATE RISK
AREA: FRONT (HIP FLEXORS, QUADRICEPS)

STARTING POSITION: Sit on ground or bench with feet toward weight stack, working leg (knee slightly bent) attached to ankle cable attachment. The unattached leg should be bent with foot flat on the floor. Lean upper body back at approximately a 45-degree angle, not below, supporting your weight on your hands (placed behind your torso, palms down, and fingers pointing away from body).

MOVEMENT: Lift the attached leg up and back, keeping the knee slightly bent throughout the entire movement. Lift as high and as far back as possible without allowing the upper body to move. Return to starting position under control. Repeat with other leg when finished.

TRAINER'S TIPS:
- Maintain stationary position with your torso.
- Focus your mind on your thighs and hip flexors as you lift your leg.
- Maintain the contraction as you return to the starting position.
- Avoid jerky motions.
- This lift is potentially dangerous for the lower back if you do not maintain a stationary position with torso. It is also important to maintain support (keeping abs tight) throughout the exercise.
- This exercise can also be performed with a rubber band and with ankle weights.

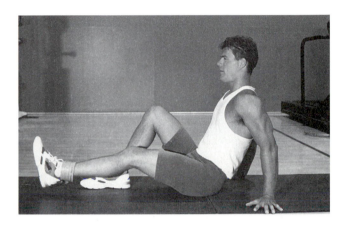

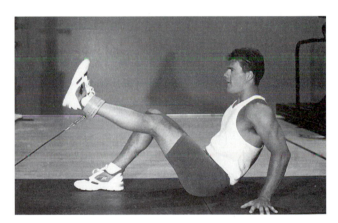

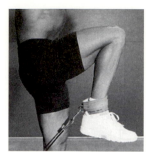

Exercise: Standing Knee-Ups

DIFFICULTY: 1
LOWER BACK: LOW RISK
AREA: FRONT (HIP FLEXORS, QUADRICEPS)

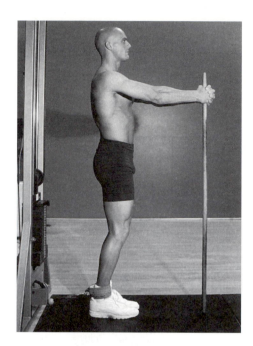

STARTING POSITION: Stand with back to weight stack and secure one leg to ankle cable attachment. Both legs should be slightly flexed at the knee. If support is available in front of you, use your hands to balance; otherwise you must balance free form.

MOVEMENT: Lift the attached knee up toward the chest, bending your leg as you lift, until the quad is parallel or higher to the ground. Return to starting position under control.

TRAINER'S TIPS:
- Maintain stationary position with your torso.
- Focus your mind on your hip flexors as you lift toward your chest, maintaining the contraction as you return to the starting position.
- Avoid jerky motions.
- This exercise can also be performed with a rubber band and ankle weights.

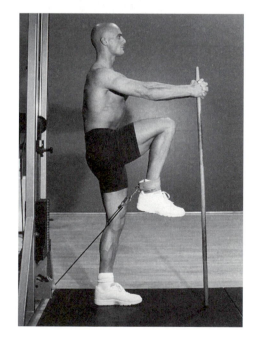

CHAPTER ELEVEN

The Inside

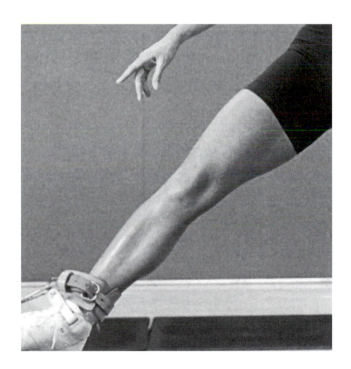

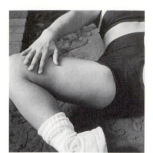

Exercise: Butterfly Inside Raises

DIFFICULTY: 1
LOWER BACK: LOW RISK
AREA: INSIDE (ADDUCTORS, QUADRICEPS)

STARTING POSITION: Lie on your back, one leg bent, foot flat on the floor, the other leg bent and dropped toward the floor (rotating hip out), with the sole of the foot (of the working leg) facing the inside of the other foot. Place your hand on the inside of the dropped knee for resistance.

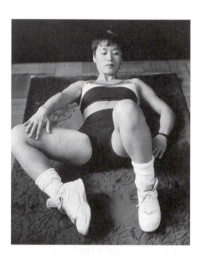

MOVEMENT: Keeping your legs bent raise the dropped knee toward your other knee, using your hand for resistance. Raise knee of the down leg up toward other leg, rotating hip in. Return to starting position. Repeat with other leg when finished.

TRAINER'S TIPS:
- Keep both legs bent throughout the motion.
- Use your hand to provide as much resistance as needed to make the dropped knee work.
- Keep lower back pressed to the ground.
- Focus your mind on the inner thigh.

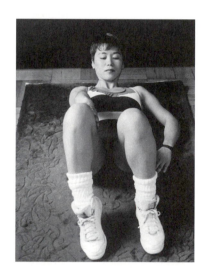

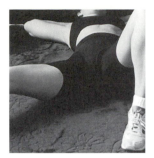

Exercise: Lying Adductions

DIFFICULTY: 1
LOWER BACK: LOW RISK
AREA: INSIDE (ADDUCTORS, QUADRICEPS)

STARTING POSITION: Lie on your back. Your working leg is extended out (slightly bent in the knee) and stretched away from other leg. Bend your non-working leg so your foot is flat to the floor. Flex the foot in the working leg and rotate it out.

MOVEMENT: Pull the working leg in and up until it is even with other leg. Return to starting position. Repeat with other leg when finished.

TRAINER'S TIPS:
• Keep lower back flat to the floor.
• Keep foot flexed and leg rotated out throughout the exercise.
• Focus your mind on the inner part of the thigh while raising.
• Control the return to the starting position.
• You may also perform this exercise using a rubber band, ankle weights, cable attachment, or body weight for resistance.

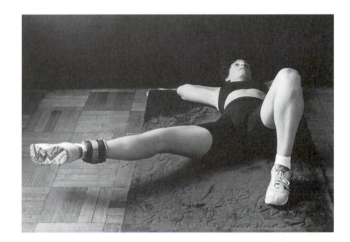

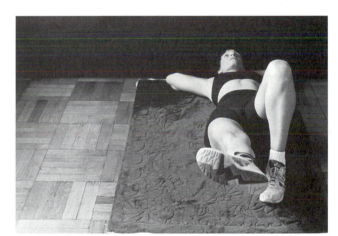

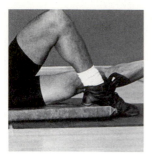

Exercise: Lying Inside Raises

DIFFICULTY: 1
LOWER BACK: LOW RISK
AREA: INSIDE (ADDUCTORS, QUADRICEPS)

STARTING POSITION: Lie on side supporting your head with your hand. Place your other hand in front of chest, palm down, for added stability. Bend your top leg and place it in front of your other leg so your foot is flat on the floor. Your bottom leg is straight (slightly bent at the knee), inner thigh is toward the ceiling, and the foot is flexed.

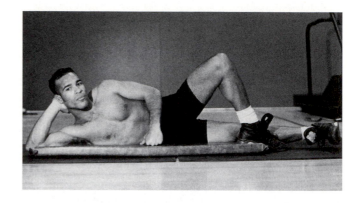

MOVEMENT: Raise bottom leg toward the ceiling as high as possible without moving the rest of your body. Return to starting position without touching the floor with your foot. Repeat with other leg when finished.

Variation: You can employ hand resistance, i.e., Lying Inside Raises (Hand Resistance), by pushing against the inner thigh (with hand) throughout range of motion.

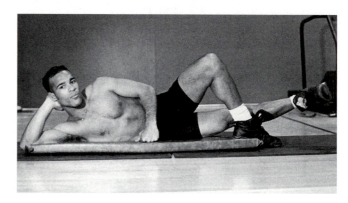

TRAINER'S TIPS:
- Keep your body stationary except for the bottom leg.
- Pause at top for a count.
- Focus on the inner part of the thigh while raising and lowering.
- Control both the raising and lowering of the leg.
- You may also perform this exercise using a rubber band, ankle weights, cable attachment, or body weight for resistance.

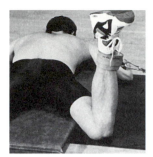

Exercise: Prone Adductions

DIFFICULTY: 2
LOWER BACK: MODERATE RISK
AREA: INSIDE (ADDUCTORS)

STARTING POSITION: Lie on stomach, side to weight stack with working leg (hooked to ankle cable attachment) nearest to the stack. The working leg should be bent at a 90-degree angle, and the foot flexed. The unattached leg can be either bent or straight. The feet should be at least shoulder width apart. Arms are extended forward and face is down.

MOVEMENT: Keeping your attached leg bent, drag it across floor to the unattached leg. Return to starting position without touching the weights to the stack. Repeat with other leg when finished.

TRAINER'S TIPS:
- Keep body flat and stationary. The only body part moving is the attached leg.
- Keep attached leg bent and foot flexed throughout the exercise.
- Focus your mind on the inner part of the thigh while pulling.
- Control the return to the starting position; don't let the cable pull leg back.
- You may also perform this exercise using a rubber band, ankle weights, or body weight for resistance.
- This has potential to bother the lower back. Don't arch back or perform jerky motions.

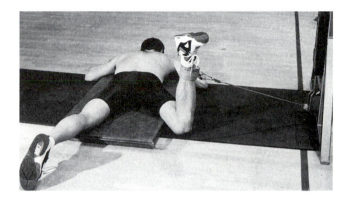

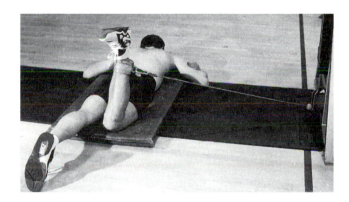

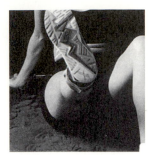

Exercise: Seated Inside Raises

DIFFICULTY: 1
LOWER BACK: LOW RISK
AREA: INSIDE (ADDUCTORS, QUADRICEPS)

STARTING POSITION: Sit with your nonworking leg bent and your foot flat to the floor. Your working leg is extended straight (slightly bent at the knee), with the foot flexed and the hip rotated out (toes pointed out). Lean your upper torso back, supporting your weight on both elbows.

MOVEMENT: Pull the working leg in and up at an angle toward the top of your nonworking bent knee. Return to starting position without touching the ground (keep it about an inch above the ground). Repeat with other leg when finished.

TRAINER'S TIPS:
- Keep body square. The only body part in movement is the leg being raised.
- Keep attached leg and foot flexed into position throughout the movement.
- Hold at top for a one count.
- Focus your mind on the inner part of the thigh while raising.
- Control the lowering of the leg; don't let the cable pull it back.
- You may also perform this exercise using a rubber band, ankle weights, cable attachment, or body weight for resistance.

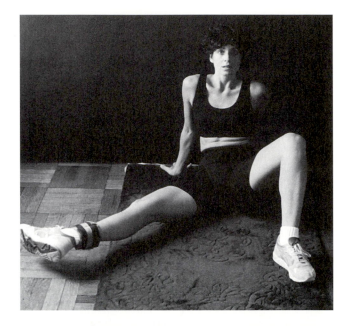

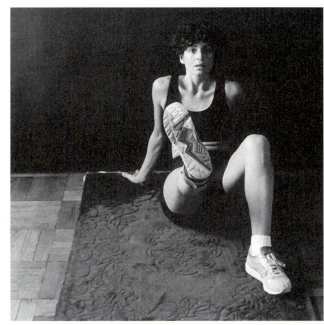

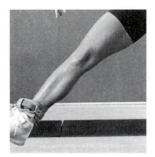

Exercise: Standing Adductions

DIFFICULTY: 1
LOWER BACK: LOW RISK
AREA: INSIDE (ADDUCTORS)

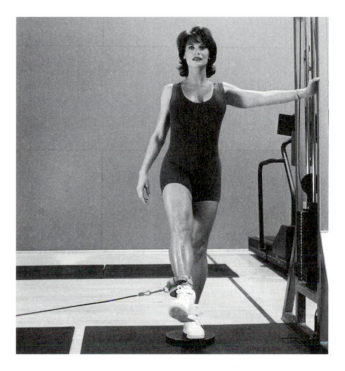

STARTING POSITION: Stand side to weight stack with working leg (hooked to ankle cable attachment) nearest to weight stack. The working leg should be straight (slightly bent at the knee) with the foot flexed and the hip rotated out (toes pointed out). Your unattached leg should also be slightly bent. Your legs should be far enough apart to allow for an approximately two-foot range of motion.

MOVEMENT: Pull the working leg even with the unattached leg. Return to starting position without letting the weights touch the stack. Repeat with other leg when finished.

TRAINER'S TIPS:
- Keep body square. The only body part to move is the working leg.
- Maintain leg and foot position throughout the exercise.
- Focus your mind on the inner part of the thigh while pulling.
- Control the return to the starting position; don't let the cable pull you back.
- You may also perform this exercise using a rubber band, ankle weights, or body weight for resistance.

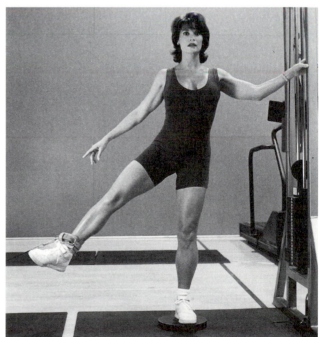

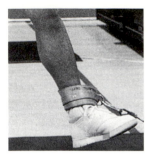

Exercise: Standing Inside Crosses

DIFFICULTY: 1
LOWER BACK: LOW RISK
AREA: INSIDE (ADDUCTORS)

STARTING POSITION: Stand holding on to a rail or bar for support. Place feet a little wider than shoulder width apart, with the working leg slightly bent and your foot flexed.

MOVEMENT: Raise working leg up and to the inside across the front of your planted leg. Return to starting position. Repeat with other leg when finished.

TRAINER'S TIPS:
- Keep body square. The only body part in movement is the working leg.
- Pause at top for a one count.
- Focus your mind on the inner part of the thigh while raising.
- Control both the raising and lowering of the leg.
- You may also perform this exercise using a rubber band or ankle weights for resistance.

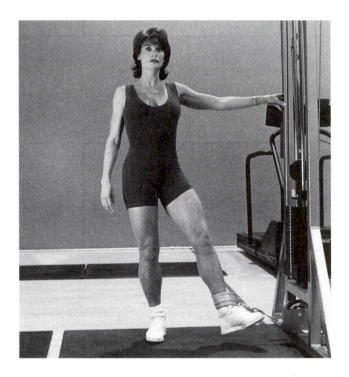

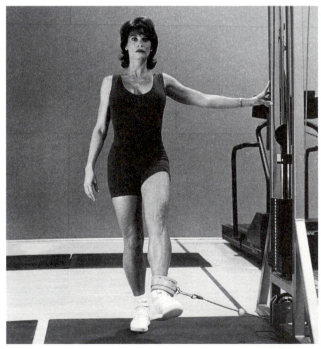

The Outside

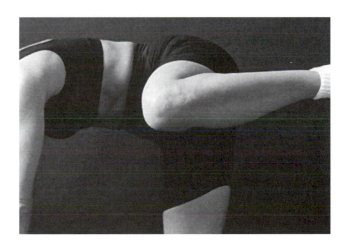

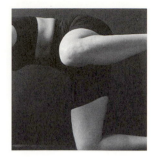

Exercise: Kneeling Side Leg Raises

DIFFICULTY: 1
LOWER BACK: LOW RISK
AREA: OUTSIDE (ABDUCTORS, GLUTES)

STARTING POSITION: Get on all fours.

MOVEMENT: Keeping your working leg bent at a 90-degree angle, raise it to the side, parallel to the ground or as high as possible without twisting your upper torso. Return to starting position. Repeat with other leg when finished.

TRAINER'S TIPS:
- Control your return to the starting position.
- Focus your mind on the outer part of the hip throughout the exercise.
- Keep head straight so that spine is aligned.
- Keep back flat.
- You may also perform this exercise using a rubber band, ankle weights, cable attachment, or body weight for resistance.

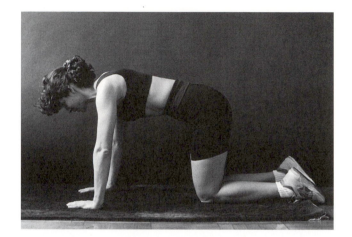

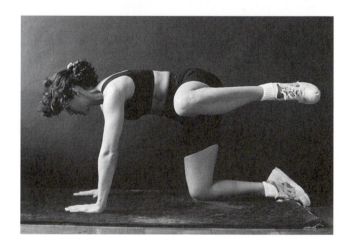

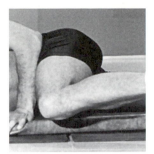

Exercise: Lying Bent-Leg Side Raises

DIFFICULTY: 1
LOWER BACK: LOW RISK
AREA: OUTSIDE (ABDUCTORS, GLUTES)

STARTING POSITION: Lie on your side with bottom leg straight, top leg perpendicular to the body, knee bent at 90 degrees, and hip rotated inward (foot pointed in). Support your head with your bottom hand and stabilize your body by placing other hand palm down in front of your chest.

MOVEMENT: Keeping your top leg perpendicular to the body throughout the exercise, raise leg up as high as you can without twisting the torso or compromising your foot position (maintain inward rotation). Return to starting position. Repeat with other leg when finished.

TRAINER'S TIPS:
- Keep top knee bent and rotated in throughout the motion.
- Maintain flexed foot position throughout the exercise.
- Maintain static upper body throughout exercise; no twisting.
- Control your return to the starting position.
- Focus your mind on the outer part of the hip throughout the exercise.
- You may use a rubber band, ankle weights, or cable attachment for added resistance.

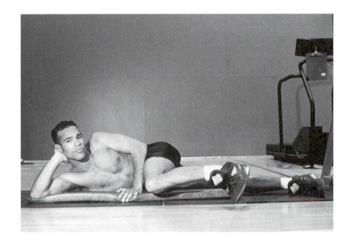

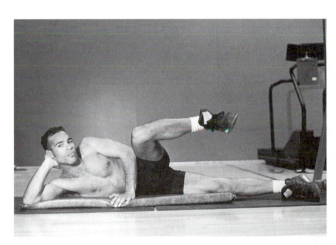

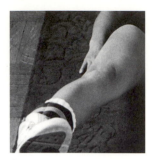

Exercise: Lying Abductions

DIFFICULTY: 2
LOWER BACK: LOW RISK
AREA: OUTSIDE (ABDUCTORS, GLUTES)

STARTING POSITION: Lie on your back. Your nonworking leg is slightly bent and your lower back should be pressed flat to the floor. Your working leg is straight (knee slightly bent) and raised perpendicular to your upper body. Your foot is flexed and pointed in so that your hip is rotated inward.

MOVEMENT: Pull directly to the side as far as you can without twisting or moving your torso. Return to vertical starting position. Repeat with other leg when finished.

TRAINER'S TIPS:
- Maintain foot position throughout exercise.
- Maintain static upper body throughout exercise; no twisting or rocking.
- Control your return to the starting position.
- Focus your mind on the outer part of the hip throughout the exercise.
- Keep your lower back pressed flat to the ground throughout the movement.
- You may also perform this exercise using a rubber band, ankle weights, cable attachment, or body weight for resistance.

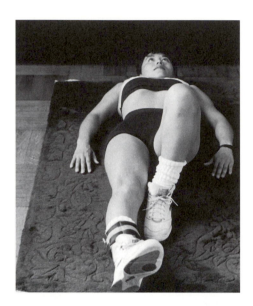

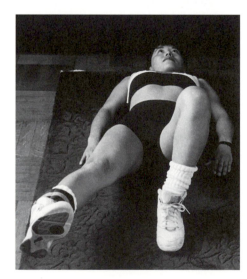

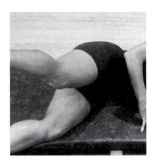

Exercise: Lying Straight-Leg Side Raises

DIFFICULTY: 1
LOWER BACK: LOW RISK
AREA: OUTSIDE (ABDUCTORS, GLUTES)

STARTING POSITION: Lie on side with legs together and forward from the upper torso (about 30 degrees) and knees slightly bent. The foot of the top leg should have the toe pointed down so the hip is rotated in. Support your head with your bottom hand and stabilize your body by placing your other hand in front of your chest with the palm down.

MOVEMENT: Keeping your top leg rotated in (toe in) and your foot flexed, raise the top leg as high as you can without moving the torso or losing your inward rotation. Return to starting position. Repeat with other leg when finished.

TRAINER'S TIPS:
- Keep top leg rotated in throughout motion.
- Maintain foot position throughout exercise.
- Maintain stable upper body throughout exercise.
- Control your return to the starting position.
- Focus your mind on the outer part of the hip throughout the exercise.
- You may use a rubber band for resistance by attaching to both legs, or an ankle weight on the working leg for resistance.

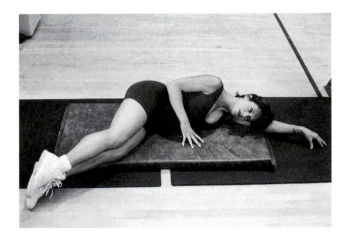

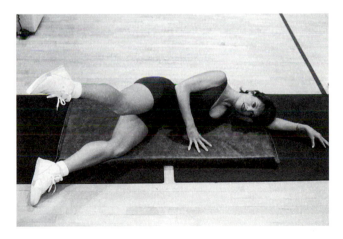

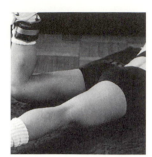

Exercise: Prone Abductions

DIFFICULTY: 1
LOWER BACK: MODERATE RISK
AREA: OUTSIDE (ABDUCTORS, GLUTES)

STARTING POSITION: Lie on stomach, nonworking leg is extended straight, head is face down. Your working leg is bent 90 degrees, foot flexed.

MOVEMENT: Keeping your working leg bent throughout the exercise, pull it to the side as far as you can without twisting or moving your upper body. Return to starting position. Repeat with other leg when finished.

TRAINER'S TIPS:
- Keep leg bent throughout the motion.
- Maintain foot position throughout exercise.
- Maintain stable torso throughout exercise; no twisting or rocking.
- Control your return to the starting position.
- Focus your mind on the outer part of the hip throughout the exercise.
- Keep head straight so as not to twist spine.
- Lie flat; do not elevate yourself on your elbows as this will place the lower back in an undesirable position.
- You may also perform this exercise using a rubber band, ankle weights, cable attachment, or body weight for resistance.

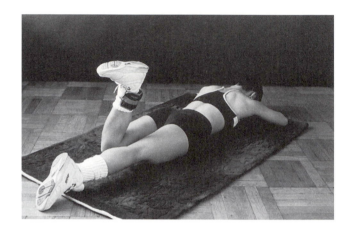

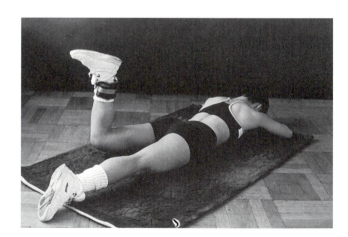

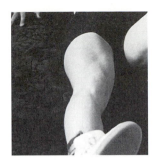

Exercise: Seated Abductions

DIFFICULTY: 1
LOWER BACK: LOW RISK
AREA: OUTSIDE (ABDUCTORS, GLUTES)

STARTING POSITION: In seated position, working leg is extended in front with knee slightly bent and foot flexed. The nonworking leg is bent with the foot flat on the floor.

MOVEMENT: Keeping your knee slightly bent and your foot flexed, pull the working leg to the side as far as you can without moving the torso. Return to starting position. Repeat with other leg when finished.

TRAINER'S TIPS:
- Keep leg slightly flexed throughout the motion.
- Maintain foot position throughout exercise.
- Maintain static upper torso throughout exercise—no swinging or rocking.
- Control your return to the starting position.
- Focus your mind on the outer part of the hip throughout the exercise.
- You may also perform this exercise using a rubber band, ankle weights, cable attachment, or body weight for resistance.

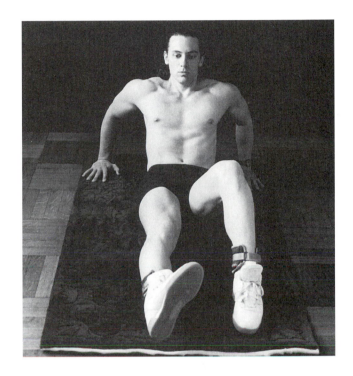

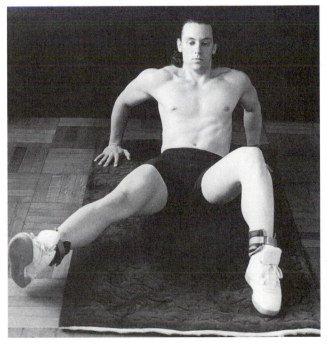

Exercise: Seated Outside Raises

DIFFICULTY: 1
LOWER BACK: LOW RISK
AREA: OUTSIDE (ABDUCTORS, GLUTES)

STARTING POSITION: Sit on floor, side to the weight stack, and bend the leg closest to the weight stack so your foot is flat on the floor. Your other leg is straight (knee slightly bent) with the hip rotated in (toe pointed in) and hooked to the ankle cable attachment. Lean back and support yourself with your elbows on the floor.

MOVEMENT: Raise the attached leg up and out at about a 20- to 30-degree angle. Raise as high and as far out as you can without twisting your torso. Return to starting position without touching the floor or the weights to the stack (lower to within about one inch of the floor). Repeat with other leg when finished.

TRAINER'S TIPS:
- Keep leg slightly rotated in throughout the motion.
- Maintain foot position throughout exercise.
- Maintain stable upper body throughout exercise—no twisting or rocking.
- Control your return to the starting position; don't let the cable pull you back.
- Focus your mind on the outer part of the hip throughout the exercise.
- This exercise may be performed as a floor exercise with no attachments. Rubber bands or ankle weights may be used for resistance if desired.

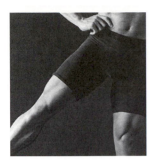

Exercise: Standing Abductions

DIFFICULTY: 1
LOWER BACK: LOW RISK
AREA: OUTSIDE (ABDUCTORS, GLUTES)

STARTING POSITION: Standing, holding on to a pole or wall for balance; both knees are slightly bent.

MOVEMENT: Keeping your legs slightly flexed and your foot flexed on working leg, pull working leg straight to the side. Pull as far as you can without moving the upper torso and return to starting position. Repeat with other leg when finished.

TRAINER'S TIPS:
- Maintain foot position throughout exercise.
- Maintain static upper torso throughout exercise— no swinging or rocking.
- Control your return to the starting position.
- Focus your mind on the outer part of the hip throughout the movement.
- You may also perform this exercise using a rubber band, ankle weight, cable attachment, or body weight for resistance.

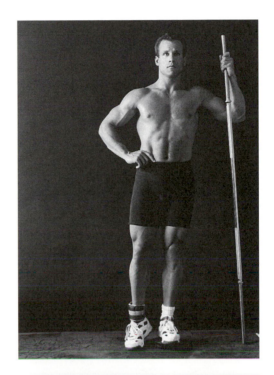

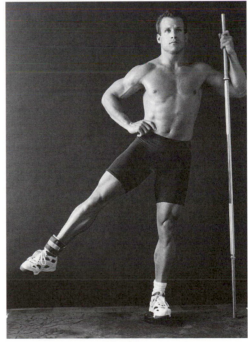

CHAPTER THIRTEEN

The Combination Exercises

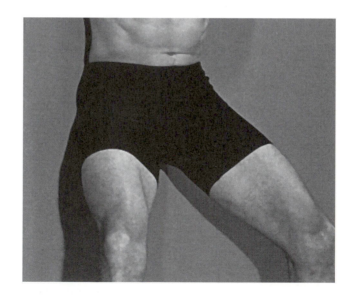

The Squat

Many people are afraid to perform the squat. This fear may arise due to a lack of information. People fear the squat basically for three reasons: (1) they think it is a difficult exercise to perform correctly; (2) it "hurts"; and (3) they have misconceptions about injury.

The squat is a very important exercise, and we hope to alleviate your fears. The benefits of squatting are substantial:

1. It improves overall performance.
2. It enhances self-esteem.
3. It reduces potential for injury.

This book provides you with an innovative way to learn the squat. Many of you will be able to perform the squat easily, and some of you won't. No worries. For those who are having, or have had, trouble squatting we suggest learning how to squat by performing the front squat. The front squat gives you several real advantages in learning how to squat in general:

1. It teaches you proper balance distribution and better kinesthetic awareness.
2. It increases hip and lower leg flexibility.
3. It teaches proper back alignment.

The front squat allows you almost no alternative but to perform the exercise correctly.

When learning the front squat, refer to the techniques on learning the squat (page 164). The techniques here are basically the same. The only difference is the two alternatives to "racking" the bar (placing the bar in a safe and operative position) while performing the front squat.

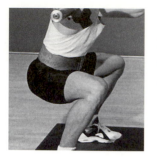

Exercise: Front Squat

DIFFICULTY: 3
LOWER BACK: HIGH RISK
AREA: BACK (HIP EXTENSORS),
FRONT (KNEE EXTENSORS),
ERECTOR SPINAE

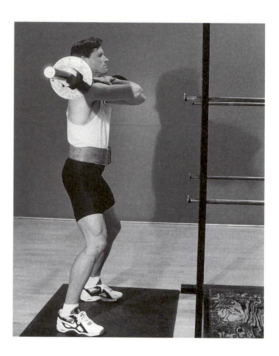

STARTING POSITION: Place barbell on a power rack or squat rack at midchest height. Facing rack, place hands evenly spaced from the center of the bar, slightly wider than shoulder width. Walk to bar placing the bar at the top of the chest. Move shoulders in front of the bar and secure bar with preferred choice of "racking" the bar (placing the bar in a safe and operative position) while performing this exercise. Rest bar on shoulders. Extending hips and legs, lift bar and back out of the rack one step. Prepare to squat by first setting your lower body: feet should be comfortably apart (shoulder width or wider in most cases), toes pointed slightly out, and weight distributed from the balls of the feet to the heel. Next, set the torso with proper exercise alignment (chest out, shoulders back, lower back straight, with a slight forward lean). Head should be aligned with spine, eyes focused straight ahead.

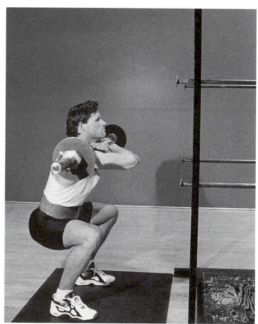

MOVEMENT: To begin the movement you need to take a deep breath and hold. Descend in a controlled manner until the tops of your thighs are parallel to the ground. As you descend, keep shins as close to perpendicular to the floor as possible; don't let your knees come out over your toes. Once bottom position is reached begin the ascent. During the ascent roll the hips slightly forward, while contracting the abdominals. The ascent should be powerful. Do not let hips shoot backwards at the beginning of the ascent, make sure heels are flat, and do not allow knees to go in front of the toes. As the movement reaches the top, exhale, decrease speed, and do not lock knees out.

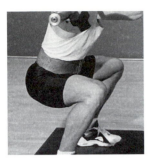

Spotting: For the front squat we recommend three spotters: one on each end of the bar, and an additional spotter in front to help pick up the elbows.

TRAINER'S TIPS:
- Bar should rest behind the front muscle of the shoulder (anterior deltoid) with either racking technique.
- Elbows should be elevated.
- Weight should be distributed from the balls of the feet back to the heels.
- Weight should be reduced when performing the front squat.
- Focus eyes straight ahead.

- During the descent the velocity of the descent should be slow and controlled (three count).
- During descent sit back on heels similar to sitting in a chair.
- No bouncing should occur at the bottom of the movement.
- The bar should travel down in a vertical path.
- Keep heels flat.
- Avoid exaggerated trunk lean.
- Do not allow hips to move backwards during the ascent.
- Focus on working muscles.
- Keep knees and toes in alignment.
- Always back out of rack, never back into the rack (when replacing the bar).

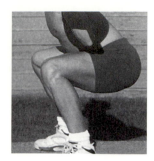

Exercise: Squat

DIFFICULTY: 3
LOWER BACK: HIGH RISK
AREA: BACK (HIP EXTENSORS); FRONT (KNEE EXTENSORS)

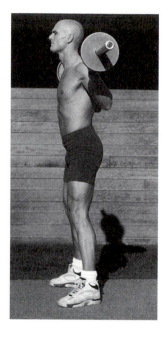 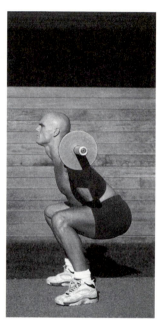

STARTING POSITION: Place barbell on a power rack or squat rack at midchest height. Facing rack, place hands evenly spaced from the center of the bar, slightly wider than shoulder width. Walk underneath the bar. Rest bar behind the neck. Extending hips and legs, while keeping torso erect, lift bar and back out of the rack one step. Prepare to squat by first setting your lower body: feet comfortably apart (shoulder width or wider in most cases), toes pointed slightly out, and weight distributed from the balls of the feet to the heel. Next, set the torso with proper exercise alignment (chest out, shoulders back, lower back straight, with a slight forward lean). Your head should be aligned with your spine, eyes focused straight ahead.

MOVEMENT: To begin the movement you need to take a deep breath and hold. Descend in a controlled manner until the tops of your thighs are parallel to the ground. As you descend, keep shins as close to perpendicular to the floor as possible; don't let your knees come out over your toes. Once bottom position is reached begin the ascent. During the ascent roll the hips slightly forward, while contracting the abdominals. The ascent should be powerful; do not let hips shoot backwards at the beginning of the ascent; make sure heels are flat; do not allow knees to go in front of the toes. As the movement reaches the top, exhale, decrease speed, do not lock knees out.

Variation: A one-quarter squat, half squat, and three-quarter squat can all be performed by varying depth of descent accordingly. The squat can also be performed using dumbbells (see Dumbbell Wide Squat, page 167).

TRAINER'S TIPS:
- Focus eyes straight ahead.
- During the descent the velocity of the descent should be slow and controlled (three count).
- During descent sit back on heels similar to sitting in a chair.
- No bouncing should occur at the bottom of the movement.
- The bar should travel down in a vertical path.
- Keep heels flat.
- Avoid exaggerated trunk lean.
- Do not allow hips to move backwards during the ascent.
- Focus on working muscles.
- Keep knees and toes in alignment.
- Always back out of rack, never back into the rack (when replacing the bar).

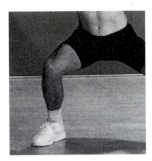

Exercise: Side Squat (Alternating)

DIFFICULTY: 3
LOWER BACK: MODERATE TO HIGH RISK
AREA: BACK (HIP EXTENSORS),
      FRONT (KNEE EXTENSORS),
      OUTSIDE (ABDUCTORS)

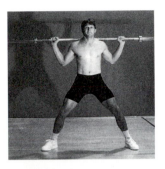

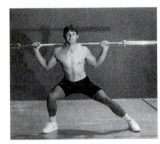

STARTING POSITION: Grasp two dumbbells, bring them to shoulder height and width, palms facing out. Or place barbell on a power rack or squat rack at mid-chest height. Facing rack, place hands evenly spaced from the center of the bar, slightly wider than shoulder width. Walk underneath the bar. Rest bar behind the neck. Extending hips and legs, while keeping torso erect, lift bar and back out of the rack one step. Prepare to squat by first setting your lower body: feet comfortably apart (shoulder width or wider in most cases), toes pointed slightly out, and weight distributed from the balls of the feet to the heel. Next, set the torso with proper exercise alignment (chest out, shoulders back, lower back straight, with a slight forward lean). Head is aligned with spine; eyes are focused straight ahead.

MOVEMENT: To begin the movement you need to take a deep breath and hold. Descend bending the right knee until top of the thigh is parallel to the ground; keep the left leg extended. Distribute weight over the right leg. During the descent sit back on the right leg, distributing the weight on the foot from the ball of the foot backwards; do not allow the knee to go over the foot. Hold for one count. Once bottom position is reached, begin the ascent. During the ascent roll the hips slightly forward while contracting the abdominals. The ascent should be powerful; do not let hips shoot backwards at the beginning of the ascent. Make sure heels are flat; do not allow knees to go in front of the toes. As the movement reaches the top, exhale, decrease speed, and do not lock knees out. Perform same movement with opposite leg.

Variations: This exercise can be performed using multiple repetitions on a single leg, or various dumbbell or barbell positions.

TRAINER'S TIPS:
- Keep torso forward.
- Do not lock out knee at the top of the movement.
- Focus eyes straight ahead.
- During the descent the velocity of the descent should be slow and controlled (three count).
- No bouncing should occur at the bottom of the movement.
- Keep heels flat.
- Avoid exaggerated trunk lean.
- Do not allow hips to move backwards during the ascent.
- Focus on working muscles.
- Keep knees and toes in alignment.
- Always back out of rack, never back into the rack (when replacing the bar).

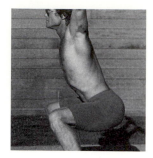

Exercise: Overhead Squat

DIFFICULTY: 3 PLUS
LOWER BACK: HIGH RISK
AREA: BACK (HIP EXTENSORS),
FRONT (KNEE EXTENSORS),
SHOULDERS, TRICEPS

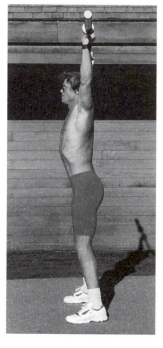
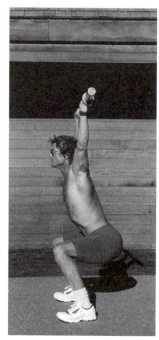

STARTING POSITION: Place bar on power rack slightly above the top of the head. Facing rack, place hands evenly spaced from the center of the bar, slightly wider than shoulder width. Walk underneath the bar. Extend bar overhead, locking elbows. Carry the bar over the back (posterior) part of the head. Back out of the rack one step. Prepare to squat by first setting your lower body: feet comfortably apart (shoulder width or wider in most cases), toes pointed slightly out, and weight distributed from the balls of the feet to the heel. Next, set the torso with proper exercise alignment (chest out, shoulders back, lower back straight, with a slight forward lean). Head is aligned with spine; eyes are focused straight ahead.

MOVEMENT: To begin the movement you need to take a deep breath and hold. Descend in a controlled manner until the tops of your thighs are parallel to the ground. As you descend, keep shins as close to perpendicular to the floor as possible; don't let your knees come out over your toes. Once bottom position is reached begin the ascent. During the ascent roll the hips slightly forward while contracting the abdominals. The ascent should be powerful; do not let hips shoot backwards at the beginning of the ascent, make sure heels are flat, and do not allow knees to go in front of the toes. As the movement reaches the top, exhale, decrease speed, and do not lock knees out.

Variation: Can be performed with dumbbells held over head.

TRAINER'S TIPS:
- Keep elbows locked, bar slightly behind head.
- Focus eyes straight ahead.
- During the descent the velocity of the descent should be slow and controlled (three count).
- During descent sit back on heels similar to sitting in a chair.
- No bouncing should occur at the bottom of the movement.
- The bar should travel down in a vertical path.
- Keep heels flat.
- Avoid exaggerated trunk lean.
- Do not allow hips to move backwards during the ascent.
- Focus on working muscles.
- Keep knees and toes in alignment.
- When replacing the bar, always back out of rack; never back into the rack.

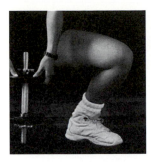

Exercise: Dumbbell Wide Squat

DIFFICULTY: 2
LOWER BACK: MODERATE RISK
AREA: BACK (HIP EXTENSORS), FRONT (KNEE EXTENSORS)

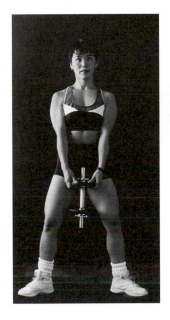 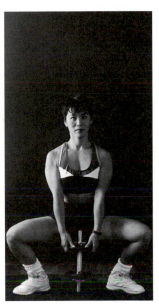

STARTING POSITION: Grasp a dumbbell by the end, arms hanging down, fully extended. Prepare to squat by first setting your lower body: feet wider than shoulder width apart, toes pointed slightly out, and weight distributed from the balls of the feet to the heel. Next, set the torso with proper exercise alignment (chest out, shoulders back, lower back straight with a slight forward lean). Head is aligned with spine; eyes are focused straight ahead.

MOVEMENT: To begin the movement you need to take a deep breath and hold. Descend in a controlled manner until the tops of your thighs are parallel to the ground. As you descend, keep shins as close to perpendicular to the floor as possible; don't let your knees come out over your toes. Once bottom position is reached begin the ascent. During the ascent roll the hips slightly forward while contracting the abdominals. The ascent should be powerful; do not let hips shoot backwards at the beginning of the ascent, make sure heels are flat, and do not allow knees to go in front of the toes. As the movement reaches the top, exhale, decrease speed, and do not lock knees out.

Variation: This exercise can be varied by widening the distance between the feet.

TRAINER'S TIPS:
- Allow dumbbell to travel between the knees.
- Push up from bottom position; concentrate on taking chest up to the ceiling.
- Focus eyes straight ahead.

- During the descent the velocity of the descent should be slow and controlled (three count).
- During descent sit back on heels similar to sitting in a chair.
- No bouncing should occur at the bottom of the movement.
- The dumbbell should travel down in a vertical path.
- Keep heels flat.
- Avoid exaggerated trunk lean.
- Do not allow hips to move backwards during the ascent.
- Focus on working muscles.
- Keep knees and toes in alignment.

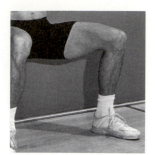

Exercise: Wall Squat

DIFFICULTY: 3
LOWER BACK: MODERATE RISK
AREA: BACK (HIP EXTENSORS),
FRONT (KNEE EXTENSORS)

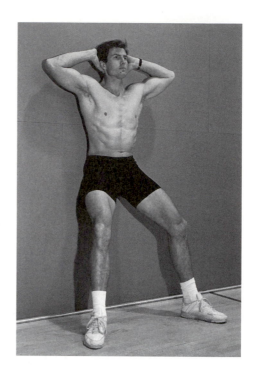

STARTING POSITION: Stand, leaning back against the wall, feet even (toes pointed slightly out), feet hip width apart or wider. Walk feet approximately eighteen inches from wall or far enough away so that shins remain perpendicular to the ground throughout the entire movement. Hands in position of choice. Torso is erect with chest out and shoulders back.

MOVEMENT: Using the wall as balance lower yourself in a three count, bending the knees and dropping the hips (flexion). Descend to a position so that the tops of the thighs of your legs are parallel to the ground. Hold for a count. During the descent keep your back against the wall and don't move knees forward over the toes. Return to the starting position by straightening out the knees and hips (extension), moving chest upward. Stop just short of locking out.

Variations: This exercise can be performed with weights (dumbbell), or with one leg. This exercise can also be done for time, holding at the bottom for a prescribed time.

TRAINER'S TIPS:
- Use wall for balance.
- Keep torso erect, chest out, shoulders back.
- Push up from bottom position, concentrating on taking chest up to the ceiling.
- Keep weight on feet from the ball of the foot to the heel.

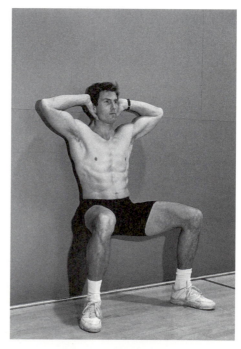

Machine Exercises

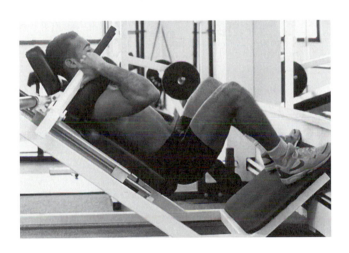

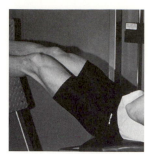

Exercise: Angle Leg Press

DIFFICULTY: 2
LOWER BACK: MODERATE
AREA: BACK (HIP EXTENSORS), FRONT (KNEE EXTENSORS)

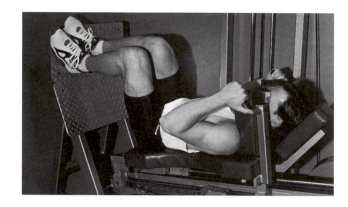

STARTING POSITION: Position yourself in leg press apparatus. Place feet evenly on the resistance plate about six inches apart. Then shift the feet at a 45-degree angle to the left. Locate feet as high on the plate as possible while leaving entire bottom portion of the foot on the plate, relieving undue stress on the knee joint. Place shoulders, lower back, and hips (torso) against the support. Release safety catch and straighten legs, but do not lock out.

MOVEMENT: From the starting position allow the sled/plate to descend in a three count by bending your knees and hips. Descend to a point where the lower leg is perpendicular to the upper part of the leg (90 degrees). During the descent keep torso firmly against the support. Once 90 degrees is reached push upward by straightening the knees and hips and return to starting position, all the time keeping torso firmly against the support. Perform for the prescribed number of repetitions and then repeat with your feet angled to the right.

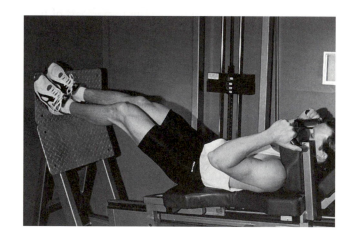

Variation: Perform this exercise in an alternating fashion, feet angled to the left one repetition then angled to the right on next repetition, as if you are parallel skiing.

TRAINER'S TIPS:
- Control your descent; don't bounce at bottom.
- Keep knees and toes in alignment.
- Keep torso against support for entire movement.
- Don't place weight on neck.
- Don't lock out knees.

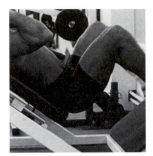

Exercise: Hack Squat (Machine)

DIFFICULTY: 2
LOWER BACK: MODERATE RISK
AREA: BACK (HIP EXTENSORS), FRONT (KNEE EXTENSORS)

STARTING POSITION: Assume position in hack squat apparatus, shoulders under pads, feet on the resistance plate. Position feet shoulder width apart or wider, toes pointed slightly out. Place feet as high on the plate as possible while leaving entire bottom of the foot on the plate. Keep torso erect and place shoulders, lower back, and hips against the back support. Straighten legs, release safety catch, but do not lock out.

MOVEMENT: Bend your knees and lower hips until the lower leg is perpendicular to the upper part of the leg (90 degrees). During the descent keep torso firmly against the support and chest expanded. Then push upward returning to starting position.

Variations: For eccentric overload, press the weight up with both legs and lower with one. This exercise can also be varied by range of motion and by emphasizing different foot and knee positions. (See Foot Positions, page 111, and knee position for squatting, page 112.)

TRAINER'S TIPS:
- Control the descent; don't bounce at bottom.
- Keep knees and toes in alignment.
- Keep torso against support and chest expanded during the entire movement.
- Eyes should be focused straight ahead.
- Don't lock out knees.

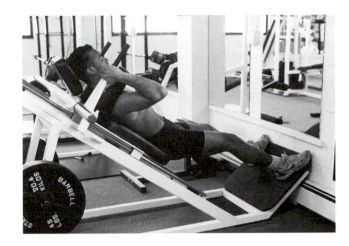

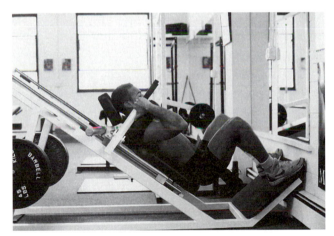

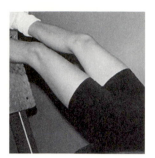

Exercise: Leg Press

DIFFICULTY: 2
LOWER BACK: MODERATE RISK
AREA: BACK (HIP EXTENSORS), FRONT (KNEE EXTENSORS)

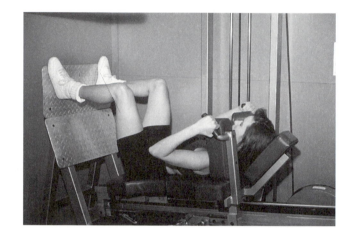

STARTING POSITION: Position yourself in leg press apparatus. Place feet on the resistance plate of the machine, shoulder width apart, toes pointed slightly out. Locate feet as high on the plate as possible while leaving the entire bottom portion of the feet on the plate, helping to relieve undue stress on the knee joint. Place shoulders, lower back, and hips (torso) against the support. Release safety catch, straighten legs, but do not lock out.

MOVEMENT: From the starting position allow the sled/plate to descend in a three count by bending your knees and hips. Descend to a point where the lower leg is perpendicular to the upper leg (90 degrees). During the descent keep torso firmly against the support. Once 90 degrees is reached, push upward by straightening the knees and hips (extension) and return to starting position, keeping torso firmly against the support.

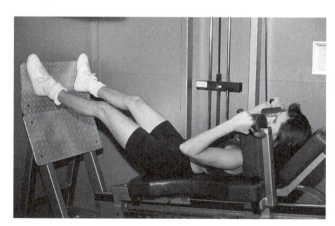

Variations: For eccentric overload, i.e., Leg Press (Negative Emphasis), raise the weight with two legs and lower with one leg. This exercise can also be varied by range of motion, and by emphasizing different foot and knee positions. (See Foot Positions, page 111, and knee position for squatting, page 112.)

TRAINER'S TIPS:
- Control the descent; don't bounce at bottom.
- Keep knees and toes in alignment.
- Keep torso against support for entire movement.
- Don't place weight on neck.
- Don't lock out knees.
- Focus your mind on the working muscles.

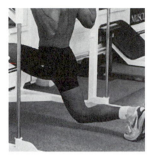

Exercise: Smith Machine Lunge

DIFFICULTY: 3
LOWER BACK: MODERATE TO HIGH RISK
AREA: BACK (HIP EXTENSORS), FRONT (KNEE EXTENSORS)

STARTING POSITION: Place bar at midchest height. Facing the rack, place hands evenly spaced from the center of the bar (slightly wider than shoulder width apart). Walk underneath the bar, placing it behind your neck. Lift bar and rotate backwards so that safety catches are released. Prepare to lunge by positioning lower body: feet placed hip width apart and toes pointed straight ahead. Next, set the torso with proper exercise alignment (chest out, shoulders back, lower back straight, with a slight forward lean), head aligned with spine, eyes focused straight ahead.

MOVEMENT: To begin the movement take a deep breath and hold. From starting position step forward (with either leg) slightly farther than average stride length, landing foot heel to toe and coming to a complete stop. Keeping torso erect (back straight, with slight forward lean) descend in a three count by bending knees, dropping hips straight down. Stop just short of the back knee touching the ground, keeping the lower portion of the front leg (shin) perpendicular to the ground. Hold for one count. Ascend by using the back leg as a fulcrum and push back (knee extension) not up with the front leg while extending hips to return to the starting position in a one count. (The plane of motion will be dictated by the Smith Machine.) Perform same movement with opposite leg and continue in an alternating fashion. As the movement reaches the top, decrease speed—do not lock knees out.

Variation: Position bar as you would for a Front Squat (see page 162) and perform as a front lunge. You can also do multiple repetitions on the same leg.

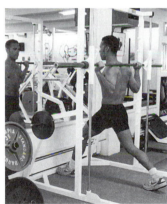

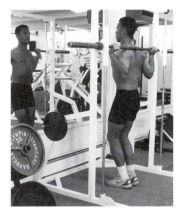

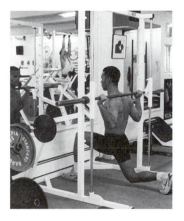

TRAINER'S TIPS:
- Focus eyes straight ahead.
- Keep back and neck aligned.
- Hips drop straight down, not forward.
- Knee should not extend over toe (shin is perpendicular to ground).
- Don't bounce back knee off the ground.

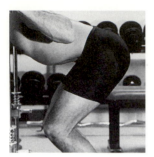

Exercise: Smith Machine Thrust

DIFFICULTY: 3
LOWER BACK: MODERATE TO HIGH RISK
AREA: BACK (HIP EXTENSORS), FRONT (KNEE EXTENSORS)

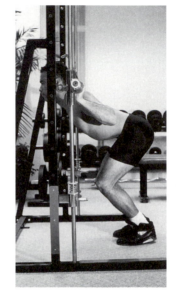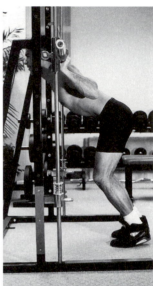

STARTING POSITION: Place bar on Smith Machine at midchest height. Facing the rack, place hands evenly spaced from the center of the bar (slightly wider than shoulder width apart). Walk underneath the bar, placing it behind your neck. Lift bar and rotate backwards so that safety catches are released. Prepare to thrust by positioning lower body: Move feet a step behind your hips so that your body is leaning slightly forward. Place feet hip width apart and point toes slightly out. Weight should be distributed on the balls of the feet. Next, set the torso with proper exercise alignment (chest out, shoulders back, lower back straight, with a slight forward lean), head aligned with spine, eyes focused straight ahead.

MOVEMENT: Take a deep breath and hold. Descend in a three count until the top of your thighs are just above parallel to the ground. From the bottom position ascend by pushing forward and up. Do not completely extend the hip. During the ascent do not let the hips shoot backwards. During the ascent the heels may come off the floor, but the knees should not go in front of the toes. As the movement reaches the top, exhale, decrease speed, and do not lock knees out.

TRAINER'S TIPS:
- Focus eyes straight ahead.
- During the descent the velocity of the descent should be slow and controlled (three count).

- No bouncing should occur at the bottom of the movement.
- Avoid exaggerated trunk lean.
- Focus on working muscles.
- Keep knees and toes in alignment.
- Do not completely extend hips.
- Concentrate on driving with your butt.
- Push forward.
- Do not allow hips to move backwards during the ascent.
- Keep shins vertical.

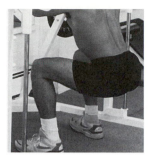

Exercise: Smith Machine Squat

DIFFICULTY: 3
LOWER BACK: MODERATE TO HIGH RISK
AREA: BACK (HIP EXTENSORS), FRONT (KNEE EXTENSORS)

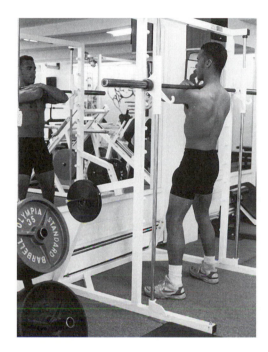

STARTING POSITION: Position barbell on Smith Machine at midchest height. Facing bar, place hands evenly spaced from the center of the bar, slightly wider than shoulder width. Walk underneath the bar, resting the bar behind your neck. Extend hips and legs, lifting bar and rotating it backwards, so that safety catches are released. Prepare to squat by first setting up your lower body, feet placed comfortably apart (shoulder width or wider in most cases), and toes pointed slightly outward. Weight should be distributed from the balls of the feet to the heel. Next, set up the torso. The chest should be expanded, shoulders back, lower back straight, with a slight forward lean. Neck should be straight and eyes focused straight ahead.

MOVEMENT: Same as Squat (see page 164).

Variation: Perform a Front Squat on the Smith Machine (as in photos) following the same movement as on page 162.

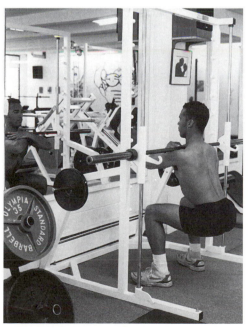

TRAINER'S TIPS:
- Look to the horizon.
- Keep heels flat.
- Do not have an exaggerated trunk lean.
- Keep torso erect.
- Do not bounce at bottom.
- Do not allow hips to move backwards during the ascent.
- Control your descent.
- Keep shins vertical.

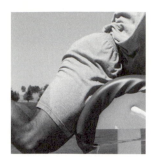

Exercise: Glute Ham Raise

DIFFICULTY: 2
LOWER BACK: MODERATE RISK
AREA: BACK (GLUTES, HAMSTRINGS)

STARTING POSITION: Position yourself in the glute ham machine as shown. Place pelvis on support pad so that your torso has full range of motion. Locate the back of your legs under the support pad so that resistance is placed on your calves. Extend torso, positioning it parallel to the ground, with your hands on your ears or across your chest.

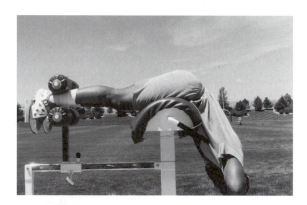

MOVEMENT: Drop your upper torso down toward the floor until you reach a 90-degree bend (or until you feel tightness in your lower back or hamstrings). Return to starting position by raising your torso to parallel to the floor, but not above parallel. Finish the Glute Ham Raise by performing knee flexion (bend knees). This will involve the hamstrings and will simulate bringing your heels toward your butt. This activation of the hamstrings will elevate your torso past parallel, as shown. To return to starting position, release contraction of the hamstring muscles.

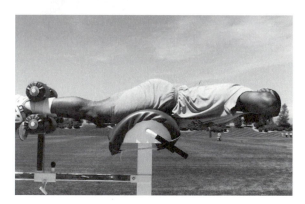

Variation: This movement may be performed with added weight.

TRAINER'S TIPS:
- Control downward phase; don't let gravity take you down.
- Concentrate on your glutes and lower back as you extend up. Pinch your buns together as you extend.
- Concentrate on hamstrings as you elevate torso past parallel.

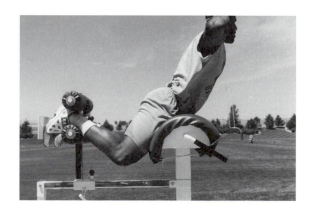

The Lunge

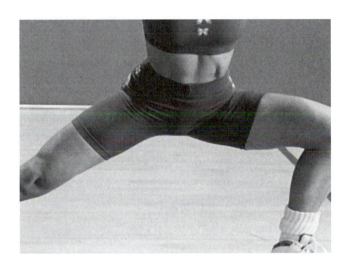

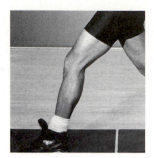

Exercise: Back Lunge Pull (Walk)

DIFFICULTY: 3
LOWER BACK: MODERATE TO HIGH RISK
AREA: BACK (HIP EXTENSORS),
FRONT (KNEE EXTENSORS, HIP FLEXORS)

STARTING POSITION: Place barbell on power rack or squat rack at midchest height. Facing the rack, place hands evenly spaced from the center of the bar (slightly wider than shoulder width apart). Walk underneath the bar, placing it behind your neck. Lift bar and back out of rack, giving yourself enough room to lunge. Prepare to lunge by positioning lower body: Place feet hip width apart and point toes straight ahead. Next, set the torso with proper exercise alignment (chest out, shoulders back, lower back straight, with a slight forward lean), head aligned with spine, eyes focused straight ahead. These guidelines apply whether you are using a barbell, dumbbells, or no weights.

MOVEMENT: Step backward (with either leg) slightly farther than average stride length, landing toe to heel, and coming to a complete stop. Keep torso erect, descending in a three count, by bending knees and dropping hips straight down. Stop just short of the back knee touching the ground, meanwhile keeping the lower portion of the front leg (shin) perpendicular to the ground. Hold for one count. Ascend by pulling back and up with the back leg while using the front leg for balance. Return to starting position. Switch legs and continue to alternate for the prescribed number of repetitions.

Variations: This movement can be performed in multiple repetitions by leading with the same leg for the prescribed number of reps, then executing with the opposite leg. This movement can be also performed in a stationary manner by stepping forward then pulling back.

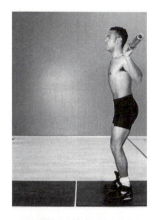

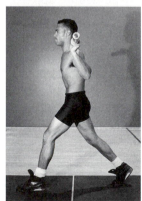

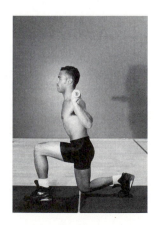

TRAINER'S TIPS:

- When pulling, roll toe to heel.
- Keep eyes focused straight ahead.
- Keep back and neck aligned.
- Hips drop straight down, not forward.
- Knee should not extend over toe (shin is perpendicular to ground).
- Don't bounce back knee off the ground.
- Once technique is perfected, no need to stop after stepping forward.

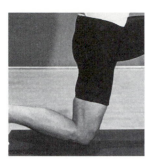

Exercise: Back Lunge Push

DIFFICULTY: 3
LOWER BACK: MODERATE TO HIGH RISK
AREA: BACK (HIP EXTENSORS), FRONT (KNEE EXTENSORS)

STARTING POSITION: Place barbell on power rack or squat rack at midchest height. Facing the rack, place hands evenly spaced from the center of the bar (slightly wider than shoulder width apart). Walk underneath the bar, placing it behind your neck. Lift bar and back out of rack, giving yourself enough room to lunge. Prepare to lunge by positioning lower body: Place feet hip width apart and point toes straight ahead. Next, set the torso with proper exercise alignment (chest out, shoulders back, lower back straight, with a slight forward lean), head aligned with spine, eyes focused straight ahead. These guidelines apply whether you are using a barbell, dumbbells, or no weights.

MOVEMENT: This lunge exercise is different in that it emphasizes the back leg in the lunging movement. Step backward (with either leg) slightly farther than average stride length, landing toe to heel, and coming to a complete stop. Keep torso erect, descending in a three count by bending knees and dropping hips straight down. Stop just short of the back knee touching the ground, meanwhile keeping the lower portion of the front leg (shin) perpendicular to the ground. Hold for one count. From the bottom position ascend by pushing forward and up with the back leg while using the front leg as a fulcrum; return to starting position. Switch legs and continue to alternate for the prescribed number of repetitions.

Variation: This movement can be performed in multiple repetitions (pump) on the same leg by not moving back to starting position, but simply to the first position of the movement.

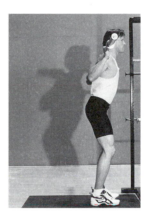

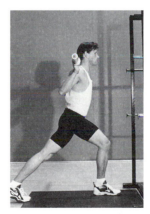

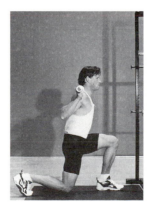

TRAINER'S TIPS:
- Emphasize pushing up with rear leg and butt.
- Keep eyes focused straight ahead.
- Keep back and neck aligned.
- Hips drop straight down, not forward.
- Knee should not extend over toe (shin is perpendicular to ground).
- Don't bounce back knee off the ground.
- Once technique is perfected, no need to stop after stepping forward.

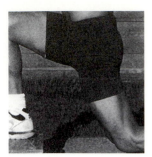

Exercise: Back Lunge Push (Descending)

DIFFICULTY: 3
LOWER BACK: MODERATE TO HIGH RISK
AREA: BACK (HIP EXTENSORS), FRONT (KNEE EXTENSORS)

STARTING POSITION: The starting position begins standing on a box eight to twelve inches high. Grasp barbell with arms fully extended to your side. Prepare to lunge by positioning lower body: Place feet hip width apart and point toes straight ahead. Next, set the torso with proper exercise alignment (chest out, shoulders back, lower back straight, with a slight forward lean), head aligned with spine, eyes focused straight ahead. These guidelines apply whether you are using a barbell, dumbbells, or no weights.

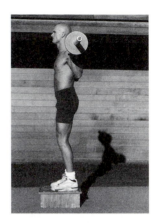

MOVEMENT: Stepping backwards off the box (with either leg) slightly farther than average stride length, land toe to heel and come to a complete stop. Keep torso erect, descending in a three count by bending knees and dropping hips straight down. Stop just short of the back knee touching the ground, while keeping the lower portion of the front leg (shin) perpendicular to the ground. Hold for one count. From the bottom position ascend by pushing forward and up with the back leg while using the front leg as a fulcrum; return to starting position. Switch legs and continue to alternate for the prescribed number of repetitions.

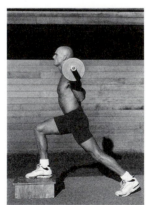

Variations: This movement can be performed in multiple repetitions on one leg or by pumping on the same leg by not moving back to starting position.

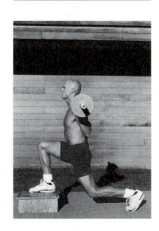

TRAINER'S TIPS:
- Emphasize pushing up with rear leg and butt.
- Keep eyes focused straight ahead.
- Keep back and neck aligned.
- Hips drop straight down, not forward.
- Knee should not extend over toe (shin is perpendicular to ground).
- Don't bounce back knee off the ground.
- Push back off lead leg, not up.
- Once technique is perfected, no need to stop after stepping forward.
- For more athletic benefits, forcefully explode from bottom position.

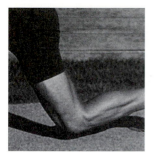

Exercise: Back Lunge Walk (Alternating)

DIFFICULTY: 3
LOWER BACK: MODERATE TO HIGH RISK
AREA: BACK (HIP EXTENSORS), FRONT (KNEE EXTENSORS)

STARTING POSITION: Grasp barbell with arms fully extended to your side. Prepare to lunge by positioning lower body: Place feet hip width apart and point toes straight ahead. Next, set the torso with proper exercise alignment (chest out, shoulders back, lower back straight, with a slight forward lean), head aligned with spine, eyes focused straight ahead. These guidelines apply whether you are using a barbell, dumbbells, or no weights.

MOVEMENT: Performance of this exercise is accomplished by moving backward. From starting position step backward (with either leg) slightly farther than average stride length, landing toe to heel and coming to a complete stop. Keep torso erect descending in a three count by bending knees and dropping hips straight down. Stop just short of the back knee touching the ground, while keeping the lower portion of the front leg (shin) perpendicular to the ground. From the bottom position, ascend by using the back leg as a fulcrum, pushing back, not up, with the front leg, returning to the starting position in a one count. Switch legs and continue to alternate (walk backward) for the prescribed number of repetitions.

Variation: This movement can be performed in multiple repetitions leading the same leg for the prescribed number of reps, then turning around and executing with the opposite leg.

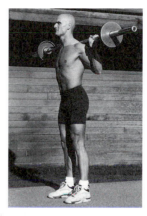

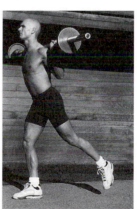

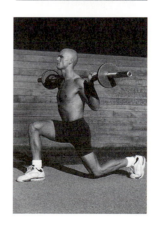

TRAINER'S TIPS:
- Distribute weight from ball of foot back toward heel on front foot.
- Perform like a wedding step, bringing feet parallel before moving backward.
- Keep eyes focused straight ahead.
- Keep back and neck aligned.
- Hips drop straight down, not forward.
- Knee should not extend over toe (shin is perpendicular to ground).
- Don't bounce back knee off the ground.
- Push back off lead leg, not up.

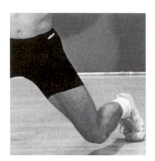

Exercise: Back Side Lunge

DIFFICULTY: 3
LOWER BACK: MODERATE TO HIGH RISK
AREA: BACK (HIP EXTENSORS),
FRONT (KNEE EXTENSORS), OUTSIDE (ABDUCTORS)

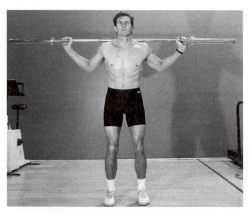

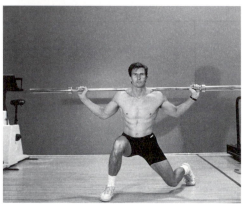

STARTING POSITION: Place barbell on power rack or squat rack at midchest height. Facing the rack, place hands evenly spaced from the center of the bar (slightly wider than shoulder width apart). Walk underneath the bar, placing it behind your neck. Lift bar and back out of rack, giving yourself enough room to lunge. Prepare to lunge by positioning lower body: Place feet hip width apart and point toes straight ahead. Next, set the torso with proper exercise alignment (chest out, shoulders back, lower back straight, with a slight forward lean), head aligned with spine, eyes focused straight ahead. These guidelines apply whether you are using a barbell, dumbbells, or no weights.

MOVEMENT: This lunge exercises the back leg in the lunging movement. From the starting position step backward at about a 45-degree angle (with either leg) slightly farther than average stride length, landing toe to heel, and coming to a complete stop. Keep torso erect, descending in a three count by bending knees and dropping hips straight down. Stop just short of the back knee touching the ground, while keeping the lower portion of the front leg (shin) perpendicular to the ground. Hold for one count. From the bottom position ascend by pushing forward (at a 45-degree angle) and up with the back leg while using the front leg as a fulcrum, returning to starting position. Switch legs and continue to alternate for the prescribed number of repetitions.

Variations: This movement can be performed in multiple repetitions (pump) on the same leg by not

moving back to starting position, but simply to the first position of the movement. This exercise can also be performed by stepping off a box.

TRAINER'S TIPS:
- Emphasize pushing up with rear leg and butt.
- Hips drop straight down, not at an angle.
- Keep torso facing forward to maintain correct angle.
- Keep eyes focused straight ahead.
- Keep back and neck aligned.
- Knee should not extend over toe (shin is perpendicular to ground).
- Don't bounce back knee off the ground.

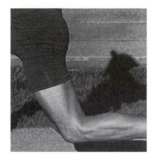

Exercise: Front Box Lunge (Pumps)

DIFFICULTY: 3
LOWER BACK: MODERATE TO HIGH RISK
AREA: BACK (HIP EXTENSORS), FRONT (KNEE EXTENSORS)

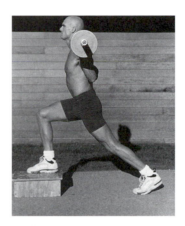

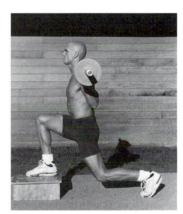

STARTING POSITION: Grasp barbell with arms fully extended to your side. Face the box, standing twelve to eighteen inches away. Prepare to lunge by positioning lower body: Place feet hip width apart and point toes straight ahead. Next, set the torso with proper exercise alignment (chest out, shoulders back, lower back straight, with a slight forward lean), head aligned with spine, eyes focused straight ahead. These guidelines apply whether you are using a barbell, dumbbells, or no weights.

MOVEMENT: Step forward (with either leg) slightly farther than average stride length, landing heel to toe and coming to a complete stop on the box. Keep torso erect descending in a three count by bending knees and dropping hips straight down. Stop just short of the back knee touching the ground, while keeping the lower portion of the front leg (shin) perpendicular to the ground. Hold for one count. From the bottom position, ascend by using the back leg as a fulcrum, pushing back, not up, with the front leg, returning to the first position of the movement (not the starting position). Perform the prescribed number of multiple repetitions with the same leg, then perform prescribed repetitions with the other leg.

Variation: You can perform these in alternating fashion by just pushing all the way back to the original starting position and alternating legs.

TRAINER'S TIPS:
- Keep eyes focused straight ahead after securing foot on the box.
- Keep back and neck aligned.

- Hips drop straight down, not forward.
- Knee should not extend over toe (shin is perpendicular to ground).
- Don't bounce back knee off the ground.
- Push back off lead leg, not up.
- Once technique is perfected, no need to stop after stepping forward.
- Strive to bring back knee close to the ground to enhance flexibility gains.
- Do not lock front knee completely when extending.
- Weight should be distributed from the ball of the foot backwards to the heel.

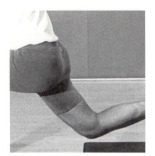

Exercise: Descending Box Lunge (Alternating)

DIFFICULTY: 3
LOWER BACK: MODERATE TO HIGH RISK
AREA: BACK (HIP EXTENSORS), FRONT (KNEE EXTENSORS)

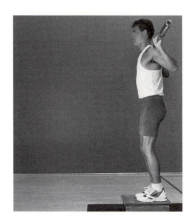

STARTING POSITION: Grasping barbell, arms fully extended to your side, stand on a box eight to twelve inches high. Prepare to lunge by positioning lower body: Place feet hip width apart and point toes straight ahead. Next, set the torso with proper exercise alignment (chest out, shoulders back, lower back straight, with a slight forward lean), head aligned with spine, eyes focused straight ahead. These guidelines apply whether you are using a barbell, dumbbells, or no weights.

MOVEMENT: Step forward off the box (with either leg) slightly farther than average stride length, landing toe to heel and coming to a complete stop. Keep torso erect, descending in a three count by bending knees and dropping hips straight down. Stop when the shin of the back leg is parallel to the ground, while keeping the lower portion of the front leg (shin) perpendicular to the ground. Hold for one count. From the bottom position, ascend by using the back leg as a fulcrum, pushing back, not up, with the front leg, returning to the starting position in a one count. Switch legs and continue to alternate for the prescribed number of repetitions.

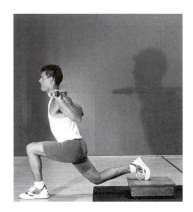

Variation: You can perform these in a pump or multiple repetition fashion by pushing back to the first position of the movement (not starting position) and repeating for the prescribed number of repetitions on one leg then repeating on the opposite leg.

TRAINER'S TIPS:
- Keep eyes focused straight ahead after securing foot on the ground.
- Keep back and neck aligned.
- Hips drop straight down, not forward.
- Knee should not extend over toe (shin is perpendicular to ground).
- Push back off lead leg, not up.
- Land toe to heel to help absorb shock.
- Push back to box explosively.

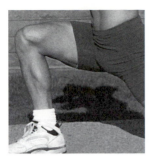

Exercise: Front Lunge (Alternating)

DIFFICULTY: 3
LOWER BACK: MODERATE TO HIGH RISK
AREA: BACK (HIP EXTENSORS), FRONT (KNEE EXTENSORS)

STARTING POSITION: Place barbell on power rack or squat rack at midchest height. Facing the rack, place hands evenly spaced from the center of the bar (slightly wider than shoulder width apart). Walk underneath the bar, placing it behind your neck. Lift bar and back out of rack, giving yourself enough room to lunge. (Barbell can also be "racked" in front position, as in photos.) Prepare to lunge by positioning lower body: Place feet hip width apart and point toes straight ahead. Next, set the torso with proper exercise alignment (chest out, shoulders back, lower back straight, with a slight forward lean), head aligned with spine, eyes focused straight ahead. These guidelines apply whether you are using a barbell, dumbbells, or no weights.

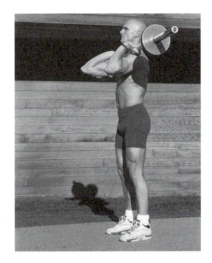

MOVEMENT: Step forward (with either leg) slightly farther than average stride length, landing foot heel to toe and coming to a complete stop. Keep torso erect, descending in a three count by bending knees and dropping hips straight down. Stop just short of the back knee touching the ground, while keeping the lower portion of the front leg (shin) perpendicular to the ground. Hold for one count. From the bottom position, ascend by using the back leg as a fulcrum, pushing back, not up, with the front leg, returning to the starting position in a one count. Switch legs and continue to alternate for the prescribed number of repetitions.

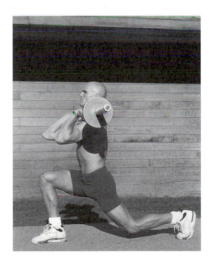

TRAINER'S TIPS:
- Keep eyes focused straight ahead.
- Keep back and neck aligned.
- Hips drop straight down, not forward.
- Knee should not extend over toe (shin is perpendicular to ground).
- Don't bounce back knee off the ground.
- Push back off lead leg, not up.
- Once technique is perfected, no need to stop after stepping forward.
- For more athletic benefits, forcefully explode from bottom position.

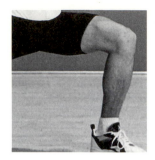

Exercise: Front Lunge Angle Pulls (Alternating)

DIFFICULTY: 3
LOWER BACK: MODERATE TO HIGH RISK
AREA: BACK (HIP EXTENSORS),
FRONT (KNEE EXTENSORS),
INSIDE (ADDUCTORS)

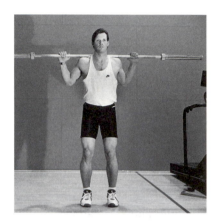

STARTING POSITION: Grasp barbell, arms fully extended to your side. Prepare to lunge by positioning lower body: Place feet hip width apart and point toes straight ahead. Next, set the torso with proper exercise alignment (chest out, shoulders back, lower back straight, with a slight forward lean), head aligned with spine, eyes focused straight ahead. These guidelines apply whether you are using a barbell, dumbbells, or no weights.

MOVEMENT: Move forward at an angle in a similar motion to a speed skater. Step forward and to the side at about a 45-degree angle (with either leg) slightly farther than average stride length, landing heel to toe (with knee and toe maintaining alignment), and coming to a complete stop. Keep torso erect, descending in a three count by bending knees and dropping hips straight down. Stop just short of the back knee touching the ground, while keeping the lower portion of the front leg (shin) perpendicular to the ground. Hold for one count. Ascend by pulling forward and up with the front leg while lifting the back leg off the ground. Bring the back leg forward and return to starting position. Switch legs and continue to alternate for the prescribed number of repetitions.

Variations: This movement can be performed in multiple repetitions by leading with the same leg for the prescribed number of repetitions, then performing the movement with the opposite leg. It can also be performed in a stationary manner (by stepping backward at an angle) in an alternating or multiple repetition fashion.

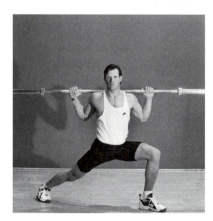

TRAINER'S TIPS:
- Distribute weight from ball of foot back toward heel.
- Space limitations may make dumbbells a better choice.
- Torso remains facing forward during the movement.
- Keep eyes focused straight ahead.
- Keep back and neck aligned.
- Hips drop straight down, not forward.
- Knee should not extend over toe (shin is perpendicular to ground).
- Don't bounce back knee off the ground.

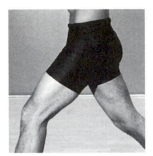

Exercise: Front Lunge (Pumps)

DIFFICULTY: 3
LOWER BACK: MODERATE TO HIGH RISK
AREA: BACK (HIP EXTENSORS), FRONT (KNEE EXTENSORS)

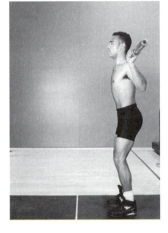

STARTING POSITION: Place barbell on power rack or squat rack at midchest height. Facing the rack, place hands evenly spaced from the center of the bar (slightly wider than shoulder width apart). Walk underneath the bar, placing it behind your neck. Lift bar and back out of rack, giving yourself enough room to lunge. Prepare to lunge by positioning lower body: Place feet hip width apart and point toes straight ahead. Next, set the torso with proper exercise alignment (chest out, shoulders back, lower back straight, with a slight forward lean), head aligned with spine, eyes focused straight ahead. These guidelines apply whether you are using a barbell, dumbbells, or no weights.

MOVEMENT: Step forward (with either leg) slightly farther than average stride length, landing foot heel to toe, and coming to a complete stop. Keep torso erect, descending in a three count by bending knees and dropping hips straight down. Stop just short of the back knee touching the ground while keeping the lower portion of the front leg (shin) perpendicular to the ground. Hold for one count. From the bottom position, ascend by using the back leg as a fulcrum, pushing back, not up, with the front leg. Do not return to starting position, but to first position of the movement. Do not fully extend knee. Perform for the prescribed number of repetitions then switch legs.

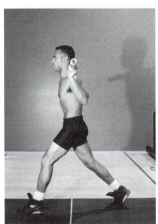

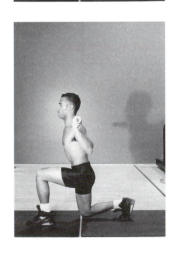

TRAINER'S TIPS:
- Hold for a count at the bottom.
- Do not extend front knee completely.
- Weight should be distributed from the ball of the foot backwards to the heel.
- Keep eyes focused straight ahead.
- Keep back and neck aligned.
- Hips drop straight down, not forward.
- Knee should not extend over toe (shin is perpendicular to ground).
- Don't bounce back knee off the ground.
- Push back off lead leg, not up.

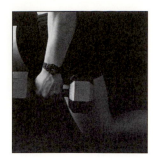

Exercise: Lunge Pulls (Walks)

DIFFICULTY: 3

LOWER BACK: MODERATE TO HIGH RISK

AREA: BACK (HIP EXTENSORS), FRONT (KNEE EXTENSORS)

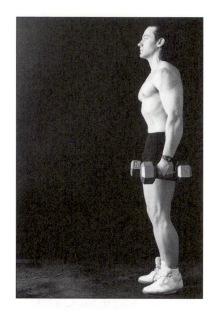

STARTING POSITION: Grasp dumbbells, arms fully extended at your side. Prepare to lunge by positioning lower body: Place feet hip width apart and point toes straight ahead. Next, set the torso with proper exercise alignment (chest out, shoulders back, lower back straight, with a slight forward lean), head aligned with spine, eyes focused straight ahead. These guidelines apply whether you are using a barbell, dumbbells, or no weights.

MOVEMENT: Step forward (with either leg) slightly farther than average stride length, landing foot heel to toe and coming to a complete stop. Keep torso erect, descending in a three count by bending knees and dropping hips straight down. Stop just short of the back knee touching the ground while keeping the lower portion of the front leg (shin) perpendicular to the ground. Hold for one count. From the bottom position, ascend by pulling forward and up with front leg. Bring the back leg forward and return to starting position. While moving forward do not allow the knee of the front leg to extend over the toe. Switch legs and continue to alternate for the prescribed number of repetitions.

Variations: This movement can be performed in multiple repetitions on one leg without alternating. It can also be performed stationary in an alternating or multiple repetition format. It can be performed with a barbell as well.

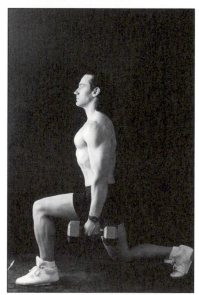

TRAINER'S TIPS:
- Knee should not extend over toe (shin is perpendicular to ground) at any time.
- Keep eyes focused straight ahead.
- Keep back and neck aligned.
- Hips drop straight down, not forward.
- Don't bounce back knee off the ground.

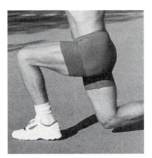

Exercise: Overhead Lunge

DIFFICULTY: 3 PLUS
LOWER BACK: HIGH RISK
AREA: BACK (HIP EXTENSORS),
FRONT (KNEE EXTENSORS), SHOULDERS, TRICEPS

STARTING POSITION: Place bar on power rack slightly above the top of the head. Facing rack, place hands evenly spaced from the center of the bar, slightly wider than shoulder width. Walk underneath the bar. Extend bar overhead, locking elbows. Carry the bar over the back part of the head. Back out of rack, giving yourself enough room to lunge. Prepare to lunge by positioning lower body: Place feet hip width apart and point toes straight ahead. Next, set the torso with proper exercise alignment (chest out, shoulders back, lower back straight, with a slight forward lean), head aligned with spine, eyes focused straight ahead. These guidelines apply whether you are using a barbell or dumbbells.

MOVEMENT: To begin the movement take a deep breath and hold. Step forward (with either leg) slightly farther than average stride length, landing foot heel to toe, and coming to a complete stop. Keep torso erect, descending in a three count by bending knees and dropping hips straight down. Stop just short of the back knee touching the ground while keeping the lower portion of the front leg (shin) perpendicular to the ground. Hold for one count. From the bottom position, ascend by using the back leg as a fulcrum, pushing back, not up, with the front leg, returning to the starting position in a one count. Switch legs and continue to alternate for the prescribed number of repetitions.

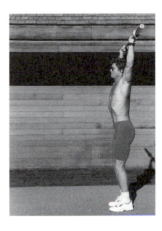 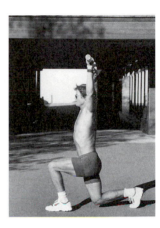

Variation: This movement can be performed with dumbbells and in a pump fashion.

TRAINER'S TIPS:
- Keep eyes focused straight ahead.
- Keep back and neck aligned.
- Hips drop straight down, not forward.
- Knee should not extend over toe (shin is perpendicular to ground).
- Don't bounce back knee off the ground.
- Push back off lead leg, not up.
- Once technique is perfected, no need to stop after stepping forward.
- For more athletic benefits, forcefully explode from bottom position.
- Keep elbows locked and carry bar slightly behind the head.

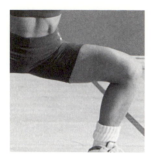

Exercise: Side Lunge (Alternating)

DIFFICULTY: 3
LOWER BACK: MODERATE TO HIGH RISK
AREA: BACK (HIP EXTENSORS), FRONT (KNEE EXTENSORS),
INSIDE (ADDUCTORS), OUTSIDE (ABDUCTORS)

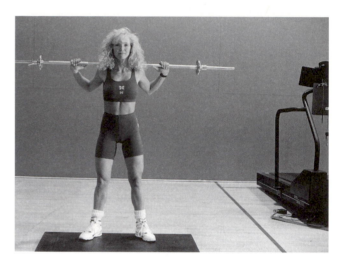

STARTING POSITION: Place barbell on power rack or squat rack at midchest height. Facing the rack, place hands evenly spaced from the center of the bar (slightly wider than shoulder width apart). Walk underneath the bar, placing it behind your neck. Lift bar and back out of rack, giving yourself enough room to lunge. Prepare to lunge by positioning lower body: Place feet hip width apart and point toes straight ahead. Next, set the torso with proper exercise alignment (chest out, shoulders back, lower back straight, with a slight forward lean), head aligned with spine, eyes focused straight ahead. These guidelines apply whether you are using a barbell, dumbbells, or no weights.

MOVEMENT: Step to the side with either leg slightly farther than average stride length, landing foot heel to toe with the toe pointing in the direction of the step (step straight to the side, knee and toe in alignment). Come to a complete stop after stepping. Torso faces forward. Descend until the top of the thigh of the lead leg is parallel to the ground while keeping the lower portion of leg (shin) perpendicular to the ground. Keep torso erect, bend knee, and drop hips straight down. Hold for one count. Ascend by using the non-working leg as a fulcrum, pushing back, not up, with the lead leg, and return to the starting position in a one count. Switch legs and continue to alternate for the prescribed number of repetitions.

Variations: This exercise can be performed in a variety of ways: multiple repetitions; ascending and/or descending (on or off a box); various angles; or side pulls.

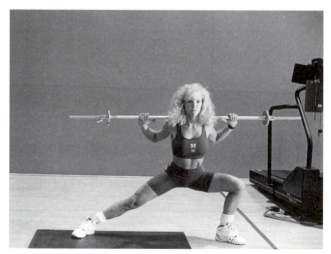

TRAINER'S TIPS:
- Keep torso forward.
- Keep eyes focused straight ahead.
- Keep back and neck aligned.
- Hips drop straight down, not forward.
- Knee should not extend over toe (shin is perpendicular to ground).
- Push back off lead leg, not up.
- Once technique is perfected, no need to stop after stepping forward.

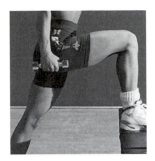

Exercise: Step-Ups

DIFFICULTY: 3
LOWER BACK: MODERATE TO HIGH RISK
AREA: BACK (HIP EXTENSORS), FRONT (KNEE EXTENSORS, HIP FLEXORS)

STARTING POSITION: Grasp dumbbells, arms fully extended at your side. Stand twelve to eighteen inches from workbench. Prepare to step up by positioning lower body: Place feet hip width apart and point toes straight ahead. Next, set the torso with proper exercise alignment (chest out, shoulders back, lower back straight, with a slight forward lean), head aligned with spine, eyes focused straight ahead. These guidelines apply whether you are using a barbell, dumbbells, or no weights.

MOVEMENT: Step up on the bench with the right leg. Place foot securely on the bench with the shin perpendicular to the ground. Keep torso erect and ascend to the top of the bench by pulling up and forward with the right leg. Do not let knee move forward over toe. Bring the left leg up and lightly tap the toe on the bench. Step back off the bench with the left leg using the right leg to control the descent. Place left foot on ground (toe to heel) and bring right leg down to the starting position. Switch legs and continue to alternate for the prescribed number of repetitions.

Variations: This movement can be performed in a multiple repetition format. Another variation would be to push with the back leg instead of pulling with the front leg.

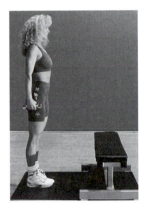

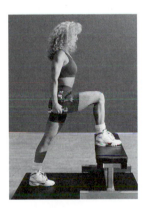

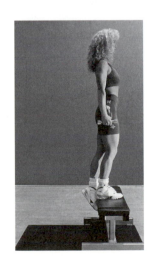

TRAINER'S TIPS:
- Emphasize pulling up with front leg.
- Knee should not extend over toe (shin is perpendicular to ground) at any time.
- Keep torso erect.
- Keep eyes focused straight ahead.
- Keep back and neck aligned.
- Control your descent.

The Balanced Movements

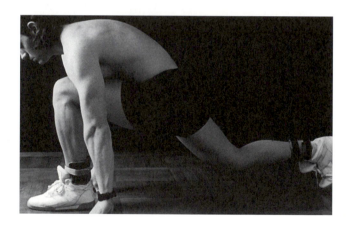

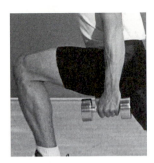

Exercise: Single-Leg Balance Squat

DIFFICULTY: 3
LOWER BACK: MODERATE RISK
AREA: BACK (HIP EXTENSORS), FRONT (KNEE EXTENSORS)

STARTING POSITION: Stand about two feet in front of a flat workbench, facing away, feet parallel, and hip width apart. Place either foot on the bench so the top portion of the foot rests on the top of the bench. Weight on the front foot should be equally distributed from the ball of the foot to the heel. Let arms hang down or place them behind your head. Torso is erect in proper exercise alignment.

MOVEMENT: Using your rear leg for balance, lower yourself in a three count. Descend to a position so your front leg is parallel to the ground. Hold for a count. During the descent make sure that the knee of the front leg doesn't move forward over the toes. Return to the starting position, stopping just short of locking out. Perform the prescribed number of repetitions, switch legs, and repeat.

Variations: This exercise can be performed with weights (dumbbell, barbell, or machine) and on a box.

TRAINER'S TIPS:
- Use rear leg for balance; do not push.
- Eyes should be focused straight ahead.
- Push up from bottom position, concentrating on coming straight up.
- Do not bend at the waist; keep torso straight.

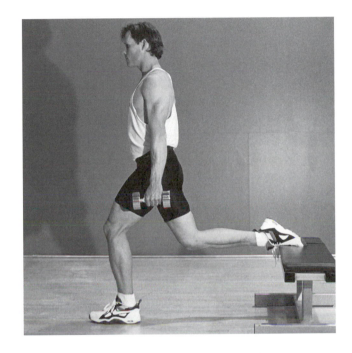

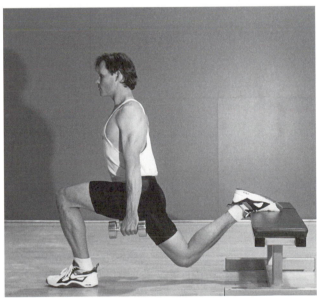

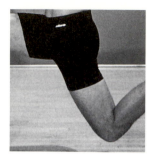

Exercise: Balance Squat (with Bench)

DIFFICULTY: 2
LOWER BACK: MODERATE RISK
AREA: BACK (HIP EXTENSORS), FRONT (KNEE EXTENSORS)

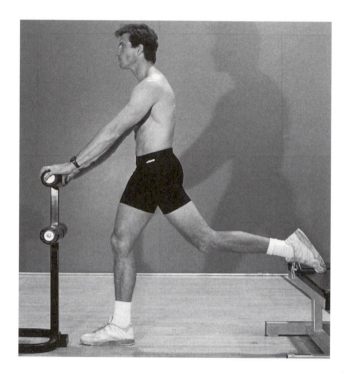

STARTING POSITION: Place a barbell on the inside of a power rack at chest level. Or use another piece of equipment for balance. Place flat bench (sideways) three feet away from the rack. Stand between bench and power rack, feet even, hip width, and toes aligned with the front edge of the power rack. Place hands on barbell, centering yourself between your arms. Place either foot back on workbench so the top portion of the foot rests on the top of the bench. Weight on the front foot should be distributed from the ball of the foot to the heel. Torso is erect with slight forward lean.

MOVEMENT: Using your hands and rear leg for balance, lower yourself in a three count by bending the forward knee and hip (flexion). Descend, sitting back (similar to sitting in a chair) so your front leg is parallel to the ground. Hold for a count. During the descent make sure that the knee of the front leg doesn't move forward over the toes. Return to the starting position, stopping just short of locking out. Perform the prescribed number of repetitions, switch legs, and repeat.

TRAINER'S TIPS:
- Use hands and rear leg for balance; do not pull or push, and don't squeeze.
- Eyes should be focused straight ahead.
- Keep torso in proper exercise alignment.
- Push up from bottom position, concentrating on coming straight up.
- Focus your mind on the working muscles.

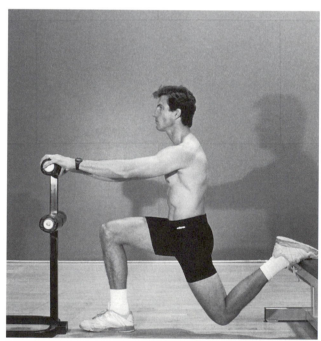

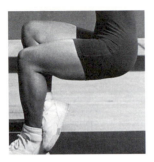

Exercise: Post Squat

DIFFICULTY: 3
LOWER BACK: MODERATE RISK
AREA: BACK (HIP EXTENSORS), FRONT (KNEE EXTENSORS)

STARTING POSITION: Position yourself facing a post or power rack, feet even and hip width apart or wider. Toes are aligned even with post and pointed slightly out. Hold post (arms fully extended at waist level). Torso is erect with chest out and shoulders back.

MOVEMENT: Using the post for balance, lower yourself in a three count by bending the knees and dropping the hips. Descend so that the top of your thighs are parallel to the ground. Hold for a count. During the descent sit back as if you're sitting in a chair, weight on your heels (to insure that the knees of the legs don't move over the toes). Return to starting position, stopping just short of locking out.

Variations: You can bring one leg forward off the ground, perpendicular to the body. Then lower yourself (Single-Leg Post Squat).

TRAINER'S TIPS:
- Use post for balance; don't pull with arms.
- Eyes should be focused straight ahead.
- Keep torso erect, chest out, and back straight.
- Push straight up from bottom position.
- Focus your mind on the working muscles.

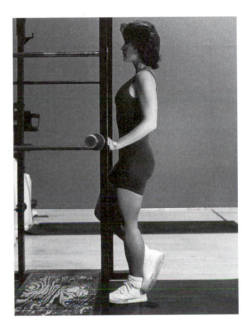

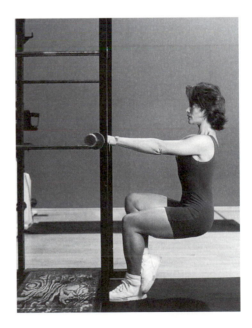

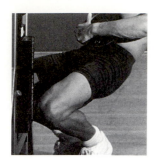

Exercise: Sissy Squat

DIFFICULTY: 3
LOWER BACK: MODERATE RISK
AREA: BACK (HIP EXTENSORS), FRONT (KNEE EXTENSORS)

STARTING POSITION: Stand facing a post, feet even with post, legs hip width apart, toes pointed out at a 45-degree angle. Hold on to post for balance and support with arms fully extended at waist level. You may hold support post with one or two hands. Torso is erect with chest out and shoulders back.

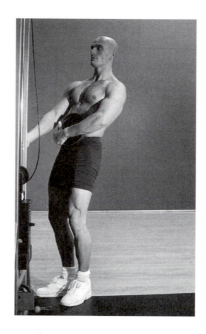

MOVEMENT: Disregard everything you have learned about squatting. Arch your back and point your chest to the ceiling; do not hyperextend your neck. Bring upper back toward the floor and lower yourself in a three count by bending the knees and dropping the hips (flexion). For this exercise, weight moves from your heels to the balls of feet, heels will come off the ground, knees will go over the toes (but not too much). Descend to a position so that the top of the thighs are parallel to the ground. Hold for a count. Return to the starting position by moving your chest upward, stopping just short of locking out.

Variations: For increased resistance, hold on to post with free hand and with the other cradle plate or dumbbell against your chest. This exercise can also be performed on one leg (Single-Leg Sissy Squat).

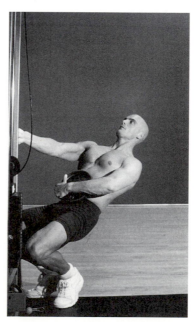

TRAINER'S TIPS:
- Use post for balance; don't pull with arms.
- Use small range of motion.
- Concentrate on taking chest up to the ceiling.
- Focus your mind on the working muscles.

Exercise: Sissy Squat (Apparatus)

DIFFICULTY: 3
LOWER BACK: MODERATE RISK
AREA: BACK (HIP EXTENSORS), FRONT (KNEE EXTENSORS)

STARTING POSITION: Position yourself in apparatus, calves against back pads, feet flat and under roller pads. Place arms in position of choice. Torso is erect with chest out and shoulders back.

MOVEMENT: Using the apparatus as balance, lower yourself in a three count bending the knees and dropping the hips. Descend so that the top of the thighs are parallel to the ground. Hold for a count. During descent, sit back as if you're sitting in a chair, keeping pressure against the pads. Place weight on your heels to insure that the knees don't move forward over the toes. Return to the starting position and concentrate on moving your chest upward.

Variation: This movement can be performed with added resistance (dumbbells, barbell, Smith Machine, etc.) or with one leg at a time.

TRAINER'S TIPS:
- Eyes should be focused on the horizon.
- Adjust back pads so that the back part of the thigh doesn't hit pads in the down position.
- Keep knees and toes aligned.
- Don't lock out.
- Keep torso erect, chest out, and back straight.
- Push up from bottom position; concentrate on taking chest up to the ceiling.
- Keep weight equally distributed on the feet.

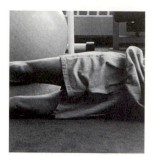

Exercise: Side Hip Extension Rotation

DIFFICULTY: 1
LOWER BACK: LOW RISK
AREA: BACK (GLUTES), OUTSIDE (ABDUCTORS)

STARTING POSITION: Lie on your side, supporting your head with your hand and forearm. Your other hand is palm down in front of chest for support. Bend bottom leg for stability. Extend your top leg and rotate hip in so that toes are pointing down at the floor in front of other leg.

MOVEMENT: Rotate your top leg out (toes moving toward ceiling) as you simultaneously move leg straight back on a horizontal plane, until you feel tightness in your butt. Return to starting position by simultaneously bringing the leg forward and rotating the leg in (toes moving toward floor) and back to the starting position. Repeat with other leg.

TRAINER'S TIPS:
- Focus your mind on the butt as you rotate and extend.
- Don't overextend on the backward motion and don't arch the back.
- Keep torso static throughout the exercise.
- Control the forward and backward motion.

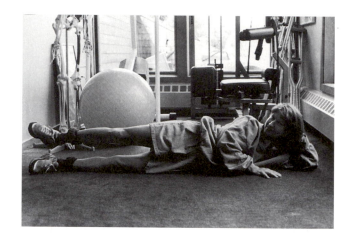

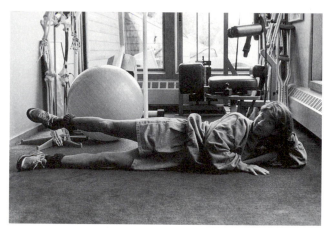

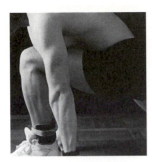

Exercise: Mountain Climbers

DIFFICULTY: 3
LOWER BACK: MODERATE TO HIGH RISK
AREA: BACK (HIP EXTENSORS), FRONT (KNEE EXTENSORS, HIP FLEXORS)

STARTING POSITION: Standing (feet hip width apart), step forward with either leg slightly farther than average stride length. Descend using correct lunging technique (drop hips straight down, keep shin of front leg perpendicular to ground). When bottom position is reached, lean forward with torso until extended arms reach the ground; distribute weight evenly between hands. From this position raise hips slightly so that back is flat.

MOVEMENT: This exercise is performed by alternating the feet as if running in place. Simultaneously step forward with back leg while bringing front leg backward, exchanging leg positions (original starting position with legs switched). During this movement keep torso still. Repeat movement so that feet move back to starting position. This equals one repetition.

Variation: This movement can be performed by attaching cables to both ankles. Be sure to control movement with cable.

TRAINER'S TIPS:
- Distribute weight evenly.
- Back should remain flat.
- Both legs should move at the same time.
- Use good lunging technique to assume proper starting position.

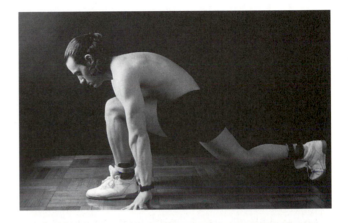

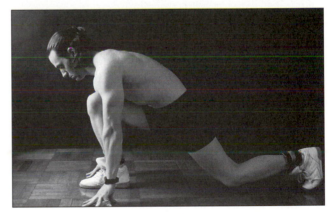

CHAPTER FOURTEEN

Water Works

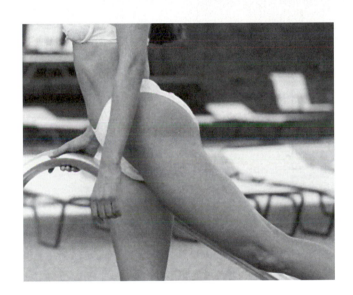

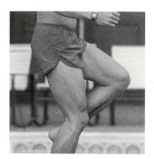

Exercise: Aqua One-Legged Tuck Jumps

DIFFICULTY: 3
LOWER BACK: MODERATE RISK
AREA: FRONT (QUADRICEPS), BACK (GLUTES, HAMSTRINGS)

STARTING POSITION: Stand in chest- to waist-deep water on one leg. Raise your other knee until thigh is perpendicular to your body. Arms are raised at your sides for balance.

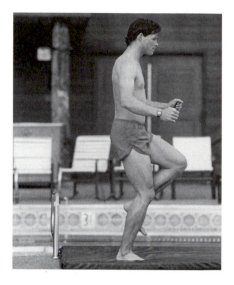

MOVEMENT: Push off the bottom with the planted leg, pulling your knee up to match the one already raised. Then push your leg back down to the starting position. Repeat with other leg when finished.

TRAINER'S TIPS:
- Exercise should be done at maximum effort.
- Hold abdominals tight throughout exercise to support the lower back.
- Don't rest between reps.
- To assist movement, pull arms down under knees as you lift.
- Be sure to exercise both legs.
- Focus your mind on the working muscles.

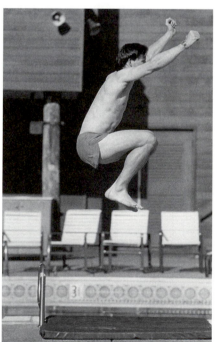

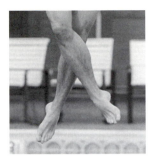

Exercise: Aqua Cross Jumps

DIFFICULTY: 2
LOWER BACK: MODERATE RISK
AREA: OUTSIDE (ABDUCTORS), INSIDE (ADDUCTORS),
FRONT (QUADRICEPS), BACK (GLUTES)

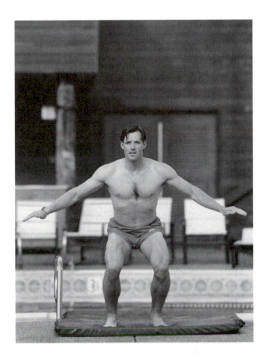

STARTING POSITION: Stand in chest- to waist-deep water with your feet hip width apart and your knees slightly bent. Chest should be open with your shoulders down. Arms should be down at your sides.

MOVEMENT: Jump up, crossing your legs one in front of the other. Return leg to starting position as you come down. Be sure to switch the leg that crosses in front.

TRAINER'S TIPS:
- Exercise should be done at maximum effort.
- Hold abdominals tight throughout exercise to support the lower back.
- Don't rest between reps.
- To assist balance, hold arms out to side.
- Be sure to alternate leg that crosses in front.

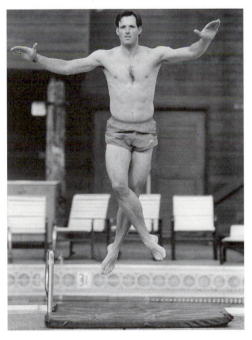

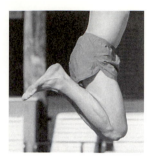

Exercise: Aqua Double-Leg Curl

DIFFICULTY: 2
LOWER BACK: MODERATE RISK
AREA: BACK (HAMSTRINGS), FRONT (QUADRICEPS)

STARTING POSITION: Stand in chest- to waist-deep water with your feet hip width apart and knees slightly bent. Arms are extended out to your sides for balance.

MOVEMENT: Jump up, pulling both heels up toward your butt. Return to starting position by pushing your legs down through the water.

TRAINER'S TIPS:
- Exercise should be done at maximum effort.
- Hold abdominals tight throughout exercise to support the lower back.
- Don't rest between reps.
- Focus the mind on the hamstrings and butt as you pull your heels up.
- Land with knees in a slightly bent position.

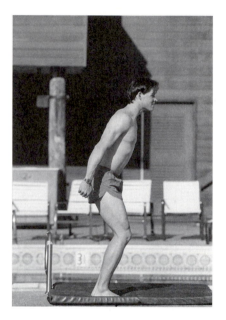

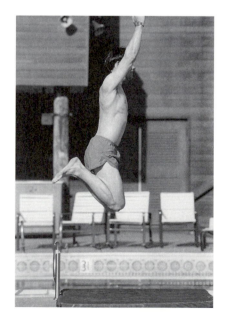

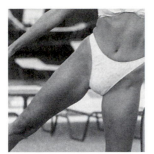

Exercise: Aqua Hip Abduction/Adduction

DIFFICULTY: 1
LOWER BACK: LOW RISK
AREA: INSIDE (ABDUCTORS), OUTSIDE (ADDUCTORS)

STARTING POSITION: In waist- to chest-deep water, stand on one leg. Place other leg slightly in front, an inch off the pool floor, both knees slightly bent. Chest should be open, shoulders down, and head up. Extend arms out for balance.

MOVEMENT: Raise leg to the side, squeezing your butt and outer hip through the movement. Pull the leg forcefully down to the starting position. Repeat with other leg when finished.

TRAINER'S TIPS:
- Maintain stationary position with your torso.
- Focus your mind on your butt and outer hip on the side kick, and your inner thigh on the return.
- Avoid jerky motions. Exercise should be done in a slow, controlled motion.
- Hold abdominals tight to support lower back.
- Don't rest between reps.

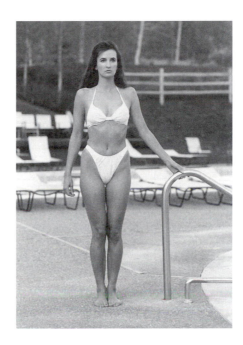

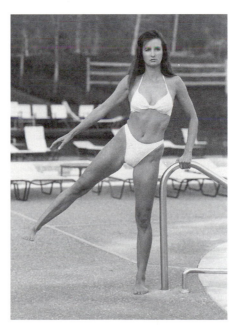

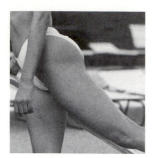

Exercise: Aqua Hip Extension

DIFFICULTY: 1
LOWER BACK: MODERATE RISK
AREA: FRONT (QUADRICEPS, HIP FLEXORS), BACK (GLUTES, HAMSTRINGS)

STARTING POSITION: Stand with side toward pool's edge (approximately six to twelve inches away) in chest- to waist-deep water with your feet hip width apart and knees slightly bent. Hold on to the side of the pool for balance. Your chest should be open, your shoulders down, and your head up.

MOVEMENT: Keeping working leg straight (knee slightly bent), push leg back behind you, lifting and squeezing with the butt. Return to starting position by pulling forward with your thighs and hip flexors. Repeat with other leg when finished.

TRAINER'S TIPS:
- Maintain stationary position with your torso.
- Focus your mind on your butt and hamstrings, lifting and squeezing on the backward movement (not throwing the leg back), and your thighs and hip flexors contracting on the forward movement.
- Avoid jerky motions. Exercise should be done in a slow, controlled motion.
- Hold abdominals tight to support lower back.
- Don't rest between reps.

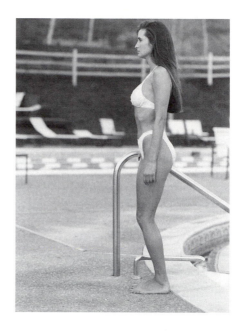

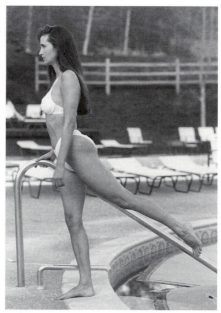

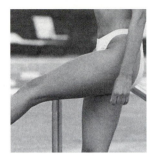

Exercise: Aqua Hip Flexion

DIFFICULTY: 1
LOWER BACK: LOW RISK
AREA: FRONT (HIP FLEXORS, QUADRICEPS), BACK (GLUTES, HAMSTRINGS)

STARTING POSITION: Stand with side toward pool's edge (approximately six to twelve inches away) in chest-deep water with your feet hip width apart, and knees slightly bent. Use hand nearest to edge to hold on for balance. Your chest should be open, your shoulders down, and your head up.

MOVEMENT: Keeping the working leg straight, raise the leg in front of you until you feel tightness in your thigh. Return to starting position by pulling leg back. Repeat with other leg when finished.

TRAINER'S TIPS:
- Maintain stationary position with your torso.
- Concentrate on your thighs and hip flexors contracting on the forward movement, and your butt and hamstrings on the backward movement.
- Avoid jerky movements. Exercise should be done in a slow, controlled motion.
- Point your toes to add frontal resistance through the water.
- Don't rest between reps.

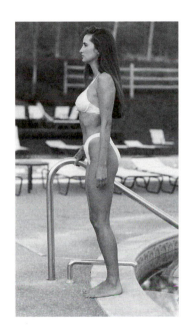

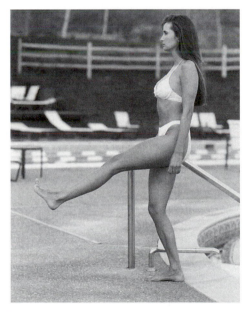

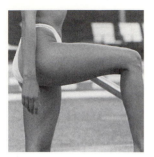

Exercise: Aqua Knee Extension

DIFFICULTY: 1
LOWER BACK: LOW RISK
AREA: FRONT (QUADRICEPS), BACK (HAMSTRINGS)

STARTING POSITION: Stand with side toward pool's edge in chest-deep water; balance on one leg. The working leg should be raised in front so that the thigh is parallel to the pool floor, and lower leg hangs straight down. Use hand nearest to edge to hold on for balance, with your support leg slightly bent. Your chest should be open, your shoulders down, and your head up.

MOVEMENT: Raise the foot of working leg until it is almost straight (leave a slight flexion). Return to starting position. Repeat with other leg when finished.

TRAINER'S TIPS:
- Maintain stationary position with your torso.
- Concentrate on lifting the lower leg forward and up by contracting the thighs. Focus on your hamstrings when you return to starting position.
- Avoid jerky movements. Exercise should be done in a slow, controlled motion.
- Hold abdominals tight throughout exercise to support the lower back.
- Don't rest between reps.
- Point toes to add frontal resistance through the water.

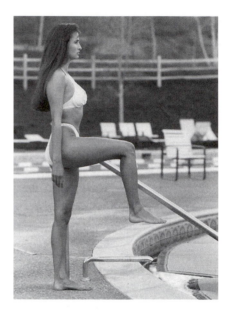

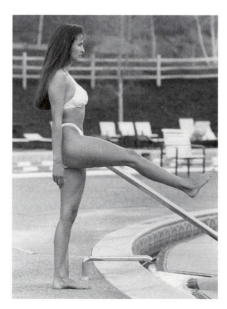

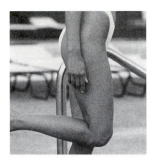

Exercise: Aqua Knee Flexion

DIFFICULTY: 1
LOWER BACK: LOW RISK
AREA: FRONT (QUADRICEPS), BACK (HAMSTRINGS)

STARTING POSITION: Stand with side toward pool's edge in chest-deep water with your feet and your knees slightly bent and together. Use hand nearest to edge to hold on for balance. Your chest should be open, shoulders down, and head up.

MOVEMENT: Pull heel of working leg up toward glutes squeezing your butt and hamstrings. Return to starting position by pushing the foot back down until it is beside your other foot. Repeat with other leg when finished.

TRAINER'S TIPS:
- Maintain stationary position with your torso.
- Focus your mind on your hamstrings, lifting and squeezing on the backward pull, and your thighs contracting on the forward push.
- Avoid jerky movements. Exercise should be done in a slow, controlled motion.
- Hold abdominals tight to support lower back.
- Don't rest between reps.
- Relax muscles of lower leg.

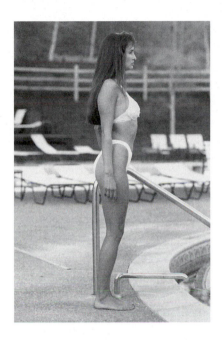

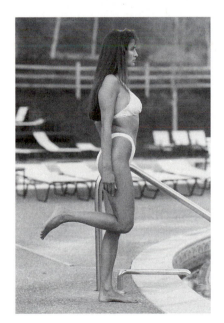

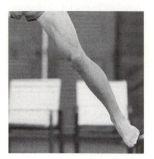

Exercise: Aqua Split Jumps

DIFFICULTY: 2
LOWER BACK: MODERATE TO HIGH RISK
AREA: FRONT (QUADRICEPS), BACK (HAMSTRINGS),
OUTSIDE (ABDUCTORS), INSIDE (ADDUCTORS)

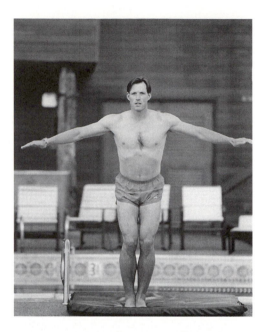

STARTING POSITION: Stand in chest- to waist-deep water with your feet together, your knees slightly bent, and arms extended out for balance.

MOVEMENT: Jump up, pushing both legs out to the sides. Return to starting position by pulling legs back together before you touch the pool bottom.

TRAINER'S TIPS:
- Exercise should be done at maximum effort.
- Hold abdominals tight throughout exercise to support the lower back. Concentrate on correct posture.
- Don't rest between reps.
- Focus mind on feeling the outside of your leg work as you extend out, and on the inside leg muscles when you bring your legs back together.

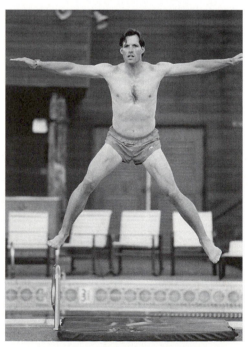

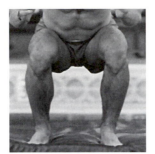

Exercise: Aqua Squat Jumps

DIFFICULTY: 2
LOWER BACK: MODERATE RISK
AREA: FRONT (QUADRICEPS), BACK (GLUTES, HAMSTRINGS)

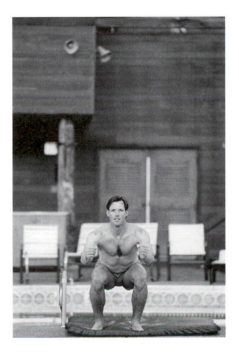

STARTING POSITION: Stand in chest- to waist-deep water with your legs hip width apart. Bend knees to a squatting position (butt parallel to pool floor). Arms at your sides.

MOVEMENT: Jump up by exploding off your heels, bringing your legs together. Return to starting position by pushing your legs back through the water to the squatting position, landing first on your toes, then the balls of your feet, and finally your heels.

TRAINER'S TIPS:
- Exercise should be done at maximum effort.
- Hold abdominals tight throughout exercise to support the lower back.
- Don't rest between reps.
- To assist movement throw arms up as you jump.
- Focus your mind on the leg muscles as you push through the movement.

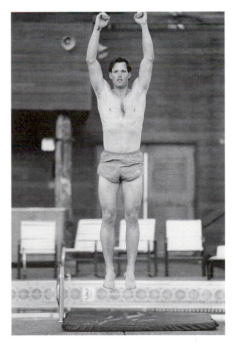

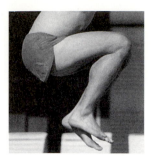

Exercise: Aqua Tuck Jumps

DIFFICULTY: 2
LOWER BACK: HIGH RISK
AREA: FRONT (QUADRICEPS), BACK (GLUTES, HAMSTRINGS)

STARTING POSITION: Stand in chest- to waist-deep water with your feet hip width apart, knees slightly bent, arms at your sides.

MOVEMENT: Push off the bottom of the pool floor with both feet, bringing your knees to your chest. Then push your legs back down through the water to the starting position.

TRAINER'S TIPS:
- Exercise should be done at maximum effort.
- Hold abdominals tight throughout exercise to support the lower back.
- Don't rest between reps.
- To assist movement, pull arms down as you jump.
- Focus your mind on the leg muscles as you push through the movement.

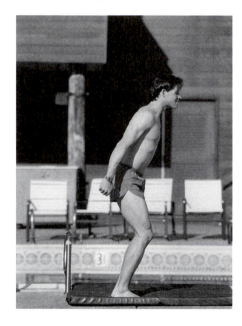

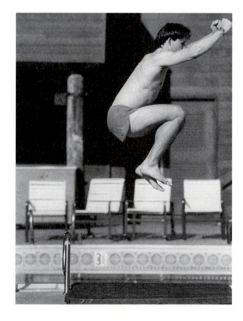

CHAPTER FIFTEEN

The Calves

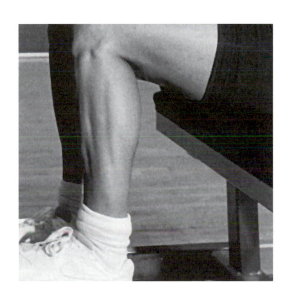

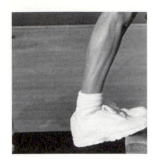

Exercise: Donkey Raises

DIFFICULTY: 1
LOWER BACK: MODERATE RISK
AREA: CALF (GASTROCNEMIUS, SOLEUS)

STARTING POSITION: Stand with legs hip width apart, toes pointed straight ahead (neutral position), heels hanging off an edge of foot support (have the balls of your feet securely placed on edge of machine). Weight is placed toward your big toe on the balls of your feet, with your knees slightly bent. Torso is bent at the waist, perpendicular to lower body, so resistance can be placed on your lower back. Arms are extended and placed against a sturdy object or support handles.

MOVEMENT: Raise feet and ankles, coming up on your toes. Make sure your weight is distributed on the balls of your feet toward your big toe. Hold for a count, then return to the starting position in a three count.

Variations: This exercise can be performed with a single leg or with toes pointed inside (inversion) or outside (eversion). It can also be performed with a partner on your back, for added resistance.

TRAINER'S TIPS:
- Extend calves through a full range of motion.
- Don't rest between steps.
- Vary toe position.
- Keep weight toward inside.
- Employ a full stretch on downward phase.

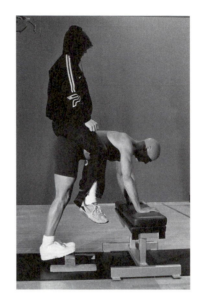

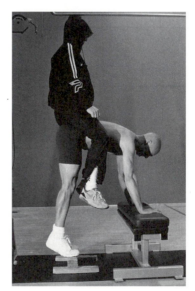

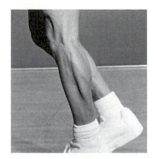

Exercise: Standing Heel Raises

DIFFICULTY: 1
LOWER BACK: MODERATE RISK
AREA: CALF (GASTROCNEMIUS, SOLEUS)

STARTING POSITION: Stand with feet hip width apart, heels hanging off platform (fully stretched), balls of feet placed securely on edge of platform and feet pointed straight ahead (neutral position). Weight should be placed toward your big toe, with your knees slightly bent.

MOVEMENT: Raise your heels off the ground as high as possible while distributing your weight toward your big toe. Hold for a count, then return to the starting position in a three count.

Variations: This exercise can be performed with a single leg, with various forms of resistance (holding one or two dumbbells, a bar across back of neck, or a machine). It can also be performed with toes pointed in (inversion) or out (eversion).

TRAINER'S TIPS:
- When using resistance, keep torso erect.
- Extend through a full range of motion.
- Control speed in downward phase.
- Always keep weight over the balls of the feet.
- Employ a full stretch in downward motion.

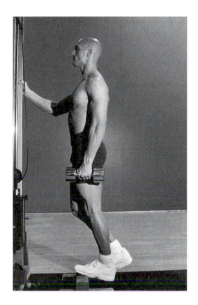

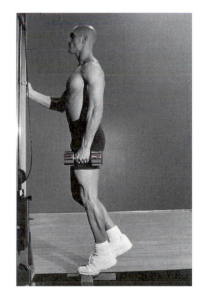

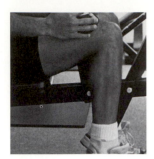

Exercise: Seated Calf Raises (Machine)

DIFFICULTY: 1
LOWER BACK: LOW RISK
AREA: CALF (SOLEUS)

STARTING POSITION: Sit on machine, bend knees, and position your feet comfortably on the platform. Feet are hip width apart, heels are hanging off (fully stretched), balls of feet are placed securely on platform, and toes are pointed straight ahead.

MOVEMENT: Raise your heels off the ground as high as possible while distributing your weight toward your big toe. Hold for a count, then return to the starting position in a three count.

Variations: This exercise can be performed with a single leg or with toes pointed inside (inversion) or outside (eversion).

TRAINER'S TIPS:
- Raise feet through a full range of motion.
- Control speed on downward phase.
- Always keep weight toward inside.
- Employ a full stretch on downward motion.

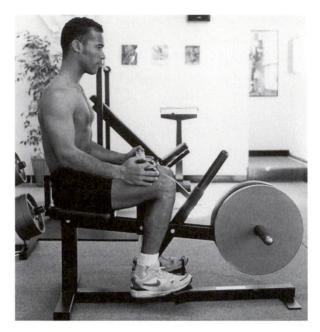

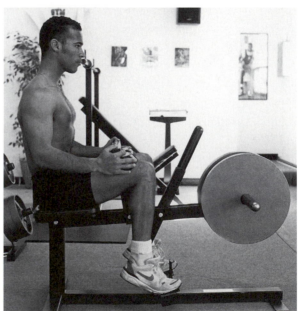

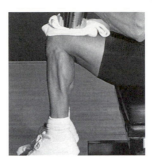

Exercise: Seated or Lying Heel Raises

DIFFICULTY: 1
LOWER BACK: LOW RISK
AREA: CALF (GASTROCNEMIUS, SOLEUS)

STARTING POSITION: Sit on a bench or lie in a hip sled or leg press. (With a machine, your heels should be suspended off the platform so that the balls of both feet are on the edge. Your knees should be slightly flexed.)

MOVEMENT: Push as high on your toes as you can. Return under control to starting position. Keep weight toward inside of foot.

Variations: This exercise may be performed with one leg. It can also be performed with toes pointed in (inversion) or out (eversion).

TRAINER'S TIPS:
- Control the downward stretch and focus on the calf as you push up.
- Maintain slight flexion in the knee throughout the exercise.

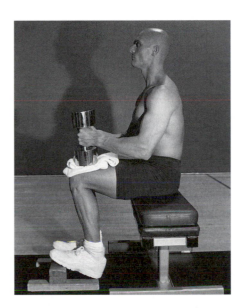

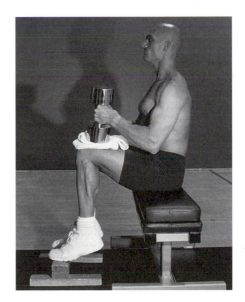

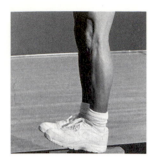

Exercise: Standing Balance Toe Raises

DIFFICULTY: 1
LOWER BACK: LOW RISK
AREA: FRONT OF CALF (ANTERIOR TIBIALUS)

STARTING POSITION: Place the heels of both feet on platform, toes suspended off the platform so that the heels (at the arch) of both feet are on the edge. Your knees should be slightly flexed and your hands should hang on to the stable object (post or wall) in front for balance.

MOVEMENT: Raise toes straight up as high as you can. Lower under control back to the starting position.

Variations: This motion can be performed using body weight, dumbbells, a barbell for resistance, or a machine that will allow you to safely execute this movement. It can also be performed with one leg. (In this case place the foot of the nonexercising leg behind the Achilles tendon of the working leg.) You can also vary the exercise by changing your foot positions—inverted and everted.

TRAINER'S TIPS:
- Control the downward stretch and focus on the front of the calf as you push up.
- Maintain slight flexion in the knee throughout the exercise.

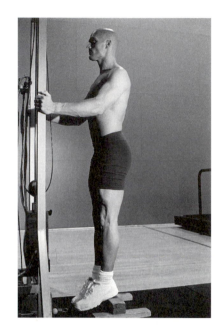

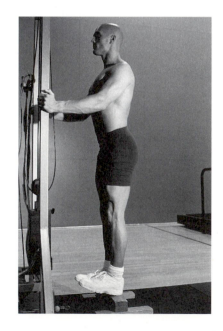

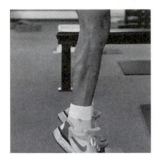

Exercise: Standing Heel Raises (Machine)

DIFFICULTY: 1
LOWER BACK: MODERATE RISK
AREA: CALF (GASTROCNEMIUS, SOLEUS)

STARTING POSITION: Adjust shoulder pads so that they are below the shoulder level. Step on platform, bend knees, and position your shoulders comfortably under the pads. Extend legs and elevate shoulder sled. Place feet hip width apart, heels hanging off (fully stretched), and feet pointed straight ahead in the neutral position (have the ball of your foot securely placed on edge of machine). Weight should be placed toward your big toe with your knees slightly bent.

MOVEMENT: Raise your heels off the ground as high as possible while distributing your weight toward your big toe. Hold for a one count, then return to the starting position in a three count.

Variations: This exercise can be performed with a single leg or with toes pointed inside (inversion) or outside (eversion).

TRAINER'S TIPS:
- When using resistance, keep torso erect.
- Extend through a full range of motion.
- Control speed.
- Always keep weight on the balls of feet.

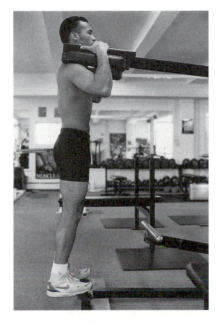

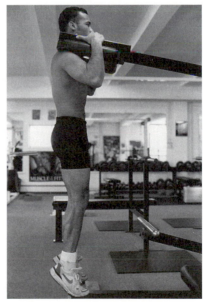

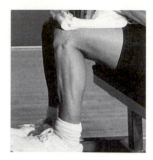

Exercise: Seated Toe Raises

DIFFICULTY: 1
LOWER BACK: LOW RISK
AREA: CALF (SOLEUS)

STARTING POSITION: Sit on a bench, toes suspended off platform.

MOVEMENT: Raise toes as high as you can off floor, and return to starting position in a controlled manner.

TRAINER'S TIPS:
- Do not let your toes rest on the floor between repetitions.
- Control upward and downward phases of the movement.
- Focus your mind on your calf muscles.

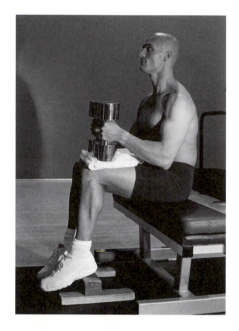

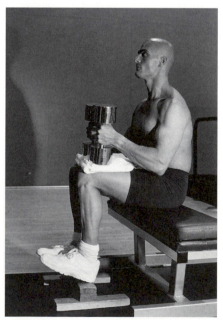

CHAPTER SIXTEEN

The Machines

DAVE JOHNSON

The purpose of this chapter is to outline the basic features of some of the popular machines found in health clubs, and to give you instructional guidelines. Sometimes it is difficult to receive personal instruction at a gym. The manufacturer's instructions and illustrations in this chapter will allow you to review at home proper machine usage. As with any of the other lower body routines, mastering the technique while using the machines is vital to insuring optimum results and safety. Be sure to read all caution labels before using any equipment and if it appears damaged or inoperable, do not attempt to use it. If possible, seek qualified instruction from a trainer at your club. But if you cannot, the following should help you on your way.

Paramount—Leg Curl

A. FEATURES

1. Solid-steel centering plate
2. Adjustable back support
3. Adjustable leg pad
4. Adjustable thigh pad
5. Padded handles

B. INSTRUCTIONS

1. From a seated position select desired weight amount.
2. Adjust the leg pad to a comfortable position.
3. Sit down and place legs on top of the leg pad, right leg first.

4. Align your knee with the pivot point and adjust the seat back to a comfortable position.

5. Adjust the thigh pad down to a comfortable position. Grip handles.

6. Flex your legs downward as far as possible at a controlled speed of movement.

7. Return to original position and repeat.

C. MUSCLES TRAINED

1. Hamstrings
2. Gastrocnemius
3. Sartorius
4. Gracilis

Paramount—Leg Extension

A. FEATURES

1. Solid-steel centering plate
2. Adjustable back support
3. Adjustable leg pad
4. Padded handles

B. INSTRUCTIONS

1. From a seated position select desired weight amount.

2. Adjust the leg pad to a comfortable position.

3. Align your knee with the pivot point and adjust the seat back to a comfortable position.

4. Grip handles. Keep back straight against the seat.

5. Extend legs forward as far as possible at a controlled speed of movement.

6. Return to original position and repeat.

C. MUSCLES TRAINED

1. Quadriceps Femoris

Paramount—Leg Press

A. FEATURES

1. Solid-steel centering plate
2. Adjustable back support
3. Adjustable shoulder pads
4. Foot platforms
5. Padded handles

B. INSTRUCTIONS

1. From the horizontal position select desired weight amount.

2. Position feet on the upper or lower section of the foot pad.

3. Adjust the carriage so that your legs are bent approximately 90 degrees at the knees.

4. Grasp the foam handles on either side of your head.

5. Relax your neck muscles and press with the legs. Do not allow the knees to lock out at full extension.

6. Return to original position and repeat.

C. MUSCLES TRAINED

1. Quadriceps
2. Hamstrings
3. Gluteus Maximus
4. Gastocnemius

Nautilus—Seated Leg Curl

A. FEATURES

1. Solid-steel centering plate
2. Adjustable back support
3. Leg pad
4. Padded handles

B. INSTRUCTIONS

1. Sit on the seat of the machine.
2. Place your lower legs between the two roller pads. The end pad should be behind your ankles and the other one should be in front of your shins, just below your knees.
3. Align your knee joints with the axis of rotation of the movement arm. The axis is marked with a red dot.
4. Pull the seat back forward until it comes in contact with your buttocks.
5. Grasp the handles lightly.
6. Curl your legs and try to touch your buttocks with your heels. Simultaneously try to raise your toes to your knees.
7. Return to the starting position, letting the weight stack barely touch and your ankles relax, then repeat.

C. MUSCLES TRAINED

1. Hamstrings

Nautilus—Leg Extension

A. FEATURES

1. Solid-steel centering plate
2. Adjustable back support
3. Leg pad
4. Optional neck support
5. Padded handles

B. INSTRUCTIONS

1. Sit on the seat of the machine.
2. Lean forward and place your shins behind the roller pad.
3. Adjust the seat back until it is securely against your buttocks.
4. Make sure your knees are aligned with the axis of rotation of the movement arm. The axis is marked with a red dot.
5. Place a small pad behind your head if you find any discomfort in the neck area.
6. Push the movement arm forward and upward. Be sure to reach full knee extension. Grasp the handles for stability during the last 45 degrees of extension.
7. Pause at full extension and evenly release your hands.
8. Lower the movement arm until the weight stack barely touches, then repeat.

C. MUSCLES TRAINED

1. Quadriceps Femoris

Nautilus—Leg Press

A. FEATURES

1. Solid-steel centering plate
2. Adjustable back support
3. Optional head support
4. Buttocks support
5. Foot platforms
6. Padded handles

B. INSTRUCTIONS

1. Sit on the machine and put your feet on the platform of the machine's movement arm. Your feet should be perfectly flat on the platform, about shoulder width apart, with your feet parallel. The seat should be adjusted so that your thighs are as close as possible to your chest. If necessary, lift the release handle thus moving the seat toward the foot pedal. Repeat to move closer. Seat is in proper position when the movement arm hits a stop in the extended position.
2. Dangle your arms and relax your upper body. Use a small pad behind your head if needed for comfort.
3. Push forward with your legs, stopping just short of the point where your knees are locked. Your feet should remain flat on the platform throughout each repetition.
4. Lower the resistance slowly and smoothly to the starting position. Slow, smooth turnarounds are mandatory at both the top and bottom positions.
5. Repeat.

C. MUSCLES TRAINED

1. Quadriceps
2. Hamstrings
3. Gluteus Maximus

Nautilus—Seated Calf

A. FEATURES

1. Solid-steel centering plate
2. Adjustable back support
3. Foot platform
4. Padded handles

B. INSTRUCTIONS

1. Adjust the seat so that when you are seated your legs are straight at the knee and your back fits firmly against the back pad. Place hands on the seat handles.
2. Position your feet on the platform so that the back of your heel rests against the bottom lip of the platform. This will align your ankles with the axis of rotation.
3. Rotate your feet downward so that full contraction of the calves is reached. If your heels come off the platform, then adjust the seat slightly forward.
4. Pause, then return slowly to the stretched position and repeat.

C. MUSCLES TRAINED

1. Gastrocnemius and soleus

Butt Blaster 990 (Plate Load)

A. FEATURES
1. State-of-the-art linear bearings
2. Heavy-duty steel-frame construction
3. Lightweight antislip foot cart
4. Steel safety shields
5. User plaque
6. Manual plate loading in rear with spare plate loader

B. INSTRUCTIONS
1. Add desired weight in two-and-a-half- to twenty-five-pound increments.
2. Position knee and elbows on pads.
3. Place foot on cart and push upward. Do not fully extend leg to lockout position.
4. Pause, then return slowly to the stretched position and repeat.

C. MUSCLES TRAINED
1. Gluteals
2. Quadriceps
3. Hamstrings

Life Circuit—Leg Extension, Leg Curl, and Leg Press

A. FEATURES
1. Setup Test—Simple test of available strength automatically programs machine for safe, maximum resistance when you select your program.
2. Manual Setup—You can override the Setup Test and punch in your own weight, in one-pound increments.
3. Optional Heavy Negative—In the Lifecircuit Program, or by entering a "2" after selecting the Regular Program, you automatically call up a negative (eccentric) resistance 15 to 40 percent heavier than the positive (concentric) resistance for each repetition.
4. Electronic Spotter—Speed sensor sounds a double beep and flashes a "Rep too fast, move more slowly" sign on message center when you use momentum, not strength. If you ignore the signals and move still faster, the movement arm locks in place, stopping your motion.
5. Repeat Set Key—After you perform one set, you can move immediately into another set by pushing this key. Machine resets to no program after thirty seconds idle.
6. "+" and "−" Keys—At any time in any set you can move weight up or down in five-pound increments by touching either key.
7. Negative Only—This provides resistance on eccentric motion only, which provides both a training option for variety and a rehabilitation tool.
8. Range of Motion Limiter—On the first repetition, concentric and eccentric arc sets program in automatically for the rest of the set.

B. INSTRUCTIONS

1. Scrolling Message Center gives a step-by-step instructional guide through every part of the workout.

C. MUSCLES TRAINED

1. Gluteals
2. Quadriceps
3. Hamstrings

Cybex—Leg Curl

A. FEATURES

1. Divergent angle between hip and chest pads to minimize possibility of back hyperextension
2. Contoured chest pad
3. Solid-steel construction
4. Padded handles

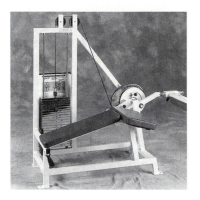

B. INSTRUCTIONS

1. Adjust the leg pad so that pad is positioned just above the Achilles tendon.
2. Adjust body position on bench so that knees are located off the bench and are aligned with the machine's axis of rotation.
3. Start movement by curling heels to buttocks with a smooth, controlled motion.
4. Slowly return to start position.

C. MUSCLES TRAINED

1. Hamstrings
2. Gastrocnemius
3. Sartorius/Gracilis

Cybex—Seated Leg Curl

A. FEATURES
1. Adjustable thigh stabilization pad
2. Range-of-motion device that adjusts in 10-degree increments
3. An adjustable back pad
4. Solid-steel construction
5. Padded handles

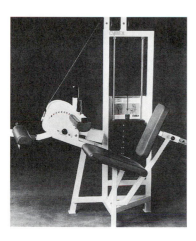

B. INSTRUCTIONS
1. Adjust the back pad so that knee is aligned with machine axis (at top of input arm).
2. Select desired resistance.
3. If range limiting is desired, use body weight to move exercise arm to start position and insert pull button in range-of-motion device on right-hand side of machine next to cam.
4. Adjust ankle pad so that the back of ankles rest comfortably on pad, just above the ankle joint.
5. Release pull button and drop thigh stabilization pad so that it is snugly against thigh; tighten lock knob to secure.
6. Start movement by curling heels back toward buttocks.
7. Slowly return to start position with a smooth, continuous motion.
8. To exit, loosen lock knob and raise thigh stabilization pad until pull button engages.

C. MUSCLES TRAINED
1. Hamstrings

Cybex—Leg Extension

A. FEATURES
1. Adjustable offset input arm allowing the pad to adjust for tibia length
2. Contoured seat pad
3. An adjustable back pad
4. Solid-steel construction
5. Padded handles

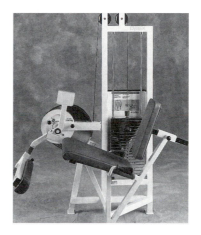

B. INSTRUCTIONS
1. Adjust shin pad so that pad rests just above the ankle.
2. Adjust back pad so that knees align with machine axis of rotation; area behind knees should lightly contact the edge of the seat pad.
3. Start movement by slowly extending legs with a smooth, controlled motion.
4. Slowly return to start position.

C. MUSCLES TRAINED
1. Quadriceps
2. Rectus Femoris

Cybex—Leg Press

A. FEATURES

1. A gravity-neutral plane back pad
2. Elbow pads
3. Large, angled foot platform for various foot placements
4. A calf block on the foot platform
5. Solid-steel construction
6. Padded handles

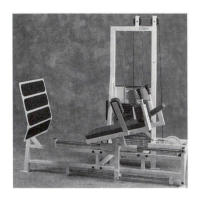

B. INSTRUCTIONS

1. Adjust starting position of sled for desired knee angle using the pull button located next to the sled.
2. Adjust body position on sled so that head, shoulders, and elbows remain in contact with pads, knees aligned with big toe.
   Note: Many foot positions are possible that may change the emphasis on muscles trained; in general, maintain a foot position that keeps toes at or above the height of knees when at start of movement.
3. Start movement by straightening legs with a smooth, controlled motion. Do not hyperextend or lock out knees.
4. Pause briefly in the lifted position.
5. Slowly return to start position.

C. MUSCLES TRAINED

1. Quadriceps
2. Hamstrings
3. Gluteal group
4. Gastocnemius
5. Soleus

Cybex—Standing Calf Raise

A. FEATURES

1. Dual foot plates
2. Adjustable input arm to accommodate height
3. A one-to-one lifting ratio
4. An optional free weight kit allowing for an addition of plates for resistance above the three hundred pounds on the weight stack
5. Solid-steel construction
6. Padded handles

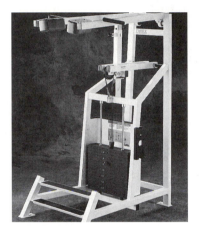

B. INSTRUCTIONS

1. Select the foot plate that allows the shoulder pads to be as close to parallel with the ground as possible.
   Note: Individuals five-feet-two or under generally use upper foot plate.
2. Adjust the shoulder pads so that the weight plates selected are in a slightly raised position when heels are in full dorsi flexion. Maintain correct posture: chin in, shoulders back, chest high, knees over toes, hips tucked in.
3. Start movement by elevating heels as far up as possible with a smooth, continuous motion.
4. Slowly return to the starting position by lowering heels.

C. MUSCLES TRAINED

1. Gastocnemius
2. Soleus
3. Plantaris

Cybex—Hip Adduction

A. FEATURES
1. Front mounted weight stack
2. An upright exercise position
3. Dual foot pegs
4. Leg pads
5. Solid-steel construction
6. Padded handles

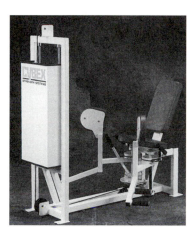

B. INSTRUCTIONS
1. Sit in machine and adjust range of motion by moving knee pads to desired start position.
2. Grip handles lightly.
3. Lift/lower weights with smooth controlled movements.
4. Exit machine by returning weights to resting position and release knee pads by pulling the release handle that is located on your right.

C. MUSCLES TRAINED
1. Hip adductors

Cybex—Hip Abduction

A. FEATURES
1. Front mounted weight stack
2. An upright exercise position
3. Dual foot pegs
4. Leg pads
5. Solid-steel construction
6. Padded handles

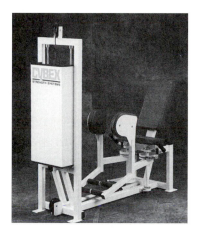

B. INSTRUCTIONS
1. Sit in machine and adjust range of motion by moving knee pads to desired start position.
2. Grip handles lightly.
3. Lift/lower weights with smooth controlled movements.
4. Exit machine by returning weights to resting position and release knee pads by pulling the release handle that is located on your right.

C. MUSCLES TRAINED
1. Hip abductors

Cybex—Multi Hip

A. FEATURES

1. A functional standing position for hip flexion/extension and abduction/adduction in one space
2. Adjustable foot platform
3. Start position adjustable in 15-degree increments
4. Leg pad
5. Solid-steel construction
6. Padded handles

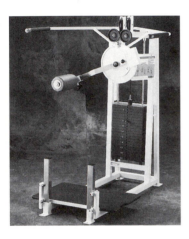

B. INSTRUCTIONS

1. Adjust platform height so that hip joint aligns with the axis of the pivot arm.
2. Adjust position of the leg pad so that the pad contact is just above the knee.
3. Select exercise. The reference chart below indicates the correct procedures for each movement.
4. Align the involved joint with the axis of the pivot arm and grasp handles for stabilization.
5. Start and end movement with smooth, controlled motions.

Hip Flexion

a. For Right Hip Flexion: Position the leg pad between 4 and 6 o'clock.
   For Left Hip Flexion: Position the leg pad between 6 and 8 o'clock.
b. Stand as indicated in machine illustration with the side to be exercised closest to the pivot arm. Align the hip with the axis of the pivot arm and grasp handles for stabilization. The leg pad should be positioned comfortably across the front of the leg, just above the knee.
c. Lift the leg bar to complete forward flexion and lower to extension with smooth, controlled motions.

Hip Extension

a. For Right Hip Extension: Position the leg pad between 7 and 9 o'clock.
   For Left Hip Extension: Position the leg pad between 3 and 5 o'clock.
b. Stand as indicated in machine illustration with the side to be exercised closest to the pivot arm. Align the hip with the axis of the pivot arm and grasp handles for stabilization. The leg pad should be positioned comfortably across the back of the leg, just above the knee.
c. Lift the leg bar to complete backward extension and lower to flexion with smooth, controlled motions.

Hip Adduction

a. For Right Hip Adduction: Position the leg pad between 3 and 5 o'clock.
   For Left Hip Adduction: Position the leg pad between 7 and 9 o'clock.
b. Stand as indicated in machine illustration with the side to be exercised aligned with the axis of pivot arm. Grasp handles for stabilization. The leg pad should be positioned comfortably across the inside of the leg, just above the knee.
c. Lift the leg bar across the standing leg to complete adduction and lower to the start position with smooth, controlled motions.

Hip Abduction

a. For Right Hip Abduction: Position the leg pad between 6 and 8 o'clock.
   For Left Hip Abduction: Position the leg pad between 4 and 6 o'clock.
b. Stand as indicated in machine illustration with the side to be exercised aligned with the axis of

pivot arm. Grasp handles for stabilization. The leg pad should be positioned comfortably across the outside of the leg, just above the knee.

c. Lift the leg bar away from the standing leg to complete abduction and lower to the start position with smooth, controlled motions.

C. MUSCLES TRAINED

1. Iliopsosas
2. Rectus Femoris
3. Pectineus
4. Gluteal group
5. Hamstrings
6. Adductor Magnus
7. Longus
8. Brevis
9. Gracilis
10. Gluteus Medius
11. Gluteus Minimus
12. Gluteus Maximus
13. Tensor Fasciae
14. Sartorius

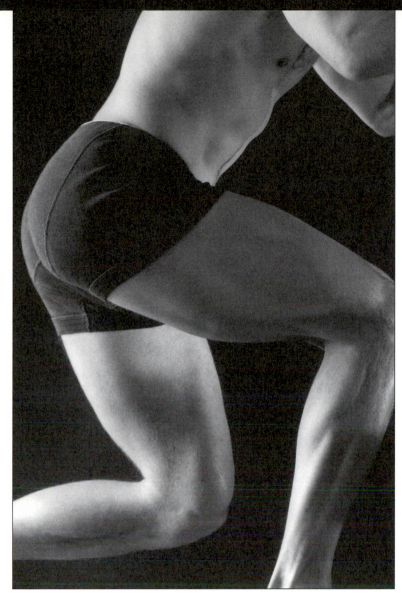

The Routines

CHAPTER SEVENTEEN

Introduction to the System

The system is divided into five programs to meet your individual needs. The programs are: Gym Men (designed for men who wish to work out in a club), Gym Women (designed for women who wish to work out in a club), Home Men (designed for men who wish to work out at home), Home Women (designed for women who wish to work out at home), and Ultimate Butt and Legs (designed to take you to your highest potential in terms of looks, endurance, strength, and power). Both of the Gym routines are six-month programs for strengthening and developing your butt, legs, and calves. The Home routines are fifteen-week programs designed to strengthen and develop your butt, legs, and calves without the use of weights (although rubber bands or ankle weights may be used). The Ultimate Butt and Legs routine is a highly advanced three-month program designed to bring your butt, legs, and calves to their full potential. You should not begin this program until you have completed all of the levels of the Gym Men or Women routines.

These programs do all of the planning for you. They incorporate the training principles discussed in chapter three into each workout. The only thing you have to do is commit to the plan.

Each level in every program stands on its own and leads progressively into the next level. Depending on your own personal needs and goals, you may complete an entire program, or stop at any level and go on a maintenance routine.

Maintenance Routines

The goal of a maintenance routine is to keep the benefits you have worked so hard to achieve. If you finish a level and don't want to move on, you need to follow a maintenance routine. You cannot just stop exercising. Consistency is the key to achieving and keeping the health benefits of exercise. You can maintain your results for each level by following the routine for the last week of the level completed. For example, if you just wanted the benefits of Level 3 for Gym Men, you would follow the workout of Week 3, three times a week. In most cases, it doesn't take as much to maintain as it does to build. If you want to increase the intensity of your maintenance routine, you can go for two options: increasing the weight (if you're doing the Gym program), or repetitions (if you're doing the Home program), or the number of sets (in either program) for each exercise. Just remember that if you increase the sets for the front part of the leg, you should also increase the sets for the back side, in the same proportion as you did for the front. The same is true for the inside and outside of the leg.

It is important to note that even though a maintenance program may be effective for a period of time, the body will ultimately grow complacent. The reasons for this are simple: A maintenance program does not adhere to the principles of progression, overload, and variety. There will be deterioration over time. You cannot sustain the same fitness level if you do not shock the body and force it to adapt.

Advancement

Everyone will progress at different speeds. Each level is designed to move you to the next level. If for some reason you do not feel ready to move on, spend another week, or two weeks if necessary, on your current level. Listen to your body. It will tell you if you feel comfortable moving on, but also keep in mind that you must shock the body to achieve growth. Don't stay too long on a level. To be what you have never been, you must do what you have never done. Therefore, you must force yourself to move on.

And don't forget, you need to follow a healthy diet, cut down on your fat content, and do some type of cardiovascular work at least three to four times a week. The combination of all these factors will create the look, feel, or other benefits you want.

Substitutions

If there is an exercise in any of the systems that you can't do for whatever reason—e.g., bad pain, lack of equipment, inability to correctly perform the exercise—then substitute. You need to choose an exercise that works the same area(s), has the same difficulty level, and isn't already in the routine. If you have exhausted all options, you can repeat an exercise that is already in the routine that fits these criteria.

Multisets

Multisets are sets comprising two or more exercises in which there is no rest period between the exercises, until the required number of repetitions for each exercise has been completed once. For example, a Squat and a Sissy Squat may be grouped in what is called a Super Set. The program may call for three sets of Super Sets, eight repetitions each. This means that you will perform eight repetitions of the Squat and then without any rest you will perform eight repetitions of the Sissy Squat. You will then rest the required time and then repeat both the Squat and Sissy Squat eight times, rest again, and repeat the Squat and Sissy Squat eight more times.

In the different programs, exercises may on occasion be grouped together. These groupings are referred to as CS, SS, TS, or GS. The following is the key to these abbreviations:

CS—*Compound Set:* A Compound Set consists of two different exercises in which opposite (agonist/antagonist) sides of a joint are worked. For example, you would do the prescribed number of reps for the Leg Extension (quads/front) immediately followed by the prescribed number of reps for Leg Curls (hamstrings/back), followed by rest. Those two exercises performed back to back equal one set. Then repeat for the prescribed number of sets.

SS—Super Set: A Super Set consists of two different exercises in which the same muscle groups are worked. For example, Standing Abductions (abductors/outside) and Lying Bent-Leg Side Raises (abductors/outside) are performed back to back, in the same fashion as the compound set, above.

TS—Tri Set: A Tri Set consists of three different exercises in which the same muscle groups are worked. For example, Seated Inside Raises (adductors/inside) are performed for the prescribed number of reps, followed by Standing Adductions (adductors/inside), and then Lying Adductions (adductors/inside), each of the latter two also performed for the prescribed number of reps. After completing all three in a row, you have done one set. Rest and repeat.

GS—Giant Set: A Giant Set consists of four or more different exercises in which the same muscle groups are worked. For example, Standing Kickbacks (glutes/back), Bent-Leg Kickbacks (glutes/back), Pelvic Lifts (glutes/back), and Backward Leg Raises (glutes/back) are performed back to back in the same manner as Super Sets, above.

Recovery Principles

It is important that you have adequate recovery for your muscles when engaged in a weight program. Current research indicates that you need a minimum of forty-eight hours recovery in between lifting the same body part; seventy-two hours is optimal; and after ninety-six hours you may start to atrophy (lose muscle size and strength). Failure to follow the above recovery guidelines will result in overtraining. It also will prevent you from obtaining the best possible results and could lead to injury. In addition, if you do not train frequently enough you will lose results that you have already attained.

Planning Your Workouts

In some levels you will work out two days a week, in others three. Remember your recovery principles when planning workouts.

The best plan for the levels in which you work out three times a week is to lift on Monday, Wednesday, and Friday. Another option would be to lift Tuesday, Thursday, and Saturday. The best plan for the levels in which you work out two times a week is to lift on Monday and Thursday, Tuesday and Friday, or Wednesday and Saturday. The most important thing is plan the days and times you know you can work out consistently, and stick with that schedule.

CHAPTER EIGHTEEN

Gym Men

Level 1: Preconditioning and the Foundation

This level is designed to build the base that will allow you to move to more sophisticated workouts down the road. It is a high-volume, low-intensity workout that will create muscle hypertrophy (increase in the cross-sectional size of the muscle fiber). This prepares you for more work down the road. It is important that you focus on proper technique. This will pay dividends for you later. Enjoy the workout. Every day you are improving yourself both mentally and physically, so give yourself credit for those victories.

WEEK 1

DAY 1 (E.G., MONDAY)

Exercises	Sets	Reps	Rest
Leg Press	1	15–20	90 seconds
Leg Curls	1	15–20	90 seconds
Post Squat	1	15–20	90 seconds
Prone Single-Leg Raises	1	15	90 seconds
Gym Calf Sequence 1 (refer to page 253)			

DAYS 2 AND 3 (E.G., WEDNESDAY AND FRIDAY)

Exercises	Sets	Reps	Rest
Leg Press	2	15–20	90 seconds
Leg Curls	2	15–20	90 seconds
Post Squat	2	15–20	90 seconds
Prone Single-Leg Raises	1	15	90 seconds
Gym Calf Sequence 1 (refer to page 253)			

WEEKS 2 AND 3

DAYS 1, 2, AND 3

Exercises	Sets	Reps	Rest
Leg Press	3	15–20	90 seconds
Leg Curls	3	15–20	90 seconds
Post Squat	3	15–20	90 seconds
Prone Single-Leg Raises	1	15	90 seconds

Gym Calf Sequence 1 (refer to page 253)

WEEKS 4, 5, AND 6

DAYS 1, 2, AND 3

Exercises	Sets	Reps	Rest
Front Lunge Pumps	3	12–15	75 seconds
Leg Curls	3	12–15	75 seconds
Balance Squat (with Bench)	3	12–15	75 seconds
Leg Press	2	12–15	75 seconds
Prone Double-Leg Raises	2	15	75 seconds

Gym Calf Sequence 1 (refer to page 253)

WEEKS 7, 8, AND 9

DAYS 1, 2, AND 3

Exercises	Sets	Reps	Rest
Front Lunge (Pumps)	3	8	75 seconds
Leg Curls	3	10	75 seconds
Front Lunge (Alternating)	3	8	75 seconds
Standing Adductions	1	10	75 seconds
Standing Abductions	1	10	75 seconds
Leg Press	3	8	75 seconds
Back Extension	1	15	75 seconds

Gym Calf Sequence 1 (refer to page 253)

Level 2: Creating Strength and Power

This level will begin to help you create the strength and power of your goals. Your base has been established and you can now begin to focus more on improving your strength and power along with bringing out the definition in your butt and legs. You will move from high volume/low intensity to low volume/high intensity in this level. Concentrate on your technique at all times, especially when your weight (intensity) increases.

WEEKS 1, 2, AND 3

DAYS 1, 2, AND 3

Exercises	Sets	Reps	Rest
Front Squat	3	15	60 seconds
Stiff-Leg Dead Lift	3	15	60 seconds
Standing Leg Curls	3	15	60 seconds
Front Lunge (Alternating)	3	15	60 seconds
Standing Adduction	2	15	60 seconds
Standing Abductions	2	15	60 seconds
Back Extension	2	15	60 seconds

Gym Calf Sequence 2 (refer to page 253)

WEEKS 4, 5, AND 6

DAYS 1, 2, AND 3

Exercises	Sets	Reps	Rest
Squat	4	8	60 seconds
Standing Leg Curls	3	8	60 seconds
Lunge Pulls (Alternating)	4	8	60 seconds
Stiff-Leg Dead Lift	3	8	60 seconds
Side Lunge (Alternating)	2	8	60 seconds
Back Extension	2	15	60 seconds

Gym Calf Sequence 2 (refer to page 253)

WEEK 7—ONE WEEK OF ACTIVE REST

WEEKS 8, 9, AND 10

DAYS 1 AND 3 (E.G., MONDAY AND FRIDAY)

Exercises	Sets	Reps	Rest
Front Squat	3	12	60 seconds
Leg Curls	3	12	60 seconds
Leg Press or Hack			
Squat (Machine)	3	12	60 seconds
Back Lunge Push	3	12	60 seconds
Standing Adduction	3	12	60 seconds
Standing Abduction	3	12	60 seconds
Back Extension	2	15	60 seconds

Gym Calf Sequence 2, Days 1 and 3 (refer to page 253)

DAY 2 (E.G., WEDNESDAY)

Exercises	Sets	Reps	Rest
Front Box Lunge (Pumps)	3	12	60 seconds
Stiff-Leg Dead Lift	3	12	60 seconds
Back Side Lunge	3	12	60 seconds
Leg Press			
(Negative Emphasis)	3	12	60 seconds
Back Extension with a Twist	1	12	60 seconds

Gym Calf Sequence 1 (refer to page 253)

WEEKS 11, 12, AND 13

DAY 1 (E.G., MONDAY)

Exercises	Sets	Reps	Rest
Squat	4	7–7–5–5	60 seconds
Stiff-Leg Dead Lift	4	7–7–5–5	60 seconds
Front Lunge (Pumps)	4	5–5–5–10	60 seconds
Leg Curls	4	5–5–5–10	60 seconds
Back Lunge Push (Alternating)	1	8	60 seconds
Side Lunge (Alternating)	1	8	60 seconds
Back Extension with a Twist	2	10 each side	60 seconds

Gym Calf Sequence 3, Days 1 and 3 (refer to pages 253–54)

DAY 2 (E.G., THURSDAY)

Exercises	Sets	Reps	Rest
Squat	3	12	60 seconds
Good Mornings	3	12	60 seconds
Front Lunge Pumps	3	12	60 seconds
Standing Leg Curls	3	12	60 seconds
Back Lunge Pull (Walk)	1	15	60 seconds
Side Lunge (Alternating)	1	15	60 seconds
Back Extension	2	20	60 seconds

Gym Calf Sequence 1 (refer to page 253)

Level 3: Achieving Strength and Power

This level will refine and increase your strength, power, and definition. It is a three-week kick-your-butt program that will send you over the top in achieving your goals. Continue to concentrate on your techniques both mentally and physically and enjoy yourself. The workouts may be hard but you'll feel the strength and power you're gaining every session. Note: Refer to pages 236–37 for explanation of CS, SS, TS, and GS.

WEEK 1

DAYS 1, 2, AND 3

Exercises	Sets	Reps	Rest
Front Squat	3	15	60 seconds
Leg Curls	3	15	60 seconds
CS—Balance Squat (with Bench), Good Mornings	3	15 each	60 seconds between each CS

Exercises	Sets	Reps	Rest
SS—Leg Extension, Sissy Squat	2	15 each	60 seconds between each SS
Standing Adduction	2	15	60 seconds
Standing Abduction	2	15	60 seconds
Back Extension	2	15	60 seconds

Gym Calf Sequence 2 (refer to page 253)

WEEK 2

DAYS 1 AND 2 (E.G., MONDAY AND THURSDAY)

Exercises	Sets	Reps	Rest
TS—Squat, Hack Squat or Leg Press, Front Lunge (Pumps)	3	8 each	60 seconds between each TS
TS—Back Lunge Push, Good Mornings, Leg Curls	3	8 each	60 seconds between each TS
TS—Standing Adduction, Standing Abduction, Back Extension with a Twist	3	8 each	60 seconds between each TS

Gym Calf Sequence 3, Days 1 and 3 (refer to pages 253–54)

WEEK 3

DAY 1 (E.G., MONDAY)

Exercises	Sets	Reps	Rest
Squat	5	5–5–5–5–12	60 seconds
Leg Curls	5	5–5–5–5–12	60 seconds
Front Lunge (Alternating)	4	5–5–5–12	60 seconds
Stiff-Leg Dead Lift	4	5–5–5–12	60 seconds
Side Lunge (Alternating)	4	5–5–5–12	60 seconds
Back Extension (Your Choice)	3	10	60 seconds

Gym Calf Sequence 4, Days 1 and 3 (refer to page 256)

DAY 2 (E.G., THURSDAY)

Exercises	Sets	Reps	Rest
Squat	3	12	60 seconds
Leg Curls	3	12	60 seconds
Front Lunge (Alternating)	3	12	60 seconds
Stiff-Leg Dead Lift	3	12	60 seconds
Side Lunge (Alternating)	3	12	60 seconds
Back Extension (Your Choice)	3	10	60 seconds

Gym Calf Sequence 4, Day 2 (refer to page 256)

CHAPTER NINETEEN

Gym Women

Level 1: Preconditioning and the Foundation

This level is designed to build the base that will allow you to move on to more sophisticated workouts. It is a high-volume, low-intensity workout that will create muscle hypertrophy (increase in the cross-sectional size of the muscle fiber). This prepares you for more work down the road. It is important that you focus on proper technique. This will pay dividends for you later. Enjoy the workout. Every day you are improving yourself both mentally and physically, so give yourself credit for those victories.

WEEK 1

DAY 1 (E.G., MONDAY)

Exercises	Sets	Reps	Rest
Leg Press	1	15 to 20	90 seconds
Leg Curls	1	15 to 20	90 seconds
Post Squats	1	15 to 20	90 seconds
Standing Adduction	1	15 to 20	90 seconds
Standing Abduction	1	15 to 20	90 seconds
Prone Single-Leg Raises	1	15	90 seconds

Gym Calf Sequence 1 (refer to page 253)

DAYS 2 AND 3 (E.G., WEDNESDAY AND FRIDAY)

Exercises	Sets	Reps	Rest
Leg Press	2	15 to 20	90 seconds
Leg Curls	2	15 to 20	90 seconds
Post Squat	2	15 to 20	90 seconds

	Sets	Reps	Rest
Standing Adduction	2	15 to 20	90 seconds
Standing Abduction	2	15 to 20	90 seconds
Prone Single-Leg Raises	1	15	90 seconds
Gym Calf Sequence 1 (refer to page 253)			

WEEKS 2 AND 3

DAYS 1, 2, AND 3

Exercises	Sets	Reps	Rest
Leg Press	3	15 to 20	90 seconds
Leg Curls	3	15 to 20	90 seconds
Post Squat	2	15 to 20	90 seconds
Standing Adduction	2	15 to 20	90 seconds
Standing Abduction	2	15 to 20	90 seconds
Prone Single-Leg Raises	1	15	90 seconds
Gym Calf Sequence 1 (refer to page 253)			

WEEKS 4, 5, AND 6

DAYS 1, 2, AND 3

Exercises	Sets	Reps	Rest
Single-Leg Post Squat	3	12–15	75 seconds
Leg Curls	3	12–15	75 seconds
Leg Press	2	12–15	75 seconds
Standing Adduction	2	15	75 seconds
Standing Abduction	2	15	75 seconds
Standing Kickbacks	1	15	75 seconds
Prone Double-Leg Raises	2	15	75 seconds
Gym Calf Sequence 1 (refer to page 253)			

WEEKS 7, 8, AND 9

DAYS 1, 2, AND 3

Exercises	Sets	Reps	Rest
Front Lunge (Pumps)	3	8	75 seconds
Leg Curls	3	10	75 seconds
Leg Press	3	8	75 seconds
Side Lunge (Alternating)	2	8	75 seconds
Standing Kickbacks	1	10	75 seconds
Back Extension	2	10	75 seconds
Gym Calf Sequence 1 (refer to page 253)			

Level 2: Creating the Dream

This level will begin to move you toward the fitter and shapelier butt and legs you've dreamed about. It becomes more intense and will move you from high-volume, low-intensity, to low-volume, high-intensity.

Keep concentrating on your technique and feel the strength and power building in your butt and legs. Notice how hard they are becoming. You're on the way.

WEEKS 1, 2, AND 3

DAYS 1, 2, AND 3

Exercises	Sets	Reps	Rest
Front Squat	3	15	60 seconds
Standing Leg Curls	3	15	60 seconds
Front Lunge (Pumps)	2	15	60 seconds
Standing Kickbacks	2	15	60 seconds
Standing Adduction	2	15	60 seconds
Standing Abduction	2	15 each	60 seconds
Pelvic Lifts	2	20	60 seconds
Back Extension	1	15	60 seconds
Gym Calf Sequence 2 (refer to page 253)			

WEEKS 4, 5, AND 6

DAYS 1, 2, AND 3

Exercises	Sets	Reps	Rest
Squat	4	8	60 seconds
Stiff-Leg Dead Lift	4	8	60 seconds
Lunge Pulls (Walks)	3	8	60 seconds
Leg Curls	3	8	60 seconds
Standing Adduction	2	8	60 seconds
Standing Abduction	2	8	60 seconds
Bent-Leg Kickbacks	1	12	60 seconds
Single-Leg Pelvic Lifts	2	15	60 seconds
Gym Calf Sequence 2 (refer to page 253)			

WEEK 7—ONE WEEK OF ACTIVE REST

WEEKS 8, 9, AND 10

DAYS 1 AND 3 (E.G., MONDAY AND FRIDAY)

Exercises	Sets	Reps	Rest
Front Squat	3	12	60 seconds
Stiff-Leg Dead Lift	3	12	60 seconds
Back Lunge Push	3	12	60 seconds
Leg Press	3	12	60 seconds
Standing Adduction	3	12	60 seconds
Standing Abduction	3	12	60 seconds
Single-Leg Pelvic Lifts	2	20	60 seconds
Bent-Leg Kickbacks	1	12	60 seconds
Back Extension	2	20	60 seconds
Gym Calf Sequence 2, Days 1 and 3 (refer to page 253)			

DAY 2 (E.G., WEDNESDAY)

Exercises	Sets	Reps	Rest
Lunge Pulls (Walks)	2	12	60 seconds
Standing Leg Curls	2	12	60 seconds
Bent Leg Kickbacks (Pulse)	3	12	60 seconds
Bent-Leg to Straight Kickbacks	3	12	60 seconds
Kneeling Side Leg Raises	3	12	60 seconds
Back Extension with a Twist	1	12 each side	60 seconds

Gym Calf Sequence 1 (refer to page 253)

WEEKS 11, 12, AND 13

DAY 1 (E.G., MONDAY)

Exercises	Sets	Reps	Rest
Squat	4	7–5–5–10	60 seconds
Stiff-Leg Dead Lift	4	7–5–5–10	60 seconds
Front Lunge (Alternating)	3	5–5–10	60 seconds
Leg Curls	3	5–5–10	60 seconds
Dumbbell Wide Squat	3	5–5–10	60 seconds
Back Lunge Push	2	8	60 seconds
Bent-Leg to Straight Kickback	1	8	60 seconds
Back Extension	2	10	60 seconds

Gym Calf Sequence 3, Days 1 and 3 (refer to pages 253–54)

DAY 2 (E.G., THURSDAY)

Exercises	Sets	Reps	Rest
Back Lunge Push	3	12	60 seconds
Good Mornings	3	12	60 seconds
Kneeling Side Leg Raises	3	12	60 seconds
Side Lunge (Alternating)	3	12	60 seconds
Single-Leg Pelvic Lifts	3	20	60 seconds
Back Extension with a Twist	2	20	60 seconds

Gym Calf Sequence 1 (refer to page 253)

Level 3: Achieving the Dream

This is what you've been preparing yourself for. Three weeks of kick-butt work that will leave your butt and legs in top shape. As always concentrate on your technique, both mind and body. Even though the work is hard it's enjoyable because you are seeing and feeling the results. Note: Refer to pages 236–37 for explanation of CS, SS, TS, and GS.

WEEK 1

DAYS 1, 2, AND 3

Exercises	Sets	Reps	Rest
CS—Front Squat, Good Mornings	3	15 each	60 seconds between each CS
CS—Standing Leg Curls, Leg Extensions	3	15 each	60 seconds between each CS
Sissy Squat	1	15	60 seconds
TS—Standing Adduction, Standing Abduction Pelvic Lifts (Weighted)	1	20	60 seconds between each TS
Back Extension	2	20	60 seconds

Gym Calf Sequence 4 (refer to page 256)

WEEK 2

DAYS 1 AND 2 (E.G., MONDAY AND THURSDAY)

Exercises	Sets	Reps	Rest
SS—Dumbbell Wide Squat, Front Lunge (Pumps)	3	8 each	60 seconds between each SS
SS—Leg Curl, Stiff-Leg Dead Lift	3	8 each	60 seconds between each SS
SS—Lunge Pulls (Walks), Sissy Squat	1	10 each	60 seconds between each SS
TS—Bent-Leg to Straight Kickback, Bent-Leg Kickback, Kneeling Side Leg Raises	2	10 each	60 seconds between each TS
Back Extension with a Twist	2	12 each side	60 seconds

Gym Calf Sequence 4, Days 1 and 3 (refer to page 256)

WEEK 3

DAY 1 (E.G., MONDAY)

Exercises	Sets	Reps	Rest
Squat	4	5–5–5–12	60 seconds
Leg Curls	4	5–5–5–12	60 seconds
Back Lunge Push (Descending) Any Machine	4	5–5–5–10	60 seconds
Do either Leg Press, Hip Sled, or Hack Squat	4	5–5–5–12	60 seconds
Back Lunge Walk (Alternating)	2	8	60 seconds

SS—Standing Adduction, Standing Abduction	2	8 each	60 seconds between each SS
Pelvic Lifts (Weighted)	2	10	60 seconds
Back Extension with a Twist	2	15 each side	60 seconds

Gym Calf Sequence 4, Days 1 and 3 (refer to page 256)

DAY 2 (E.G., THURSDAY)

Exercises	Sets	Reps	Rest
Squat	3	12	60 seconds
Standing Leg Curls	3	12	60 seconds

Back Lunge Push (Descending) Any Machine	3	12	60 seconds
Do either Leg Press, Hip Sled, or Hack Squat	3	12	60 seconds
Back Lunge Walk (Alternating)	1	12	60 seconds
SS—Standing Adduction, Standing Abduction	1	8 each	60 seconds between each SS
Pelvic Lift (Weighted)	1	10	60 seconds
Back Extension with a Twist	2	15 each side	60 seconds

Gym Calf Sequence 2, Day 2 (refer to page 253)

Home Men

Level 1: Preconditioning and the Foundation

This level is designed to build the base that will allow you to move to more sophisticated workouts down the road. It is a high-volume, low-intensity workout that will create muscle hypertrophy (increase in the cross-sectional size of the muscle fiber). This prepares you for more work later on in your progression. It is important that you focus on proper technique. This will pay dividends for you later. Enjoy the workout. Every day you are improving yourself both mentally and physically, so give yourself credit for those victories. The following routine will require a step box, and will be enhanced by dumbbells.

WEEK 1

DAY 1 (E.G., MONDAY)

Exercises	Sets	Reps	Rest
Post Squat	1	10–12	90 seconds
Front Lunge (Pumps)	1	10–12	90 seconds
Good Mornings	1	10–12	90 seconds
Back Lunge Push	1	10–12	90 seconds
Home Calf Sequence 1 (refer to page 255)			

DAYS 2 AND 3 (E.G., WEDNESDAY AND FRIDAY)

Exercises	Sets	Reps	Rest
Post Squat	2	10–12	90 seconds
Front Lunge (Pumps)	2	10–12	90 seconds
Good Mornings	2	10–12	90 seconds
Back Lunge Push	2	10–12	90 seconds
Home Calf Sequence 1 (refer to page 255)			

WEEK 2

DAYS 1, 2, AND 3

Exercises	Sets	Reps	Rest
Post Squat	3	10–12	90 seconds
Front Lunge (Pumps)	3	10–12	90 seconds
Good Mornings	3	10–12	90 seconds
Back Lunge Push	3	10–12	90 seconds
Home Calf Sequence 1 (refer to page 255)			

WEEKS 3 AND 4

DAYS 1, 2, AND 3

Exercises	Sets	Reps	Rest
Squat (Body Weight)	3	12–15	80 seconds
Front Lunge (Pumps)	3	12–15	80 seconds
Good Mornings	3	12–15	80 seconds
Back Lunge Push	3	12–15	80 seconds
Home Calf Sequence 1 (refer to page 255)			

WEEKS 5 AND 6

DAYS 1, 2, AND 3

Exercises	Sets	Reps	Rest
Single-Leg Post Squat	3	12–15	70 seconds
Balance Squat (with Bench)	3	12–15	70 seconds
Good Mornings	3	12–15	70 seconds
Back Lunge Push	3	12–15	70 seconds
Home Calf Sequence 1 (refer to page 255)			

Level 2: Creating Strength and Endurance

This level will begin to improve your strength and endurance significantly. Now that you've established your base, the workouts will become more intense by adding more volume and decreasing your rest time. Concentrate on your technique and work hard at making the mind-muscle link so that your workouts will be as effective as possible. Note: Refer to pages 236–37 for explanation of CS, SS, TS, and GS.

WEEKS 1 AND 2

DAYS 1, 2, AND 3

Exercises	Sets	Reps	Rest
Single-Leg Post Squat	3	15–20	60 seconds
Balance Squat (with Bench)	3	15–20	60 seconds
Side Lunge (Alternating)	1	15–20	60 seconds
Stiff-Leg Dead Lift	3	15–20	60 seconds
Back Lunge Push	3	15–20	60 seconds
Home Calf Sequence 1 (refer to page 255)			

WEEKS 3 AND 4

DAYS 1 AND 3 (E.G., MONDAY AND FRIDAY)

Exercises	Sets	Reps	Rest
SS—Balance Squat (with Bench), Back Lunge Walk (Alternating)	3	15 each	50 seconds between each SS
CS—Side Lunge (Alternating), Stiff-Leg Dead Lift	3	20 each	50 seconds between each SS
Sissy Squat	2	20	50 seconds
Home Calf Sequence 2, Days 1 and 3 (refer to page 255)			

DAY 2 (E.G., WEDNESDAY)

Exercises	Sets	Reps	Rest
TS—Front Lunge (Alternating), Good Mornings, Back Lunge Pull (Walk)	3	15 each	50 seconds between each TS
Bent-Leg Kickbacks	3	20	50 seconds
Home Calf Sequence 1 (refer to page 255)			

WEEKS 5 AND 6

DAYS 1 AND 3 (E.G., MONDAY AND FRIDAY)

Exercises	Sets	Reps	Rest
CS—Step Ups, Stiff-Leg Dead Lift	3	25 each	40 seconds between each SS
CS—Side Lunge (Alternating), Bent-Leg Kickbacks	1	25 each	40 seconds between each SS
CS—Front Lunge (Pumps), Back Side Lunge	3	20 each	40 seconds between each SS
Home Calf Sequence 2, Days 1 and 3 (refer to page 255)			

DAY 2 (E.G., WEDNESDAY)

Exercises	Sets	Reps	Rest
GS—Back Side Lunges, Good Mornings, Front Lunge (Alternating), Single-Leg Post Squat	3 each	20 each	40 seconds between each GS

Home Calf Sequence 1 (refer to page 255)

Level 3: Achieving Strength and Endurance

This level is designed to help you peak in attaining your strength, endurance, and definition. In this phase you are going to perform exercises for certain periods of time rather than in numbers of reps, so you will want to exercise where you can watch a clock or your watch's second hand. Continue to concentrate on both your mental and physical techniques. Enjoy the workout even though it's difficult. You've come a long way since Week 1. Note: Refer to pages 236–37 for explanation of CS, SS, TS, and GS.

WEEK 1

DAYS 1 AND 3 (E.G., MONDAY AND FRIDAY)

Exercises	Sets	Reps	Rest
Single-Leg Post Squat	3	30 seconds	30 seconds
Balance Squat (with Bench)	3	30 seconds	30 seconds
Back Lunge Push	3	30 seconds	30 seconds
Good Mornings	3	30 seconds	30 seconds
Front Lunge (Pumps)	3	30 seconds	30 seconds

Home Calf Sequence 3, Days 1 and 3 (refer to pages 255–56)

DAY 2 (E.G., WEDNESDAY)

Exercises	Sets	Reps	Rest
Lunge Pulls (Walks)	3	30 seconds	30 seconds
Back Lunge Walk (Alternating)	3	30 seconds	30 seconds
Kneeling Side Leg Raise	3	30 seconds	30 seconds
Mountain Climber Leg Curls	3	30 seconds	30 seconds

Home Calf Sequence 1 (refer to page 255)

WEEK 2

DAYS 1 AND 3 (E.G., MONDAY AND FRIDAY)

Exercises	Sets	Reps	Rest
CS—Back Lunge Walk, Good Mornings (Alternating)	3	45 seconds each	20 seconds between each SS
SS—Front Lunge (Alternating), Lunge Pulls (Walks)	3	45 seconds each	20 seconds between each SS
SS—Squat, Side Lunge (Alternating)	3	45 seconds each	20 seconds between each SS

Home Calf Sequence 3, Days 1 and 3 (refer to pages 255–56)

DAY 2 (E.G., WEDNESDAY)

Exercises	Sets	Reps	Rest
CS—Step-Ups, Stiff-Leg Dead Lift	3	45 seconds each	20 seconds between each SS
TS—Bent-Leg Kickbacks, Kneeling Side Leg Raises, Sissy Squat	3	45 seconds each	20 seconds between each TS

Home Calf Sequence 1 (refer to page 255)

WEEK 3

DAYS 1 AND 3 (E.G., MONDAY AND FRIDAY)

Exercises	Sets	Reps	Rest
TS—Squat, Front Lunge (Alternating), and Back Lunge Push (Descending)	3	60 seconds each	15 seconds between each TS
GS—Back Side Lunge, Front Lunge (Pumps), Sissy Squat, Mountain Climber Leg Curls	3	60 seconds each	15 seconds between each GS

Home Calf Sequence 3, Days 1 and 3 (refer to pages 255–56)

DAY 2 (E.G., WEDNESDAY)

Exercises	Sets	Reps	Rest
GS—Mountain Climbers, Good Mornings, Lunge Pulls (Alternating), Kneeling Side Leg Raises, Sissy Squat, Bent-Leg Kickbacks	3	60 seconds each	15 seconds between each GS

Home Calf Sequence 1 (refer to page 255)

Home Women

Level 1: Preconditioning and the Foundation

This level is designed to build the base that will allow you to move to more sophisticated workouts down the road. It is a high-volume, low-intensity workout that will create muscle hypertrophy (increase in the cross-sectional size of the muscle fiber). This prepares you for more work later on in your progression. It is important that you focus on proper technique. This will pay dividends for you later. Enjoy the workout. Every day you are improving yourself both mentally and physically, so give yourself credit for those victories. The following routine will require a step box, and can be enhanced by the use of dumbbells.

WEEK 1

DAY 1 (E.G., MONDAY)

Exercises	Sets	Reps	Rest
Post Squat	1	10–12	90 seconds
Good Mornings	1	10–12	90 seconds
Kneeling Side Leg Raises	1	10–12	90 seconds
Seated Inside Raises	1	10–12	90 seconds
Home Calf Sequence 1 (refer to page 255)			

DAYS 2 AND 3 (E.G., WEDNESDAY AND FRIDAY)

Exercises	Sets	Reps	Rest
Post Squat	2	10–12	90 seconds
Good Mornings	2	10–12	90 seconds
Kneeling Side Leg Raises	2	10–12	90 seconds
Seated Inside Raises	2	10–12	90 seconds
Home Calf Sequence 1 (refer to page 255)			

WEEK 2

DAYS 1, 2, AND 3

Exercises	Sets	Reps	Rest
Post Squat	3	10–12	90 seconds
Good Mornings	3	10–12	90 seconds
Kneeling Side Leg Raises	2	10–12	90 seconds
Seated Inside Raises	2	10–12	90 seconds

Home Calf Sequence 1 (refer to page 255)

WEEKS 3 AND 4

DAYS 1, 2, AND 3

Exercises	Sets	Reps	Rest
Squats	3	15	80 seconds
Front Lunge (Pumps)	3	15	80 seconds
Good Mornings	3	15	80 seconds
Lying Straight-Leg Side Raises	3	15	80 seconds
Seated Inside Raises	3	15	80 seconds

Home Calf Sequence 1 (refer to page 255)

WEEKS 5 AND 6

DAYS 1, 2, AND 3

Exercises	Sets	Reps	Rest
Single-Leg Post Squats	3	12–15	70 seconds
Front Lunge (Pumps)	3	15–20	70 seconds
Good Mornings	3	15–20	70 seconds
Lying Straight-Leg Side Raises	2	25	70 seconds
Seated Inside Raises	1	25	70 seconds

Home Calf Sequence 1 (refer to page 255)

Level 2: Creating Shape and Fitness

This level will begin to take you toward the goals you have for your own personal fitness and the image you have of what you want to look like. You've established your base in the first six weeks and now your workouts will become increasingly more intense. Concentrate on both your mental and physical techniques and have fun. Note: Refer to pages 236–37 for explanation of CS, SS, TS, and GS.

WEEKS 1 AND 2

DAYS 1, 2, AND 3

Exercises	Sets	Reps	Rest
Single-Leg Post Squats	3	20	60 seconds
Front Lunge (Pumps)	3	20	60 seconds
Stiff-Leg Dead Lift	3	20	60 seconds
Bent-Leg Kickbacks	2	15–20	60 seconds
Kneeling Side Leg Raises	1	25–30	60 seconds
Lying Inside Raises	1	30	60 seconds

Home Calf Sequence 2 (refer to page 255)

WEEKS 3 AND 4

DAYS 1 AND 3 (E.G., MONDAY AND FRIDAY)

Exercises	Sets	Reps	Rest
Single-Leg Post Squat	3	20	50 seconds
Lunge Pulls (Walks)	3	20	50 seconds
Back Side Lunges	3	20	50 seconds
Stiff-Leg Dead Lifts	3	25	50 seconds
Kneeling Side Leg Raises	1	30	50 seconds
Lying Inside Raises	1	30	50 seconds

Home Calf Sequence 2, Days 1 and 3 (refer to page 255)

DAY 2 (E.G., WEDNESDAY)

Exercises	Sets	Reps	Rest
GS—Front Lunge (Pump), Bent-Leg to Straight Kickbacks, Bent-Leg Kickbacks, Lying Inside Raises	3	20 each	50 seconds between each GS

Home Calf Sequence 1 (refer to page 255)

WEEKS 5 AND 6

DAYS 1 AND 2 (E.G., MONDAY AND FRIDAY)

Exercises	Sets	Reps	Rest
CS—Balance Squat (with Bench),	3	20	
Stiff-Leg Dead Lift	3	25	40 seconds between each SS
CS—Lunge Pulls (Alternating),	2	15	
Side Lunge (Alternating)	2	20	40 seconds between each SS
CS—Bent-Leg Kickbacks,	2	25 each	
Dumbbell Wide Squat			40 seconds between each SS
Sissy Squat	1	30	40 seconds

Home Calf Sequence 2, Days 1 and 3 (refer to page 255)

DAY 2 (E.G., WEDNESDAY)

Exercises	Sets	Reps	Rest
GS—Step-Ups,	3	20	
Bent-Leg to Straight Kickbacks,	3	20	
Bent-Leg Kickbacks (Pulse),	3	20	
Kneeling Side Leg Raise	3	30	40 seconds between each GS

Home Calf Sequence 1 (refer to page 255)

Level 3: Achieving Shape and Fitness

This level will increase in intensity by designating certain time intervals for each exercise and by decreasing the rest time. You should have a clock or watch with a second hand available so that you can time yourself. Even though the workout is difficult, enjoy it, because you are achieving the goals you have set for how you want to look and feel. As always, concentrate on your technique.

WEEK 1

DAYS 1 AND 2 (E.G., MONDAY AND FRIDAY)

Exercises	Sets	Reps	Rest
Lunge Pulls (Walks)	3	30 seconds	30 seconds
Back Lunge Walk (Alternating)	3	30 seconds	30 seconds
Back Side Lunge	3	30 seconds	30 seconds
Side Lunge (Alternating)	3	30 seconds	30 seconds
Sissy Squat	3	30 seconds	30 seconds
Mountain Climber Leg Curl	1	30 seconds	30 seconds

Home Calf Sequence 3, Days 1 and 3 (refer to pages 255–56)

DAY 2 (E.G., WEDNESDAY)

Exercises	Sets	Reps	Rest
GS—Dumbbell Wide Squat, Pelvic Lifts, Lying Straight-Leg Side Raises, Seated Inside Raises	3	30 seconds each	30 seconds between each GS

Home Calf Sequence 1 (refer to page 255)

WEEK 2

DAYS 1 AND 3 (E.G., MONDAY AND FRIDAY)

Exercises	Sets	Reps	Rest
SS—Balance Squats (with Bench), Mountain Climber Leg Curls	3	45 seconds each	20 seconds between each SS

Exercises	Sets	Reps	Rest
SS—Front Lunge (Alternating), Back Lunge Push	3	45 seconds each	20 seconds between each SS
CS—Pelvic Lifts, Good Mornings	3	45 seconds each	20 seconds between each SS

Home Calf Sequence 3, Days 1 and 3 (refer to pages 255–56)

DAY 2 (E.G., WEDNESDAY)

Exercises	Sets	Reps	Rest
GS—Mountain Climbers, Single-Leg Pelvic Lift, Bent-Leg Kickbacks, Kneeling Side Leg Raises, Lying Inside Raises (Hand Resistance)	3	45 seconds each	20 seconds between each GS

Home Calf Sequence 1 (refer to page 255)

WEEK 3

DAYS 1 AND 3 (E.G., MONDAY AND FRIDAY)

Exercises	Sets	Reps	Rest
GS—Front Lunge (Alternating), Back Lunge Push (Descending), Sissy Squat, Dumbbell Wide Squat	3	60 seconds each	15 seconds between each GS
GS—Back Side Lunge, Pelvic Lifts, Front Lunge, Lunge Pulls (Walks), Back Lunge Walks (Alternating)	3	60 seconds each	15 seconds between each GS

Home Calf Sequence 4, Days 1 and 3 (refer to page 256)

DAY 2 (E.G., WEDNESDAY)

Exercises	Sets	Reps	Rest
TS—Mountain Climbers, Bent-Leg to Straight Kickbacks, Single-Leg Pelvic Lifts	3	60 seconds each	15 seconds between each TS
TS—Lunge Pulls (Alternating), Kneeling Side Leg Raises, Bent-Kick Crosses	3	60 seconds each	15 seconds between each TS

Home Calf Sequence 1 (refer to page 255)

CHAPTER TWENTY-TWO

Ultimate Butt and Legs

This is the top of the line. Do not use this system unless you have completed Gym Men or Women. Remember, technique is still the core to everything you do. Enjoy yourself and bust your butt. Refer to pages 236–37 for an explanation of CS, SS, TS, and GS.

WEEKS 1, 2, AND 3

DAYS 1 AND 2 (E.G., MONDAY AND THURSDAY)

Exercises	Sets	Reps	Rest
Front Squat	3	15	60 seconds
Leg Curls	3	15	60 seconds
CS—Front Lunge (Pumps), Good Mornings	3	15 each	60 seconds between each CS
CS—Leg Press, Glute Ham Raise	3	15 each	60 seconds between each CS
Prone Adductions	3	15	60 seconds

Gym Calf Sequence 4, days 1 and 3 (refer to page 256)

WEEKS 4, 5, AND 6

DAYS 1 AND 2 (E.G., MONDAY AND THURSDAY)

Exercises	Sets	Reps	Rest
TS—Leg Extension, Squat, Sissy Squat	3	8 each	75 seconds between each TS
TS—Leg Curl (Two Legs Up and One Leg Down), Stiff-Leg Dead Lift, Back Extension with a Twist	3	8 each	75 seconds between each TS
CS—Leg Press, Good Mornings	2	10 each	75 seconds between each CS
Standing Adduction	3	8	75 seconds

Standing Abduction	3	8	75 seconds

Gym Calf Sequence 2, Days 1 and 3 (refer to page253)

WEEKS 7, 8, AND 9

DAY 1 (E.G., MONDAY)

Exercises	Sets	Reps	Rest
Squat	6	5–5–5–5–5–12	90 seconds
Standing Leg Curls	3	8	90 seconds
Leg Press	5	5–5–5–5–12	90 seconds
Stiff-Leg Dead Lift	6	5–5–5–5–5–12	90 seconds
CS—Front Lunge (Pumps), Back Extension	3	8 each	90 seconds between each CS

Gym Calf Sequence 3, Days 1 and 3 (refer to pages 253–54)

DAY 2 (E.G., THURSDAY)

Exercises	Sets	Reps	Rest
Squat	3	12	90 seconds
Standing Leg Curl	3	12	90 seconds
Leg Press	3	12	90 seconds
Stiff-Leg Dead Lift	3	12	90 seconds
CS—Front Lunge (Pumps), Back Extension	3	12 each	90 seconds between each CS

Gym Calf Sequence 1 (refer to page 253)

WEEKS 10, 11, AND 12

DAY 1 (E.G., MONDAY)

MORNING

Exercises	Sets	Reps	Rest
Leg Extension	3	12	60 seconds
Single-Leg Sissy Squat	3	8	60 seconds
Squat	6	8–5–5–3–2–10	60 seconds
Side Lunge (Alternating)	3	8	60 seconds
Leg Press (Two Legs Up and One Leg Down)	3	12	60 seconds

EVENING

Exercises	Sets	Reps	Rest
Back Extensions with a Twist	3	10 each way	60 seconds
Leg Curls (Two Legs Up and One Leg Down)	3	8	60 seconds
Stiff-Leg Dead Lift	6	8–5–5–3–2–10	60 seconds
Single-Leg Pelvic Lifts	3	12	60 seconds
Prone Adductions	3	10	60 seconds
Prone Abductions	3	10	60 seconds

Gym Calf Sequence 4, Days 1 and 3 (refer to page 256)

DAY 2 (E.G., THURSDAY)

MORNING

Exercises	Sets	Reps	Rest
Leg Extension	3	15	60 seconds
Single-Leg Sissy Squat	3	15	60 seconds
Squat	6	15	60 seconds

EVENING

Exercises	Sets	Reps	Rest
Back Extension with a Twist	3	15 each way	60 seconds
Leg Curls (Two Legs Up and One Leg Down)	3	15	60 seconds
Stiff-Leg Dead Lift	6	15	60 seconds

Gym Calf Sequence 2, Days 1 and 3 (refer to page 253)

Gym Calf Sequence

Calf Sequence 1

DAYS 1, 2, AND 3 (OR AS SPECIFIED IN ANY OF THE PROGRAMS FOR THE BUTT AND LEGS)

Exercises	Sets	Reps	Rest
Standing Heel Raises (Eversion)	1	15	No Rest
Standing Heel Raises (Neutral)	1	15	No Rest
Standing Heel Raises (Inversion)	1	15	No Rest

Calf Sequence 2

Refer to page 237 for an explanation of TS.

DAYS 1 AND 3 (OR AS SPECIFIED IN ANY OF THE PROGRAMS FOR THE BUTT AND LEGS)

Exercises	Sets	Reps	Rest
Standing Single-Leg Heel Raises (Eversion)	2	15	No Rest
Standing Single-Leg Heel Raises (Neutral)	2	15	No Rest
Standing Single-Leg Heel Raises (Inversion)	2	15	No Rest

Perform all three exercises back to back on one leg, then perform on the other.

DAY 2 (OR AS SPECIFIED IN ANY OF THE PROGRAMS FOR THE BUTT AND LEGS)

Exercises	Sets	Reps	Rest
TS—Standing Heel Raises (Eversion), Standing Heel Raises (Neutral), Standing Heel Raises (Inversion)	2	8 each	60 seconds between each TS

Calf Sequence 3

Refer to page 237 for an explanation of TS.

DAYS 1 AND 3 (OR AS SPECIFIED IN ANY OF THE PROGRAMS FOR THE BUTT AND LEGS)

Exercises	Sets	Reps	Rest
TS—Seated Heel Raises (Eversion), Seated Heel Raises (Neutral), Seated Heel Raises (Inversion)	3	8 each	60 seconds between each TS

DAY 2 (OR AS SPECIFIED IN ANY OF THE PROGRAMS FOR THE BUTT AND LEGS)

Exercises	Sets	Reps	Rest
TS—Standing Single-Leg Heel Raises (Eversion), Standing Single-Leg Heel Raises (Neutral), Standing Single-Leg Heel Raises (Inversion)	2	12 each	60 seconds between each TS

Calf Sequence 4

Refer to page 237 for an explanation of TS.

DAYS 1 AND 3 (OR AS SPECIFIED IN ANY OF THE PROGRAMS FOR THE BUTT AND LEGS)

Exercises	Sets	Reps	Rest
TS—Lying (Hip Sled) Heel Raises (Eversion), Lying (Hip Sled) Heel Raises (Neutral), Lying (Hip Sled) Heel Raises (Inversion)	3	5	60 seconds between each TS
TS—Seated Heel Raises (Eversion), Seated Heel Raises (Neutral), Seated Heel Raises (Inversion)	3	8 each	60 seconds between each TS
TS—Standing Heel Raises (Eversion), Standing Heel Raises (Neutral), Standing Heel Raises (Inversion)	3	15 each	60 seconds between each TS

DAY 2 (OR AS SPECIFIED IN ANY OF THE PROGRAMS FOR THE BUTT AND LEGS)

Exercises	Sets	Reps	Rest
TS—Lying (Hip Sled) Single-Leg Heel Raises (Eversion), Lying (Hip Sled) Single-Leg Heel Raises (Neutral), Lying (Hip Sled), Single-Leg Heel Raises (Inversion)	1	12 each	60 seconds between each TS
TS—Seated Single-Leg (Bent Leg) Heel Raises (Eversion), Seated Heel Raises (single leg) Heel Raises (Neutral), Seated Heel Raises (single leg), Heel Raises (Inversion)	1	12 each	60 seconds between each TS
TS—Standing Single-Leg Heel Raises (Eversion), Standing Single-Leg Heel Raises (Neutral), Standing Single-Leg Heel Raises (Inversion)	1	12 each	60 seconds between each TS

Home Calf Sequence

Calf Sequence 1

DAYS 1, 2, AND 3 (OR AS SPECIFIED IN ANY OF THE PRO-
GRAMS FOR THE BUTT AND LEGS)

Exercises	Sets	Reps	Rest
Standing Heel Raises (Eversion)	1	15	No Rest
Standing Heel Raises (Neutral)	1	15	No Rest
Standing Heel Raises (Inversion)	1	15	No Rest

Calf Sequence 2

Refer to page 237 for an explanation of TS.

DAYS 1 AND 3 (OR AS SPECIFIED IN ANY OF THE PROGRAMS
FOR THE BUTT AND LEGS)

Exercises	Sets	Reps	Rest
Standing Single-Leg Heel Raises (Eversion),	2	15	No Rest
Standing Single-Leg Heel Raises (Neutral),	2	15	No Rest
Standing Single-Leg Heel Raises (Inversion)	2	15	No Rest

DAY 2 (OR AS SPECIFIED IN ANY OF THE PROGRAMS
FOR THE BUTT AND LEGS)

Exercises	Sets	Reps	Rest
Standing Heel Raises (Eversion)	1	15	No Rest
Standing Heel Raises (Neutral)	1	15	No Rest
Standing Heel Raises (Inversion)	1	15	No Rest

Calf Sequence 3

DAYS 1 AND 3 (OR AS SPECIFIED IN ANY OF THE PROGRAMS
FOR THE BUTT AND LEGS)

Exercises	Sets	Reps	Rest
TS—Donkey Raises (Eversion),	3	8 each	60 seconds

Donkey Raises (Neutral),   between
Donkey Raises (Inversion)   each TS

DAY 2 (OR AS SPECIFIED IN ANY OF THE PROGRAMS
FOR THE BUTT AND LEGS)

Exercises	Sets	Reps	Rest
TS—Standing Single-Leg Heel Raises (Eversion), Standing Single-Leg Heel Raises (Neutral), Standing Single-Leg Heel Raises (Inversion)	2	15 each	60 seconds between each TS

Calf Sequence 4

DAYS 1 AND 3 (OR AS SPECIFIED IN ANY OF THE PROGRAMS
FOR THE BUTT AND LEGS)

Exercises	Sets	Reps	Rest
TS—Single-Leg Donkey Raises (Eversion), Single-Leg Donkey Raises (Neutral), Single-Leg Donkey Raises (Inversion)	3	8 each	60 seconds between each TS

DAY 2 (OR AS SPECIFIED IN ANY OF THE PROGRAMS
FOR THE BUTT AND LEGS)

Exercises	Sets	Reps	Rest
TS—Donkey Raises (Eversion), Donkey Raises (Neutral), Donkey Raises (Inversion)	3	12 each	60 seconds between each TS

Specialized Routines from the Pros

Aqua Power Moves
by Georgia L. Norgren

Georgia L. Norgren instructs all levels of aquatic fitness. She is also a fully certified ski instructor and has designed Ski I.T. (interval training), which is an aquatic ski-conditioning program utilizing sport-specific moves, plyometrics, and interval training. Georgia is certified by ACE, AEA, and the Cooper Institute of Aerobics Research.

AQUA POWER MOVES
This is an intermediate to advanced routine that offers a challenge in a different environment. The water provides resistance that is beneficial for muscular strength and endurance, while the relatively impact-free quality reduces the risk of injury potential. In utilizing this routine you should adhere to the following guidelines: (1) The routine should be started with a thermal warmup and a prestretch, and concluded with a poststretch; (2) The exercises should be performed in chest-depth water. Shallower water increases the impact, and deeper water makes it difficult to control moves due to buoyancy; (3) All of the standing exercises should be executed through a full range of motion, at a speed to maintain control and proper body position, and with equal force in both directions to create muscular symmetry; and (4) All of the power moves should be done with maximum effort. Allow one to two minutes between exercises.

THE EXERCISES
STANDING
THREE TIMES PER WEEK

	Sets	Reps	Rest	Remarks
Aqua Hip Flexion	2	20	45 seconds	Build to 3 sets.
Aqua Hip Extension	2	20	45 seconds	Build to 3 sets.
Aqua Knee Extension	2	20	45 seconds	Build to 3 sets.
Aqua Knee Flexion	2	20	45 seconds	Build to 3 sets.
Aqua Hip Abduction/ Adduction	2	20	45 seconds	Build to 3 sets.

POWER MOVES
THREE TIMES PER WEEK

	Sets	Reps	Rest	Remarks
Aqua Tuck Jumps	1	15–20	90 seconds	Build to 30 reps.
Aqua Split Jumps	1	15–20	90 seconds	Build to 30 reps.
Aqua Cross Jumps	1	15–20	90 seconds	Build to 30 reps.
Aqua Squat Jumps	1	15–20	90 seconds	Build to 30 reps.
Aqua Double-Leg Curl	1	15–20	90 seconds	Build to 30 reps.
Aqua One-Legged Tuck Jumps	1	15–20	90 seconds	Build to 30 reps.

Lower Back Routine
by Jaclynn Parks

Jaclynn Parks is a physical therapist at the Snowmass Lodge and Club through the Aspen Valley Hospital.

LOWER BACK

One aspect of lower back dysfunction is muscle weakness. The gluteal muscles provide support and stability for the lower back. It is important to start slowly and build a strength base gradually. You do not need to use a lot of weight to develop the muscles that support the lower back. Endurance is also necessary as you want your postural muscles to support your back throughout the day. If you have a history of lower back dysfunction you need to exercise with care. It is possible to injure your lower back further by using too much resistance too fast. It is also very important not to exercise through

pain. These exercises are not a substitute for professional medical advice. Before you put any of these recommendations to practical use, consult your doctor or therapist if you experience lower back pain.

THE EXERCISES
WEEKS 1–2, THREE TIMES PER WEEK

	Sets	Reps	Remarks
Leg Press	2	30	Single leg
Standing Adductions	2	30	Standing—balance on unattached leg. Do not hang on with hands.
Standing Abductions	2	30	Standing—balance on unattached leg. Do not hang on with hands.
Standing Kickbacks	2	30	Standing—balance on unattached leg. Do not hang on with hands.
Dumbbell Wide Squat or Post Squat	1	30–50	Start with both legs and move to single leg on Post Squat when possible
Front Lunge (Pumps)	1	30–50	
Pelvic Lifts	1	30–50	Start with both legs and move to single leg when possible
Side Hip Extension Rotation	1	30	

WEEKS 3–6, THREE TIMES PER WEEK

	Sets	Reps	Remarks
Leg Press	2	20	Single leg
Dumbbell Wide Squats or Post Squat or Front Lunge (Pumps)	Choose one of these three for two sets of twenty.		Single leg on Post Squat
Front Lunge (Alternating)	2	20	
Back Lunge Push	2	20	
Side Lunge (Alternating)	2	20	
Leg Curls	2	20	Single leg
Back Extension	2	10 to 15	

Preseason Ski Routine
by Coulter Bright
and Mike Brungardt

Coulter Bright received his bachelor of science degree in Physical Education with a concentration in Sports Management from James Madison University in

Virginia. He also received the Fitness Instructor Education and Training Course Certification, "The Cutting Edge," from the University of Colorado Health Science Center in Denver, Colorado. Coulter started at the Midvalley Sports Medicine Clinic in Basalt, Colorado, as an assistant to the physical therapist and a fitness trainer. He spent three years working at the Aspen Club in Aspen, Colorado, as a one-on-one trainer and fitness tester. He is currently working at the Snowmass Lodge and Club as fitness trainer. Coulter is a member of the National Strength and Conditioning Association and is also a ski instructor.

Mike Brungardt (see credits, page 283)

PRESEASON SKI

Many people go into the ski season without any physical preparation. This is an invitation to disaster. Without a proper strength and conditioning base you will be much more susceptible to injury. Your performance will probably also suffer. This program is designed to prepare you so that you can perform in the manner you wish to. Realize that this program won't improve your skills, but it will help you to achieve the physical status that will allow you to perform these skills more effectively.

This program is designed to strengthen areas that are the most susceptible to injury while skiing. It is also designed to enhance your performance by training the muscle groups used in skiing in a manner specific to skiing. The second part of the program (two to three weeks prior to season) is a peaking cycle. You should spend about four weeks previous to this program establishing a strength base.

THE EXERCISES
PREP PHASE (STRENGTH BASE)—4 WEEKS, THREE TIMES PER WEEK

	Sets	Reps	Remarks
Dumbbell Wide Squats	3	12–15	
Leg Extension	3	12–15	Do not use if you have a history of knee problems.
Leg Press, Hip Sled, or Hack Squat	3	12–15	
Leg Curls	3	12–15	
Standing Heel Raises	3	12–15	

PEAKING PHASE—2 TO 3 WEEKS PRIOR TO SEASON, THREE TIMES PER WEEK

	Sets	Reps	Remarks
Back Lunge Walks (Alternating)	3–4	6–8	
Front Lunge Angle Pulls (Alternating)	3–4	6–8	
Angle Leg Press	3–4	6–8	
Leg Curls	3–4	6–8	
Standing Heel Raises	3–4	8–10	

Tennis Routine
by Jim Landis

Jim Landis has been a personal trainer for thirteen years. He specializes in strength and conditioning. He works with business executives, television personalities, and professional athletes. He trains such top Indy car drivers as Danny Sullivan and Emerson Fittipaldi, tennis champions Chris Evert, Martina Navratilova, and Pam Shriver, and Olympic gold-medalist ice-skater Scott Hamilton, to name a few. Jim has worked with the Arizona Heart Institute and the Aspen Institute for Fitness and Sports Medicine, and he is a member of the National Strength and Conditioning Association.

TENNIS

When designing a program for a specific sport such as tennis, the main concern is to employ a workout that will most effectively enhance the playing performance. Basically, the workout should enhance a player's power and speed. This will be reflected in the relatively low repetitions and explosive type of contractions in this program.

Although professional women's tennis has no real off-season, there are short periods during which the players have down time where there is no match play. This workout is for these training times. Adjustments would have to be made for the in-season training period. A preparatory phase of 3 to 4 weeks is required before this level of intensity should be attempted.

THE EXERCISES
2 TO 3 WEEKS, THREE TIMES PER WEEK

	Sets	Reps	Remarks
Step-Ups	3	5–6	Perform explosively
Leg Press (Cybex)	3	5–6	Perform explosively in relatively short range of motion (90 degrees)
Front Lunge (Alternating) or Side Lunge (Alternating)	3	5–6	
Balance Squat (with Bench)	2–3	5–6	
Leg Curls	4	6–8	
Hip Abduction	3	8–10	
Hip Adduction	3	8–10	
Standing Heel Raises	3	8–12	

Golf Routine
by Brett Brungardt

THE EXERCISES
OFFSEASON—6 WEEKS

Routine should be performed three times a week, ideally after golf practice. Routine should be performed in conjunction with abs routine for golf (see *The Complete Book of Abs*).

Week	Day	Exercises	Sets	Reps
1	1, 2, and 3	Front Lunge (Pumps)	1	10
		Back Extension	1	10
		Standing Heel Raises	1	10
2	1, 2, and 3	Front Lunge (Pumps)	2	12
		Back Extension	2	12
		Back Side Lunge	1	12
		Standing Heel Raises	1	12 each way
3 and 4	1 and 2	Front Lunge (Alternating)	3	15
		Back Extension	3	15
		Back Side Lunge	2	15
		Heel Raises (in, out, and str)	1	15 each way
	2	Front Lunge Pumps	1	12
		Hip Extension	1	12
		Back Side Lunge	1	12
		Standing Heel Raises	1	12 each way
5 and 6	1 and 3	Front Lunge Alternates	3	8
		Pelvic Lifts	3	15
		1/4 squats	3	8
		Standing Leg Curls	3	10

PRESEASON—6 WEEKS

Twice a week, with 72 hours' recovery between workouts (perform after golf practice).

Week	Day	Exercises	Sets	Reps
		Heel Raises (3-way)	1	8 each way
	2	Leg Press	1	15
		Back Extension with a Twist	1	10 each way
		Back Side Lunge	1	12
		Stiff-Leg Dead Lift	1	10
7 and 8	1	1/4 Squat	3	5
		Stiff-Leg Dead Lift	3	8
		Leg Press	3	8
		Back Extension with a Twist	2	10 each way
		Calf Sequence 1		
	2	same exercises	1	15
9 and 10	1	Lunge Pulls (Alternating)	3	12
		Leg Curls	3	12
		Side Squats	3	12
		Pelvic Lifts	3	12
		Calf Sequence 2		
	2	TS 1/4 Squat		
		Leg Extension		
		Front Lunge (Pumps)	2	8
		TS Stiff-Leg Dead Lift		
		Standing Leg Curls		
		Back Extension with a Twist	2	8
		Standing Heel Raises	1	15
11 and 12	1	Back Lunge Walk (Alternating)	3	8
		Stiff-Leg Dead Lifts	3	8
		Sissy Squat	3	8
		Leg Curls (2 up, 1 down)	3	8
		Calf Sequence 3		
	2	1/4 Side Squat	3	15
		Descending Box Lunge	1	15
		Leg Press	2	15
		TS Standing Leg Curls		
		Back Extension with a Twist		
		Pelvic Lifts	3	12

Woman Tone and Shape Routine by Charisse D. Layne

Charisse D. Layne has experience in the health and fitness industry in both managerial and consulting roles. She is well recognized as one of the top fitness consultants, and exercise and dance instructors, in the country. Among her experiences in the fitness field are: consulting for Reebok, Inc., on industry trends and strategic planning; choreographing and performing for the video *Back Aid;* personal trainer to Janet Jones-Gretsky; and personal trainer and cast member for the video *The Firm,* vol. 2. Ms. Layne is a 1984 National Fitness Aerobics champion. She is presently an aerobics instructor and personal trainer at the Maroon Creek Club in Aspen and the Snowmass Lodge and Club in Snowmass, Colorado.

TONE AND SHAPE

I like isolating the hamstrings first because I have experienced that most people, including myself, are a little weaker in this area as opposed to the quadriceps. Therefore, I will have more energy for this area if I work it first.

WARM-UP

Warm up at least ten minutes with an easy jog or bike pedaling. A standing warm-up could be done with rhythmic movements such as marches, pliés, knee lifts, half squats, etc. Thoroughly stretch hamstrings and quads before beginning.

THE EXERCISES
3 TIMES PER WEEK

	Sets	Reps	Remarks
Leg Curls	6	20	Use at least 15 pounds—3 sets on flat and 3 sets on incline.
Leg Extension (Single Leg)	3	20	Poundage should be adjusted to make last 5 reps of each set really burn.
Leg Extension (Both Legs)	3	20	
Front Lunge Angle Pulls (Alternating)	4	30	Add weight as you get stronger.
Squats	3	20	Use at least one-third your body weight.
Single-Leg Post Squat	3	20	Hand position—hang on above head. Your weight should be behind knees. Dig your weight through heels on way up. Motion should be slow and controlled.

To top off the leg/butt workout, I like to do some sort of fine limbering and isolated body weight work.

Lying Straight-Leg Side Raises	3	2 minutes	Slow and controlled with good form. *Stay in the contraction!*

As you finish on the floor move into static stretching for the lower back. Take each stretch to the point of tightness and then hold for twenty seconds.

1. Knees-to-Chest Hug.
2. Hamstring Stretch.
3. Quadriceps Stretch.

Power Lifting Routine by Vernon Banks

Vernon Banks is the current strength and conditioning coach for the Denver Broncos of the NFL. He has also been the head strength coach at the University of Wyoming and the assistant strength coach at the University of Colorado, the University of Wyoming, and Stanford. Vernon is a graduate of Texas A&M (in Parks and Recreation Management), where he also played cornerback for the Aggies. He received his master's in Exercise Science from the University of Houston. Vernon is a three-time state champion power lifter, winning titles in Wyoming (1987) and California (1989 and 1990).

POWER LIFTING

The following is a ten- to twelve-week squat/lower body training routine for a novice to intermediate-level power lifter. There are three phases:

1. Phase I: *Hypertrophy Phase*—Proper squatting/lifting technique is emphasized during this phase, along with muscular endurance and stamina development. This phase lasts approximately two and a half to three weeks. The core lifts are done at three to four sets, between eight and ten reps, and at 60 to 73 percent of your one-repetition max. Conditioning of the connective tissue occurs to promote joint stability.

2. Phase II: *Base Strength Phase*—Base strength is developed in this phase for the heavier lifting to be done later on along with continued hypertrophy. This phase will last three weeks. The core exercises are done at four to six sets, between five and eight reps, at 73 to 85 percent of your one-repetition maximum.

3. Phase III: *Peak Strength Phase*—Maximum strength is developed during this phase. The goal is to establish a new one-repetition maximum at the completion of this phase. The overall volume of the workout decreases (the number of exercises, sets, and repetitions) but near maximum training intensity is expected. Four to six weeks is the length of this phase. The core exercises are done at five to seven sets, between one and five reps, at 82 to 100-plus percent.

This leg routine is to be performed twice a week. There is a designated heavy workout day and a designated light workout day. Following this weekly routine is important for maximum strength gains. Quality rest and recovery between intense training sessions is a must.

During Phase I on the light leg workout day, you will perform one-half of the sets and repetitions on each leg lift. During Phase II and III on the designated light leg workout day you will decrease the exercises, sets, and repetitions even more.

Incorporate flexibility training (five to eight minutes) before and after strength training, along with low to moderate cardiovascular work two to three times a week. Good nutrition plays a key role in maximizing your strength gains also.

THE EXERCISES

PHASE I: HYPERTROPHY

WEEK 1, DAY 1, MONDAY (HEAVY)

	Sets	Reps	Remarks
Weighted Sit-Ups	3	15–18	Use 10-pound weights.
Squat	3	10	Do first set at 60 percent of your one-rep max. Do second set at 63 percent, third set at 67 percent.
Leg Curls	3	10	
Leg Extension	3	10	
Standing Heel Raises	3	10	
Back Extension	2	10	

WEEK 1, DAY 2, THURSDAY (LIGHT)

	Sets	Reps	Remarks
Weighted Sit-Ups	3	15	Use 10-pound weights.
Squat	2	10	Do first set at 60 percent of your one-rep max. Do second set at 63 percent.
Leg Curls	2	10	
Leg Extension	2	10	
Standing Heel Raises	2	10	
Back Extension	2	10	

WEEK 2, DAY 1, MONDAY (HEAVY)

	Sets	Reps	Remarks
Weighted Sit-Ups	3	15–18	Use 10-pound weights.
Squat	4	10–10–8–8	Do first set at 63 percent of your one-rep max. Do second set at 67 percent, and last two sets at 70 percent.
Leg Curls	4	10–10–8–8	
Leg Extension	3	10–10–8	
Standing Heel Raises	4	10–10–8–8	
Back Extension	2	10	

WEEK 2, DAY 2, THURSDAY (LIGHT)

	Sets	Reps	Remarks
Weighted Sit-Ups	3	15	Use 10-pound weights.
Squat	2	10	Do first set at 60 percent of your one-rep max. Do second set at 63 percent.

Exercise	Sets	Reps	Notes
Leg Curls	2	10	
Leg Extension	2	10	
Standing Heel Raises	2	10	
Back Extension	2	10	

WEEK 3, DAY 1, MONDAY (HEAVY)

Exercise	Sets	Reps	Notes
Weighted Sit-Ups	3	18	Use 10-pound weights.
Squat	4	10–10–8–8	Do first set at 63 percent of your one-rep max. Do second set at 67 percent, third set at 70 percent, and fourth set at 73 percent.
Leg Curls	3	10–10–8	
Leg Extension	3	10–10–8	
Standing Heel Raises	4	10–10–8–8	
Back Extension	2	10	

WEEK 3, DAY 2, THURSDAY (LIGHT)

Exercise	Sets	Reps	Notes
Weighted Sit-Ups	3	15	Use 10-pound weights.
Squat	2	10	Do first set at 60 percent of one-rep max. Do second set at 63 percent.
Leg Curls	2	10–8	
Leg Extension	2	10–8	
Standing Heel Raises	2	10	
Back Extension	2	10	

PHASE II: BASE STRENGTH

WEEK 4, DAY 1, MONDAY (HEAVY)

Exercise	Sets	Reps	Notes
Weighted Sit-Ups	3	18	Use 25-pound weights.
Squat	4	8	Do first set at 63 percent of your one-rep max. Do second set at 70 percent, and last two sets at 73 percent.
Leg Curls	3	8	Use heavy weights.
Leg Extensions	3	8	Use heavy weights.
Standing Heel Raises	3	8	
Back Extension	2	10–8	

WEEK 4, DAY 2, THURSDAY (LIGHT)

Exercise	Sets	Reps	Notes
Weighted Sit-Ups	3	15	Use 10-pound weights.
Squat	2	10–8	Do first set at 60 percent of your one-rep max. Do second set at 63 percent.
Leg Curls	2	10–8	
Leg Extension	2	10–8	
Standing Heel Raises	2	10–8	
Back Extension	2	10–8	

WEEK 5, DAY 1, MONDAY (HEAVY)

Exercise	Sets	Reps	Notes
Weighted Sit-Ups	3	18	Use 25-pound weights.
Squat	4	8–8–6–6	Do first set at 60 percent of your one-rep max. Do second set at 70 percent, and last two sets at 80 percent.
Leg Curls	3	8–6–6	Use heavy weights.
Leg Extension	3	8–6–6	Use heavy weights.
Standing Heel Raises	3	8	
Back Extension	2	8	

WEEK 5, DAY 2, THURSDAY (LIGHT)

Exercise	Sets	Reps	Notes
Weighted Sit-Ups	3	15	Use 10-pound weights.
Squat	2	8	Do first set at 60 percent of your one-rep max. Do second set at 70 percent.
Leg Curls	2	8	
Leg Extension	2	8	
Standing Heel Raises	2	10–8	
Back Extension	2	10–8	

WEEK 6, DAY 1, MONDAY (HEAVY)

Exercise	Sets	Reps	Notes
Weighted Sit-Ups	3	20	Use 25-pound weights.
Squat	5	5	Do first set at 63 percent of your one-rep max. Do second set at 70 percent. Do third set at 75 percent, and last two sets at 83 to 85 percent.
Leg Curls	3	6	Use heavy weights.
Leg Extension	3	6	Use heavy weights.
Standing Heel Raises	3	8	
Back Extension	2	8	

WEEK 6, DAY 2, THURSDAY (LIGHT)

Exercise	Sets	Reps	Notes
Weighted Sit-Ups	3	15	Use 10-pound weights.
Squat	2	4–5	Do first set at 60 percent of your one-rep max. Do second set at 70 percent.
Leg Curls	2	8	
Leg Extension	2	8	
Standing Heel Raises	2	8	
Back Extension	2	8	

PHASE III: PEAK STRENGTH

WEEK 7, DAY 1, MONDAY (HEAVY)

Exercise	Sets	Reps	Notes
Weighted Sit-Ups	3	20	Use 25-pound weights.
Squat	5	4–5–5–5–5	Do first set at 60 percent of your one-rep max. Do second set at 70 percent. Do third set at 78 percent, and last two sets at 85 to 88 percent.
Leg Curls	4	5	Use heavy weights.
Leg Extension	3	5	Use heavy weights.
Standing Heel Raises	3	8–6–6	
Back Extension	1	12	

WEEK 7, DAY 2, THURSDAY (LIGHT)

Exercise	Sets	Reps	Notes
Weighted Sit-Ups	3	15	Use 10-pound weights.
Squat	2	5	Do first set at 60 percent of your one-rep max. Do second set at 63 percent.
Leg Curls	2	10–8	
Leg Extension	2	10–8	
Standing Heel Raises	2	8	
Back Extension	2	10–8	

WEEK 8, DAY 1, MONDAY (HEAVY)

Exercise	Sets	Reps	Notes
Weighted Sit-Ups	3	20	Use 25-pound weights.
Squat	5	4–5–5–5–5	Do first set at 60 percent of your one-rep max. Do second set at 70 percent. Do third set at 80 percent, and last two sets at 88 percent.
Leg Curls	4	5	Use heavy weights.
Leg Extension	3	5	Use heavy weights.
Standing Heel Raises	3	8–6–6	
Back Extension	1	12	

WEEK 8, DAY 2, THURSDAY (LIGHT)

Exercise	Sets	Reps	Notes
Weighted Sit-Ups	3	15	Use 10-pound weights.
Squat	2	4–5	Do first set at 60 percent of your one-rep max. Do second set at 73 percent.
Leg Curls	2	10–8	
Leg Extension	2	10–8	
Standing Heel Raises	2	8	
Back Extension	2	10–8	

WEEK 9, DAY 1, MONDAY (HEAVY)

Exercise	Sets	Reps	Notes
Weighted Sit-Ups	3	20	Use 25-pound weights.
Squat	5	5–5–3–3–3	Do first set at 63 percent of your one-rep max. Do second set at 73 percent. Do third set at 82 percent, and last two sets at 90 percent.
Leg Curls	3	5	Use heavy weights.
Leg Extension	3	5	Use heavy weights.
Standing Heel Raises	2	8–6	
Back Extension	1	12	

WEEK 9, DAY 2, THURSDAY (LIGHT)

Exercise	Sets	Reps	Notes
Weighted Sit-Ups	3	15	Use 10-pound weights.
Squat	2	5	Do both sets at 60 percent of your one-rep max.
Leg Curls	2	8	
Leg Extension	2	8	
Standing Heel Raises	2	8	
Back Extension	2	8	

WEEK 10, DAY 1, MONDAY (HEAVY)

Exercise	Sets	Reps	Notes
Weighted Sit-Ups	2	20	Use 25-pound weights.
Squat	6	5–5–3–3–3–3	Do first set at 63 percent of your one-rep max. Do second set at 70 percent. Do third set at 82 percent, and last three sets at 92 percent.

Leg Curls	2	5	
Seated Leg Extension	2	5	
Standing Heel Raises	2	8	
Back Extension	2	12 to 10	

WEEK 10, DAY 2, THURSDAY (LIGHT)

Weighted Sit-Ups	2	15	Use 10-pound weights.
Squat	2	5	Do both sets at 60 percent of your one-rep max.
Leg Curls	10	10	
Leg Extension	10	10	
Standing Heel Raises	10	10	
Back Extension	10	10	

WEEK 11, DAY 1, MONDAY (HEAVY)

Weighted Sit-Ups	2	20	Use 25-pound weights.
Squat	6	5–5–3–2–2–2	Do first set at 63 percent of your one-rep max. Do second set at 73 percent. Do third set at 82 percent, and last three sets at 95 to 98 percent.
Leg Curls	2	5	Use heavy weights.
Leg Extension	3	5	Use heavy weights.
Standing Heel Raises	2	8 to 6	
Back Extension	2	10 to 8	

WEEK 11, DAY 2, THURSDAY (LIGHT)

Weighted Sit-Ups	2	15	Use 10-pound weights.
Squat	2	5	Do both sets at 63 percent of your one-rep max.
Leg Curls	2	10	
Leg Extension	2	10	
Standing Heel Raises	2	10	
Back Extension	2	10	

WEEK 12, DAY 1, MONDAY (HEAVY)

| Weighted Sit-Ups | 2 | 15 | Use 25-pound weights. |
| Squat | 6 | 5–5–2–1–1–1 | Do first set at 63 percent of your one-rep max. Do second set at 73 percent. Do third set at 85 percent, and last three sets at 98 to 102 percent. |

Leg Curls	2	5	Use heavy weights.
Leg Extension	3	5	Use heavy weights.
Standing Heel Raises	2	8	
Back Extension	2	12 to 10	

WEEK 12, DAY 2, THURSDAY (LIGHT)

Weighted Sit-Ups	2	15	Use 10-pound weights.
Squat	2	5	Do both sets at 63 percent of your one-rep max.
Leg Curls	2	10	
Leg Extension	2	10	
Standing Heel Raises	2	10	
Back Extension	2	10	

Peaking the Mind and Body Routine by Kumiko Yamashita

Kumiko Yamashita is the owner of a personal training company in New York City specializing in one-to-one body sculpting for women. She is a top young prospect in women's competitive bodybuilding. Originally from Japan, she is known for her use of Eastern philosophies and movement techniques for training the mind and body.

Using the Peaking the Mind and Body Routine for all of your training should be helpful. As you continue to train and as the muscle becomes more and more identifiable, the mind will begin to concentrate more and more on the muscle. This will create a cyclical developmental process. The mind will help the body "peak" and the body will help the mind "peak."

LOWER BODY WISDOM
Lower body training is essentially the same as training other body parts. All of the muscles must be warmed up and stretched properly before beginning a strength and conditioning routine. Each muscle must be completely isolated during contraction.

THE MIND
The mind must be concentrated on the muscle you are working. With each repetition you must focus all energy into isolating that particular muscle and hold it at the

top of the movement, i.e. "the peak." You will feel the muscle begin to pump up. Many of my clients come to me overweight or having never trained at all. One typical question is "If I can't see my muscle, how can I make it contract at the 'peak'?" As many early Eastern philosophers taught, you must visualize something in order to make it a reality.

THE BODY

The body must be warm before attempting any exercises in order to avoid injury. Typically, I do at least ten minutes of cardiovascular training at a low level to warm up my lower body. I enjoy using the step machines for this because it tends to apply less pressure on my knee joints than running, although I recommend being flexible and changing your type of cardiovascular training from time to time. After warm-up the use of light weights and proper technique will help you on your way to visualizing your "peak."

THE EXERCISES

QUADRICEPS

Leg Extension: Work up to five sets total. I begin with a warm-up and gradually move up in weight, and finish with a low-weight, high-repetition set. I allow up to sixty seconds of rest between sets. Particularly with this exercise I do high repetitions because it tightens up the quadriceps like no other exercise I have used.

> *First Set*—maximum reps (to failure)
> *Second Set*—12 reps
> *Third Set*—10 reps
> *Fourth Set*—8 reps
> *Fifth Set*—maximum repetitions (to failure)

Sissy Squat: This is an exercise that should be renamed, because it is anything but "sissy." This exercise works buttocks, hamstrings, and quads. I usually do Sissy Squats (for 20 reps) between sets of Heavy Leg Extension (5 to 6 reps) and Leg Press (5 to 6 reps). I have found doing this at high repetition, especially before competition, helps to cut, shape, and tighten my legs. While doing this you should use "peak" contraction, holding the buttocks tight at the top of the move-

ment and holding the quads tight at the bottom of the movement. You will be surprised that even when using no weights at all this exercise will pump and tighten the muscle. Guys, don't be too upset if you can't do too many of these; no one will really think you are a sissy!

HAMSTRINGS

Leg Curls: Also with this exercise I work up to five sets total. I begin with a warm-up and gradually move up in weight, and finish with a low-weight, high-repetition set. I allow up to sixty seconds of rest between sets. In my later sets, when I am using heavier weight, I always use a spotter in order to pull my heels all the way up to my buttocks and hold the contraction for at least two counts. With heavier weights, sometimes my spotter must help me hold the weight at the top of the movement, and this is okay because it allows for the maximum stretch of the muscle. For me this exercise is the toughest one. Since you are lying face down in this exercise, you cannot see the muscle. So visualizing the muscle and its growth requires all of my focused energy on every repetition.

> *First Set*—maximum reps (to failure)
> *Second Set*—12 reps
> *Third Set*—10 reps
> *Fourth Set*—8 reps
> *Fifth Set*—maximum reps (to failure)

BUTTOCKS

Straight-Leg Dead Lift: Begin with light weights. I also advise using a high-quality weight belt: This gives added support for the lower back. I usually do four sets with heavy weight and low repetition, increasing weight with each set. At the "peak" I suggest squeezing the buttocks together as if "pinching a penny" between the cheeks of the buttocks. Each repetition should be done slowly with proper technique in order to avoid any injuries.

> *First Set*—maximum reps (to failure)
> *Second Set*—8 reps
> *Third Set*—6 reps
> *Fourth Set*—4 reps

CALVES

Stair-Step Calf Raises: Although nothing beats heavy-weighted donkey raises and seated calf raises to increase muscle mass for the calves, most women do not want large calves; rather, they prefer a tight diamond-shaped lower leg. To create quality cut and shape in the calves I suggest using a simple staircase without weights. One leg at the time, go up contracting the muscle at its "peak" and hold it for two counts. This will stretch the muscle to its maximum level. As you come down allow the heel to drop as far below the step as possible. This will help develop the symmetry of the muscle. I generally do three sets of twenty repetitions using three different foot positions. Make sure that you are always pushing off on your big toe to minimize any stress on the ankle.

> *First Position*—Feet Straight
> (neutral)   2 sets × 20 reps
> *Second Position*—Eversion
> Toes (pointed outward
> like a ballerina)   2 sets × 20 reps
> *Third Position*—Inversion
> Toes (pointed inward
> as if pigeon-toed)   2 sets × 20 reps

If you find you have done these and have extra energy, using both feet at once, point the toes outward as in the second position while clenching the cheeks of the buttocks. Go up and down on the toes using a flat surface (floor) to a maximum number of repetitions (to failure). This will tighten both the buttocks and the calves.

The Huskies Lower Body Balance, Coordination, and Foot Quickness Routine by Rick Huegli

Rick Huegli is strength and conditioning coach at the University of Washington. He was National Strength and Conditioning Coach of the Year in 1992.

Our objective is to develop the complete athletic qualities for each person on each team at the University of Washington. As a result, footwork, lower body coordination, and speed are characteristics upon which every athlete can continue to improve.

The first thing the athletes do when they come into the weight room for training is their warm-up. This is done by using a variety and combination of foot quickness and footwork drills.

One day will incorporate from three to five minutes of jumping rope. This is alternated with a day of foot quickness and agility drills that we call the Dot Drills and the Hexagon Drill.

THE JUMP ROPE ROUTINES

The jump rope routines aim to enhance the most basic footwork patterns with the jump rope and then to progress to more complex movements, emphasizing coordination, foot speed, and endurance. A conditioning objective is achieved by advancing from one routine to the next with only slight rest intervals so there is a continuous three to five minutes of jumping.

Coaching Point 1: Choose three to five different exercises and complete fifty to one hundred turns of the rope.

Coaching Point 2: Choose a jump rope by standing in the middle of the rope. The handles should not quite come up to the armpits.

Coaching Point 3: Position the elbows close to the body with the lower arm turned out and palms up. Turn the rope with the wrists.

Coaching Point 4: If you are a beginner, have patience and keep a good attitude. Your footwork will get better.

Coaching Point 5: Each jump should be done without a rope if being done for the first time.

Double Foot Jumps: 100 turns of the rope. This is the most basic of the jump rope routines. Turn the rope at a rhythmic rate with one ground contact for each turn of the rope.

Alternate Foot Jumps or Boxer Shuffle: 100 turns minimum. This can also be done on a length-of-time interval. Turn the rope, making ground contact with the right foot for two turns, then cycling through the left foot for two turns.

Single Leg Hops: 50 to 100 consecutive turns for each foot, one ground contact for each turn of the rope.

Jumping Jack Jumps: 50 to 100 turns. Begin with a Double Foot Jump for a turn, then laterally widen the feet for a turn. Repeat the movements, feet together and feet laterally apart for each turn.

Forward-Together-Back Split Jump: 50 to 100 turns. Begin with a Double Foot Jump followed with the right foot split forward and the left foot split directly backward. This is followed by both feet together, then the left foot split forward and the right foot split directly backward. Continue to jump in this pattern for the prescribed number of jumps or length of time.

Forward and Back Split: 50 to 100 turns. The skill is executed like the previous exercise except that both feet do not come together; rather, the right foot and left foot alternate split positions for each turn of the rope.

Jumping Jack/Split Combo: 50 to 100 turns. Begin with a Double Foot Jump then laterally widen for a Jumping Jack Jump repetition, followed by another Double Foot Jump. This is followed by two Split Jumps—right foot in front for one, left foot in front for the second—then return to the initial Double Foot position. Below is an overhead illustration of one complete cycle of the footwork:

First Position:	❣ ❣		(Double Foot)
Second Position:	❣ ❣		(Jumping Jack)
Third Position:	❣ ❣		(Double Foot)
Fourth Position:	❣	(Split)
Fifth Position:	❣	(Split)
Sixth Position:	❣ ❣		(Double Foot)

Foot Crossover Jumps: 50 turns. Begin with a Double Foot Jump followed by crossing the right foot across the body and the left foot behind. This is followed by a Double Foot Jump and then the left foot across the body with the right foot behind.

SPEED JUMPS

Double Jump with Bounce: 50 times. The rope clears the feet twice on first jump and then clears the feet one time on second jump (Bounce).

Double Jump in Succession: 50 times. The rope clears the feet twice for each jump.

Bonus Jumps: As many Double Foot Jumps as you can get in 30 to 60 seconds.

Running in Place Jumps: As many alternate foot jumps as you can get in 30 to 60 seconds.

Quadrant Jumps: These are based on a cross layout. (You can use tape on the floor.) See below.

1		2
4		3

Coaching Point: These jumps can be done as a circuit and should progress from 1 through 8.

1. Side to Side: (4 to 3 and back)—50 times with both feet.
2. Up and Back: (4 to 1 and back)—50 times with both feet.
3. Up and Back, One Foot: (4 to 1 and back)—25 times each foot.
4. Side to Side, One Foot: (4 to 3 and back)—25 times each foot.
5. Triangle: (1–2–4)—50 times both feet.
6. One Foot Triangle: (1–2–4)—25 times each foot.
7. Four Square: (1–3–2–4)—50 times both feet.
8. Four Square, One Foot: (1–3–2–4)—25 times each foot.

THE DOT DRILLS

The Dot Drills are designed to develop balance, coordinated footwork, and foot quickness. They are performed at the beginning of a weight workout paired with the Hexagon Drill and are done on alternate days with the jump rope.

You can purchase Dot Drill pads from a number of equipment companies or you can make your own dots on a floor. We use basketball/volleyball court tape.

The Dot Drill pad dimensions are:

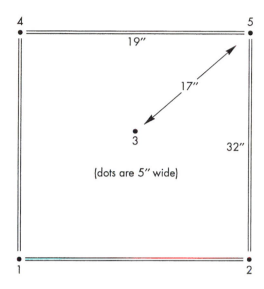

The Dot Drills consist of seven movements. We have standardized our Dot Drill routine to a twenty-second exercise interval with fifteen-second rest between exercises. The Dot Drills are as follows:

1. Both Feet Apart, Both Feet Together, Both Feet Apart. Using the numbered diagram:

    A. Begin with left foot on 1 and right foot on 2.
    B. Bring both feet to 3.
    C. Shift simultaneously, the left foot to 4 and the right foot to 5.
    D. Continue back with both feet to 3.
    E. Shift both feet, the left to 1 and the right to 2.

Repeat sequence for twenty seconds.

Coaching Points: First, the athlete should maintain a bent-knee balanced position. We emphasize that the athlete stay low. Second, to make the drill competitive, have a partner count the number of contacts made on the center dot (3) for each twenty-second set. You want to move the feet as quickly as possible.

2. Both Feet Apart, Right Foot Middle, Both Feet Apart.

    A. Left foot on 1, right foot on 2.
    B. Shift right foot only to 3.
    C. Simultaneously shift the left foot to 4 and the right foot to 5.
    D. Return right foot only to 3.
    E. Simultaneously shift the left foot to 1 and the right foot to 2.
    F. Continue the pattern for twenty seconds.

3. Both Feet Apart, Left Foot Middle, Both Feet Apart.

    A. Same footwork as the previous drill except the left foot makes contact with the center dot.

4. Two-Foot Figure 8.
    A. Begin with both feet on dot 1.
    B. Quickly shift both feet to dot 3.
    C. Both feet to dot 5.
    D. Both feet to dot 4.
    E. Both feet to dot 3.
    F. Both feet to dot 2.
    G. Both feet to dot 1.
    H. Continue the 1–3–5–4–3–2–1 pattern.

5. Right-Foot Figure 8.
    A. Same footwork as previous drill (4), using the right foot only.

6. Left-Foot Figure 8.
    A. Same footwork as previous drills (4 and 5), using the left foot only.

7. Feet Apart, Feet Together, Feet Apart, Turn Clockwise, Feet Apart, Feet Together, Feet Apart, Turn Counterclockwise.
    A. Same footwork pattern as drill 1 with a 180-degree turn clockwise, then counterclockwise.

Coaching Points: First, the athlete should move the feet quickly, staying low and balanced. Second, stay with the drill. Coordination, balance, and dot contact are points of concentration. You will get better with practice and repetition.

THE HEXAGON DRILL

The Hexagon Drill is done before or following the Dot Drills. Its objective, like the Dot Drills, is to develop lower body balance, coordination, and foot quickness, while serving as a training warm-up.

Using tape (we use court tape), mark a 24-inch-per-side hexagon on the floor with angles of 120 degrees.

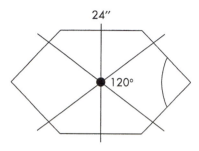

Coaching Point 1: Have the athlete stand in the middle of the hexagon facing forward. The athlete must face the same direction for the duration of the drill.

Coaching Point 2: The athlete begins by jumping forward over the tape with both feet and immediately back into the hexagon.

Coaching Point 3: The athlete continues to face forward and jump over the next side and back to the middle, until he or she has performed three full revolutions.

Coaching Point 4: The athlete should stay low and move both feet across the lines.

Coaching Point 5: When timing this drill or using it as a test, begin the clock with a "ready-set-go" command. When the feet enter the hexagon after three full revolutions, stop the clock. If using the Hexagon Drill as a test, deduct .5 second for each line touched and deduct 1 second for failure to follow proper sequence.

Dancin' Grannies:
These Grannies Don't Bake No Pies
Thighs Routine
by Beverly Gemigniani

Beverly Gemigniani is founder and director of Dancin' Grannies. She is a four-time gold medal aerobic winner in the Senior Olympics and was named a National Master in aerobics by the President's Council. Ms. Gemigniani is certified through ACE. She has performed at the White House and in the Macy's Thanksgiving Day Parade, is listed in *Who's Who International,* and has produced four mature exercise videos and a walking and relaxation audiotape.

PART ONE—THREE TIMES A WEEK

Take a two-and-a-half-inch telephone book, put three lines of duct tape one way and three lines the other way.

1. Lie on your back—elbows out and bent—hands in line with head, palms up. With knees bent, place book against shins, legs together, and raise legs so that thighs are at a 90-degree angle to floor and shins are parallel to floor, with book held level by shins. Knees should be over your hips, not the stomach.
2. Slide feet away slowly about 8 inches and return slowly to thighs perpendicular position.

Note: Back must stay flat, so never let feet go too far away as this puts pressure on the back. If knees are over the stomach no work is being accomplished.

Start with 10 reps and work up to 20 reps. Works the quadriceps and the abdominals.

PART TWO—THREE TIMES A WEEK

1. Stand with one foot on the taped book, knee soft or slightly bent. Make sure the body is upright with stomach tight and shoulders relaxed.
2. Step opposite foot to front slowly as far as you can and land flat footed. Return slowly. Do this same technique out to the side and then to the rear. The pattern is front-in-side-in-rear-in and repeat on same leg for 10 reps. Stretch out the hamstring and the quadricep and then do other leg. Work up to 20 reps.

Note: Moving foot should always be flat and out from the book as far as an upright body will allow. Do all of this slowly.

This exercise works the hamstrings, the adductors and abductors, and the thighs, and if you will move your arms out and in and up and in and out-front and in as you do the footwork, you will feel the stomach muscles work also.

Suggested Hip and Thigh Exercises for the Older Population by Deborah M. Holmes, M.S.

CONCERNS FOR THE ELDERLY

In most cases there are very limited concerns associated with the elderly population. However, as the body ages there are a few prevention concerns that become important when performing any exercise program. When designing an exercise program, you should avoid all contraindicated exercises. Contraindicated exercises are those exercises that place undue stress on any part of the body. Knees and hips are the most susceptible areas for these kinds of exercises.

For seniors it is extremely important to pay special attention to the hip area. This particular area is extremely susceptible to injury with increased aging. For seniors who exercise it is valuable to use a variety of hip exercises that allow the hip to strengthen and move throughout its entire range of motion. It is also important to consider the functions needed. Concentrate on exercises that help these functions of daily life, for example: getting up and down out of a chair, going up and down stairs, bending over, stepping over an object. These are basic functions that become more difficult as our joints and muscles age, and therefore we need routines that will strengthen our function in these kinds of activities.

In order to assure safety we advise that you concentrate on duration of exercise rather than intensity. Aim for increased numbers of repetitions instead of increasing the difficulty levels of the exercises. However, if you are strong and have no joint or muscle difficulties there are no increased dangers with any routine designed for seniors. Always employ a program that focuses on "full body" strength training and protects all muscular and skeletal structures.

Here's what we recommend for seniors who wish to strengthen their hips and thighs.

IN WEIGHT ROOM

LEG EXTENSION: 60 TO 75 PERCENT IF MAXIMUM STRENGTH

	SETS	REPS
Beginners:	1	12 to 15
Intermediate:	2	15 to 20
Advanced:	2	12 to 15 (or to failure)

LEG CURL: (SEATED LEG CURL PREFERRED)

	SETS	REPS
Beginners:	1	12 to 15
Intermediate:	2	15 to 20
Advanced:	2	12 to 15 (or to failure)

LEG PRESS: 60 TO 75 PERCENT IF MAXIMUM STRENGTH

	SETS	REPS
Beginners:	1	12 to 15
Intermediate:	2	15 to 20
Advanced:	2	12 to 15 (or to failure)

Note: Avoid weighted squat exercises; use caution with lunges.

CALF RAISES: (USE CAUTION WITH SHOULDER WEIGHTED MACHINES)

	SETS	REPS
Beginners:	1	25
Intermediate:	2	25
Advanced:	3	25 (or to failure)

CALISTHENIC EXERCISES

STANDING LEG WORK: These kinds of exercises are extremely valuable for hip strengthening and balance work.

Side Leg Lifts: Balance on one leg; use chair for balance. Lift opposite leg directly out to the side.

Front Knee Lifts: Balance on one leg; use chair for balance. Lift opposite knee directly to the front and lift as high as possible.

Rear Leg Raises: Balance on one leg; use chair for balance. Lift opposite leg directly to the back while maintaining upright posture.

Squats to Chair: Standing in front of chair, with proper form squat back into chair and then stand.

Standing Pelvic Tilts: Standing with hands on hips, tilt pelvis forward and concentrate on squeezing gluteal muscles and tightening abdominal muscles.

	SETS	REPS
Beginners:	1	15 to 20
Intermediate:	1	25
Advanced:	1	25 (or to failure)

FLOOR LEG WORK: These exercises are designed for specific strengthening of the hip joint. Depending on routine and time, these exercises can be done all together two to three times a week. Or split up routine and do a different set each day.

SIDE LEG WORK

Side Leg Lifts: Lying on side, keep alignment of hips-knees-ankles in straight line. Lift upper leg straight up and down.

In-and-out: Lying on side, bend bottom leg slightly for balance. Bring top knee in toward chest and then extend leg out straight, pushing through heel.

90-degree Lift: Lying on side, bend both knees up to 90 degrees in front of you. Lift top knee and ankle up and down in front of you.

	SETS	REPS
Beginners:	1	15 to 20
Intermediate:	1	25
Advanced:	1	25 (or to failure)

REAR/GLUTEAL LEG WORK

Rear Straight Leg: Lying on stomach, relax upper body. Lift one leg directly up to the back.

Rear Bent Knee: Lying on stomach, relax upper body. Keep knee bent to 90 degrees, with toes pointed to ceiling. Lift toe up directly to ceiling.

Fire Hydrants (for intermediate and advanced routines only): On knees and elbows, lift one leg directly out to the side. Try to get knee up to hip level.

	SETS	REPS	REMARKS
Beginners:	1	15 to 20	
Intermediate:	1	15 to 20	Take exercises up to elbows/hands and knees.
Advanced:	1	25 (or to failure)	Keep up on elbows/hands and knees.

INNER THIGH

"V" Squeeze: Lying on back, support your lower back with hands slightly under hips. Start with legs directly up in the air. Let legs open wide and then bring together. Focus on bringing heels together.

Froggies: Lying on back, support lower back with hands slightly under hips. Start with legs directly up in the air. Attempt to put bottoms of feet together. Let knees drop toward chest and then squeeze knees together as you push feet back up into air.

Inner-Side Lifts: Lying on side, rest upper leg in front of lower leg or place behind lower leg. Keep lower ankle flexed as you lift lower leg up and down.

	SETS	REPS
Beginners:	1	15 to 20
Intermediate:	1	25
Advanced:	1	25 (or to failure)

Lower Body Training by John Buzzerio

John Buzzerio is the fitness supervisor for New York Health and Racquet Clubs. He trains the fitness instructors for all locations. John specializes in corporate fitness planning and does private consultations in the areas of business management, exercise programming, and club design. He is a member of the American College of Sports Medicine and is certified as an exercise test technologist, exercise specialist, and program director. John has a B.A. in physical education and a master's in exercise physiology.

BUILDING A LOWER BODY FOUNDATION

I'm sure you've heard of an hourglass figure, but how about a lollipop figure? Those with the latter are people who spend hours training their upper bodies, and little time, if any, working their legs. For health and wellness you need a balance between your upper and lower bodies. It is like building a house: You need a strong foundation. This routine is designed to work the lower body with minimal stress on the lower back. Be sure to warm up properly and focus your mind during the workout. This workout should be done three times a week.

THE EXERCISES

	SETS	REPS
Leg Press	3	15
Leg Extensions	3	15
Leg Curls	3	15
Seated Calf (Machine)	3	15

The Cable Routine
by Eugenie Tartell

Eugenie Tartell, BS, RN, DC, FIACA, is the founder and director of the Upper Westside Chiropractic. She is the staff chiropractor for the Equinox Performance Center. Her practice has a broad-based clientele, which includes many performing artists (dancers, actors, and musicians). She is also a fitness and sports enthusiast.

EXERCISES
ON A BENCH

	SETS	REPS	REST	REMARKS
1. Bent-Leg Kickbacks	1 to 3	up to 20	30 seconds or less	For all, after you achieve 20 reps, increase weight.
2. Bent-Leg to Straight Kickbacks	1 to 3	up to 20	30 seconds or less	

STANDING

	SETS	REPS	REST	REMARKS
1. Standing Kickbacks	1 to 3	up to 20	30 seconds or less	For all, after you achieve 20 reps, increase weight.
2. Standing Adduction	1 to 3	up to 20	30 seconds or less	
3. Standing Abduction	1 to 3	up to 20	30 seconds or less	

Bulls Lunge and Up
by Al Vermiel

Al Vermiel is the strength and conditioning coach for the Chicago Bulls. He is the only professional strength coach with both an NBA and Super Bowl ring.

Exercise: This movement is a combination of a lunge and a step-up.

Starting Position: Stand with barbell resting on back or holding dumbbells at your side, feet even and shoulder width apart. Position yourself approximately two yards from bench or box.

Movement: Lunge forward with left foot, then bring right leg all the way through and on top of the box or bench. Drive left leg through and to the top of the box or bench, so you are standing on it. Bring left leg down and reverse motion, bringing right leg back and through to lunge position, then bring your left leg back, returning to starting position.

Training Wisdom:
- Start out with light weight.
- This is a great exercise to improve running and jumping.
- Use this as an alternative to the squat.
- Lighter weights reduce spine compression.
- Single-leg movements are sport specific.

Exercising Pregnant
by Deborah M. Holmes, M.S.

There are a few special concerns that must be recognized with exercise and pregnancy. Pregnancy is a time when your body undergoes chemical, physical, and structural changes. There is no hard evidence that someone who is pregnant should not exercise; in fact, most of the evidence indicates that there are benefits to exercise during pregnancy. However, if you have not been exercising prior to your pregnancy, it is not advisable to begin now. Individuals who have already established an exercise routine, however, can continue their exercise but should pay extra attention to their bodies each and every exercise session.

The pregnant body will begin to develop limitations. Some occur early in pregnancy with the changes in hormones; for example, increased nausea, increased fatigue, and the need for more sleep. You may find that the energy you used to receive from exercise will not have the same effect on you anymore. Oftentimes it would be advisable to take a "power nap" insead of a power workout. Your body is demanding sleep for a reason, so listen to your body. Another suggestion would be to change your workouts to the time of day where you have more energy; you might want to change evening training to morning training. If you are experiencing nausea, remember that you cannot have an effective training session if you are unable to keep nutrients down. Don't get discouraged during this time. These early signs usually only last for ten to fourteen weeks, after which the hormones will change slightly and you will again feel more energy. Remember that these first few months are the most critical to assure a healthy pregnancy, so pay particular attention to your body and consult your physician about any concerns.

There are no real restrictions for an "exercise-fit" person. In the past it was recommended that you keep your exercise heart rate below 140. Recent studies indicate, however, that physically fit individuals have no increased dangers exercising in their normal target heart rate zone. The most important precaution is watching your body temperature: You do not want to overheat your body temperature during an exercise session. (This is why pregnant women are advised not to soak in hot tubs or baths for long durations.) Avoid increased body temperatures by exercising during cooler hours of the day, shortening your exercise session, keeping properly hydrated, and wearing appropriate "cool and comfortable" clothing.

When strength training, always exercise with proper form and concentrate on your breathing. As you get further into your pregnancy, your circulatory system (along with everything else) will begin experiencing more stresses, so you will need to modify your training to allow for the changes happening within your body. Remember that you will be carrying more weight on your body, so moving in general requires more energy, not to mention the increased efforts to strength train. Your body will be releasing a hormone called relaxin, which softens your ligaments and bones all over your body, so pay particular attention to increasing weights. In fact, you may find that you don't need to increase any of your weights; just maintaining your workout is more than enough to get all the benefits during your pregnancy. If you are using the system simply maintain the level you are on, or switch to an easier level.

THE EXERCISES:

MONTHS 1–3 (FIRST TRIMESTER)
- Maintain all exercises.
- Listen to your body!

MONTHS 4–6 (SECOND TRIMESTER)
- You may find that you are experiencing some physical aches and pains. Modify accordingly.
- Maintain weights and sets as much as possible. Avoid exercises that leave you feeling any increased strains in the pelvic or abdominal regions.
- Do wide-stance squats or bench squats (placing a bench or chair underneath hips to limit range of motion and add support). Avoid putting weights on shoulders if experiencing lower back pain.
- Lunges will become more difficult, so modify as needed.
- Modify Leg Curls to Seated Leg Curl or Standing Leg Curl. It will become difficult to do anything lying on stomach or back.
- Modify gluteal work up to hands and knees (Donkey Kicks, etc.), as opposed to Glute Tucks lying on your back.

MONTHS 7–9 (THIRD TRIMESTER)
- Avoid exercises that leave you completely unsupported. Your body has increased amount of

relaxin, so potential injury becomes more of a concern.

- This is a good time to change your workout to include mostly exercise machines.
- Maintain training weights, decrease sets (one to two sets are plenty):

    Squat machine (if possible)

    Leg Extension

    Leg Curls

    Calf Raises

    Abduction/Adduction machines or Side Leg Raises (lying on side with pillow supporting lower back and abdomen)

Kegal exercises (often included with inner thigh exercises or abdominal exercises)

Note: Always contact your physician at the onset of any spotting, cramping, pain, or any other concern.

POST-PARTUM

- Remember that you will continue to have relaxin in your body for up to one year after delivery.
- Begin slowly, preferably with exercise machines.
- One set per body part, full body training.
- Increase your training according to your recovery.

CHAPTER TWENTY-SIX

Creating Your Own

The time will come when you have to leave the nest and create your own training routine. This may cause anxiety, and that's expected. Don't worry. This chapter will give you the tools you need to design your own routine so you can become your own personal trainer.

We are going to outline the principles you need to design your own personal routine. What is good for one individual may not be as good for another. We want you to find your ultimate lower body routine.

Part One: The Design Model

When creating a lower body routine you need a basic design model or blueprint from which to work. You need to divide the lower body into five separate areas: front, back, outside, inside, and lower.

To build a routine you need to think about how you want to shape and strengthen each area. This will depend on your individual needs and goals; keep in mind such things as weak areas, aesthetics, and sport-specific training. It is always important to remember that you must create a balance and symmetry between these areas, not only in the area of appearance, but also in strength. Since the exercises in this book are categorized according to the five basic lower body areas, you'll find it easy to plug in exercises and personalize your routine.

Part Two: Basic Concepts

Setting up a lower body training program requires preparation and attention to detail. An understanding of the basic concepts of training is necessary for the design to be successful. It is also necessary to conform these principles to the specifics of lower body training.

The following are key concepts (along with the principles in Chapter 3) you will need to consider when building your routine.

VOLUME

Volume, as it relates to lower body training, can be described most simply as the number of repetitions performed. Fifteen repetitions is a higher volume than ten reps. Total volume for a workout can be defined by total sets times repetitions. When creating a progressive series of routines, you want to keep an eye on total volume, making sure you're doing enough but not too much. Volume is also important as it relates to intensity. These two components are inversely related: If volume goes up, intensity goes down—and vice versa.

INTENSITY

Intensity can most easily be measured by the weight lifted. Intensity is dependent upon the goals, specificity, training stage, and experience or maturity of the individual. The intensity that different people can handle will vary greatly. Beginners or novices should not attempt to handle high-intensity training until they have established a training base. Intensity can also be affected by total volume of work. Intensity in training is the key to successful training. *An individual should use an intensity that will produce momentary muscular fatigue in the prescribed number of repetitions.*

VARIATION

Variation is often the most neglected training principle. Training needs to be varied for the following reasons: to prevent overtraining, to avoid training plateaus, to alleviate the boredom of monotonous training, and to bring about the best possible training effect.

The most important aspect of variation is related to intensity and volume. When you first start working your lower body, it is easier to shock your muscles and cause adaptations. As you become more advanced you will need to change your workouts more frequently. An example of how to do this is to increase your intensity (weight) and decrease your repetitions (volume). Another way to create variety is to do the opposite:

Increase volume (repetitions) and decrease intensity (weight). When you're considering variations in volume and intensity, you may want to vary similar training days within a training week. You will have a day of high-intensity training (heavy) and one of low-intensity training (light). The terms *heavy* and *light* can be misnomers. For the optimal training effect, overloading (i.e., momentary muscular fatigue) should always occur on both "heavy" and "light" days.

INJURY PREVENTION AND REHABILITATION

The greatest benefit of strength training (including lower body training) is that of injury prevention. By strengthening the muscles and connective tissue (done by proper strength training), a specific area of the skeletal structure is better supported. Bone density is also improved through increased retention of calcium. This decreases the potential for injury in that area.

If an individual is unlucky enough to be injured and has been involved in a proper strength training program, that person will recover from that injury faster than a person who was not involved in a strength-training program.

With obvious benefits such as injury prevention, quicker recovery, and more complete rehabilitation, you should choose exercises that address these purposes and include them in your training routine. On the other hand, you should avoid exercises that aggravate specific areas.

ENERGY SYSTEMS

Exercises are not all created equal. To insure the best overall lower body development you'll need to include three kinds: (1) exercises of high intensity and short duration; (2) exercises of medium intensity and medium duration; and (3) exercises of low intensity and longer duration. In other words, you need to include exercises that are arduous and that exhaust you quickly, and exercises that are less strenuous and that allow you to train for longer intervals.

Including exercises or training protocols that encompass these three basic energy systems will insure the best overall lower body development. Designing this type of training will guarantee that you will be using a variety of muscle fiber types as you introduce variety and specificity into your training regimen. To take best advantage of this concept, you should train for each of these levels of intensity in periodization (see "Part Three: Periodization," this chapter).

PERFORMANCE

All of us want to improve ourselves; that is the premise of this book. Exercise improves us whether in everyday activities or in some recreational pursuit.

When formulating a lower body training program you need to analyze performance needs. Is there a specific sport or activity in which you wish to improve performance? Remember, the lower body is at the core of the body's strength and power system. Power is most often initiated by the lower body. Examine the movements of the sport or activity. Is there running, jumping, stabilization, change of direction, and/or power transference? I'll bet there is. From this analysis choose and incorporate the lower body exercises in Part 3 of this book that will enhance these specific movements.

MUSCLE BALANCE

Muscle balance is another consideration when choosing exercises. Lower body muscles work together in a variety of movements and also work in a supportive and structural alignment capacity. The movements used in lower body training need to include all the muscle groups (see Chapter 2) while working these muscle groups at a variety of angles (refer to parts three and four).

All muscles should be trained in an effort to maintain muscular balance. When a muscle, or muscle group, becomes considerably stronger than others it works with, the potential for injury is greatly increased.

In the same respect, never completely neglect one muscle area to work on weaker areas. If you have strong areas, still train these areas, but work on more of a maintenance regimen (less intensity or volume, or possibly both).

Movements should also include combination exercises (exercises that work two or more muscle groups at the same time).

The training routines included in this book incorporate these movement patterns to produce optimal gains,

while maintaining muscular balance and symmetry. Pick and choose or create your own.

SPECIFICITY

Specificity, or the S.A.I.D. principle (Specific Adaptations to Imposed Demands), is an important training concept. Choose exercises to fit your specific needs. For example:

Training Stage: Your exercise choice will affect your training stage: a preconditioning stage, a maintenance stage, a peak performance stage, etc.

Sport or Activity: The specific needs of your sport are a major consideration in exercise selection. You need to train for specific kinds of movements as well as the type of energy output you use in that sport. Chapter 25 may include routines for your sport, designed by professionals in that field.

Personal Goals: When choosing exercises, you have to be aware of your specific goals: what you want and how much time you are willing to spend. If you are a bodybuilder, your goals are going to be much different from someone who wants to firm up a little and improve his or her general fitness level.

EXERCISE ORDER

In general, the best order for exercises is from largest muscles to the smallest (see Chapter 2). But the order can also be affected by individual goals and the need for variety. If your primary goal is to shape your calf muscles, then you will want to target them first. But staying with the same exercise order for extended periods of time will cause muscle complacency (no adaptations), which means less than optimal gains.

Part Three: Periodization

Periodization is a systematic and progressive training method designed to aid in planning and organization. This cyclical training encompasses all of the basic training principles and helps bring performance to a peak. It is utilized by the greatest athletes and strength coaches in the world (many of whom are included in this book).

The scope of this book does not allow for a detailed discussion of the many intricacies of periodization, but the following summary will help you in creating your own lower body routines.

The basis for periodization is derived from the General Adaptation Syndrome (GAS), which was developed during the 1930s. It was intended to describe a person's ability to adapt to stress. There are three distinct phases to the GAS:

1. *Alarm Stage*—This relates to the individual's initial response to training. This could manifest as a temporary drop in performance due to stiffness or soreness.
2. *Resistance Stage*—This stage manifests as the period when the athlete or individual adapts to the training stimulus by making certain adjustments. These adjustments might include physiological, mechanical, structural, and psychological adaptations.
3. *Exhaustion or Overwork Stage*—If total stress placed upon the athlete is too great, the third stage sets in. Overtraining can present itself in the following ways: by a loss of, or plateauing of, performance; by chronic fatigue; by loss of appetite; by loss of body weight or lean body mass; by increased incidence of illness; by increased injury; and by decreased motivation and low self-esteem.

During this stage, desired training adaptations are not likely to occur. You should also consider outside stresses from your social life, poor nutrition, recovery, and work to avoid overtraining.

The goal then is to remain in the resistance stage of training, where your body is making the compensations to the stresses applied and is continually improving. This is where the concepts of periodization apply.

This is done by careful manipulation of certain training principles and planning. You *can* accomplish your training objectives.

OBJECTIVES

Defining your objectives is the first key step in creating your own lower body program.

First, identify areas of importance. Obviously, the muscles that constitute those of the lower body (see Chapter 2) are of primary importance. Individual muscles within this group may take priority, but remember: Do not neglect any muscle group. If an area is being rehabilitated, this area will take precedence.

Second, distinguish between training that is effective and ineffective. In many cases this comes down to a mental attitude. You must perform the exercises that are most effective, not the ones that are fun and comfortable to perform.

Third, define optimal performance. You have to learn where your optimal performance level is. You have to define how much training is enough, what is too much, how frequently to train, etc.

Fourth, work with a set time within which your lower body should peak. This may be for a competition or just for looking good at the beach. This relates to goal setting and helps you plan out your program. During this "peak" time, all facets of your endeavor should be peaking: training, diet, etc.

Remember, very few things are set in stone, especially when it comes to fitness training. Periodic evaluation and changing of objectives and methods is essential to make any long-term program successful.

THE CYCLES

Once your goals and objectives have been defined, the next step is planning. This can be divided into four training phases.

Macrocycle: The macrocycle is the longest of the training phases. Its length varies, depending on your goals. In general, the macrocycle lasts from the end of one peaking period to another. The macrocycle defines long-term goals and a specific time frame in which you want to peak: six weeks, six months, or one year. The macrocycle contains three components: preparation, peaking, and transition.

Mesocycle: The next largest phase is the mesocycle. Mesocycles make up a macrocycle. A mesocycle is a phase that has very specific goals that are aimed at achieving the objectives. (The three levels of each routine in Chapter 17 are examples of mesocycles.) For example, the goal of the first mesocycle may be that of preparation. This would include training with high volume and fairly low intensity to build a base of strength and muscular endurance. The next mesocycle's goal would be to increase to medium intensity (increased weight, more difficult exercises, shorter rest periods, etc.). This action would necessitate a lowering of volume prescriptions. The next mesocycle's goal may be oriented for strength (increase in intensity and decrease in volume). The final mesocycle space (in which you reach peak condition) might include more intensive evaluation: what areas are weak and need extra work, what areas are strong, what has worked best in the past, your diet, your mental state, etc.

Depending upon specific goals, peaking for the lower body will differ for each individual. Individuals whose goal is strength and power may continue to increase intensity and lower volume, while concentrating on optimal recovery for competition. Bodybuilders may increase volume and lower intensity while peaking for competition. Sport-specific athletes may spend more time on sport-specific movements, metabolic specificity, and skill acquisition when peaking for a competitive season (there may be several peaking phases within a competitive season). The better your preparation and the better the condition you are in, the longer you will be able to maintain your peak.

The Peaking Period: This is the phase where all your training culminates, bringing out the best possible results. This will, of course, be different for everybody. For the elite athlete, this can be very complicated, because several variables have to come together at once: strength, endurance, sport-specific skill, diet, mental state, etc. The same is true for a bodybuilder. Things become somewhat more simplified if it's just the lower body you're concerned about. If you want your lower body to reach a peak for a vacation on the beach, you should be focusing on three variables: your lower body routine, diet, and cardiovascular training. Again, the peaking period is when you bring all these elements together at their highest level.

Microcycle: Within each mesocycle are smaller units called microcycles. Microcycles further refine the objectives by manipulating training variables on a daily basis. One day may include training of high intensity and low volume, while the next day may include training of low intensity and high volume. Or it may become even more complex as in our ultimate lower body section (see Chapter 22) varying day to day from specific muscle groups and also varying in the training stimulus (volume, intensity, and specificity). In most cases, a microcycle will last from one week to four weeks.

TRANSITION

Unfortunately, maintaining peak anything for a long period of time can be very difficult. The cycle or period of time following a peaking period is the transition phase.

Transition is designed to introduce variety into the program while bringing about recovery and recuperation, both mentally and physically. As the term *transition* implies, this phase allows you to start at a higher training level for the next macrocycle or whatever your goals may entail.

We also don't want to infer that your lower body can't look great all the time. The transition phase will help insure this. Ultimately, the rigors of continuing to peak will lead us into the third stage of the GAS, which is overtraining and exhaustion. The body needs some time off from the peaking phase and from training in general, where diet restriction and the high intensity of training can eventually lead to overstraining.

When most people think of recuperation they think of sitting on their butt and doing nothing. With the transition phase the opposite is quite true. You will continue to engage in activities but at low volumes and intensities. These activities can be anything physically active that you like to do. In conjunction with these activities light lower body training once a week may be undertaken (following correct training guidelines). Depending upon your goals and the next peaking period the transition phase will usually last from one to two weeks.

Taking the Guesswork Out of Training

Correct application of the concepts of periodization takes the guesswork out of training. Periodization allows you to identify and isolate the variables necessary to obtain the ultimate lower body. Using the design model of front, back, inside, outside, and calves, and following the basic concepts outlined here and in Chapter 3, you can choose exercises from the book to create your own customized routine. Then, following the natural cycles of periodization, you can create a series of progressive routines, staying as long as possible in the growth and peaking phases, to achieve the lower body you want.

Good luck with your advanced principles. The applications of these principles will lead to your ultimate success and longevity in training.

A Case Study

It is the first of June and you want to be peak out for a tennis tournament over the Labor Day weekend (the club championship). You need to plan a three-month macrocycle.

You would probably break this down into one-month mesocycles, with two-week microcycles for the first two months and one-week microcycles the last month as you prepare to peak. If you plan to play other tournaments during the summer, that is okay. But let's say that this tournament is the most important one of the summer and this is when you want your lower body to peak.

Your breakdown would go something like this:

First Month: This is your preparation period. You build a safe foundation doing low-intensity training with high volume. Your first microcycle would include basic strength training exercises that would promote joint integrity. Your second microcycle might include more combination exercises. At this point in time before you are fine-tuning your tennis skills it is very important that weight training is undertaken when you are fresh.

Second Month: During this period the primary goal is to increase the intensity of your training; consequently your volume is going to drop. You may add some more specific exercises during the first two-week microcycle. During the second microcycle you want to introduce sport-specific movements while cycling to higher volume (increased from last microcycle) and less intensity. Skill acquisition on the court and fine-tuning your tennis technique is increasing in importance and is starting to demand more practice time.

Third Month: You now move into one-week microcycles for this month. The first-week intensity is once again increased (higher than the first microcycle of the second month) while volume is decreased. The second week you move into more specific peaking by performing a circuit routine. Court time is now taking precedence. The third week would be the same with slightly shorter rest periods.

During these three weeks pursue an ever-increasing intensity in your sport-specific training. If during this time you have scheduled to play other tournaments, consider the last tournament played to be training days; consider any previous tournaments to be off days.

The last week should consist of one training day at least seventy-two hours before the tournament. Your plyometric training should coincide with this schedule also. Skill acquisition and practice on the court is now paramount.

Kurt Brungardt has been a writer and personal trainer in New York for the last eight years. He is the author of the best-selling fitness classic *The Complete Book of Abs*. He is also the host of one of the top-selling exercise videos, *Abs of Steel for Men*. He has written for and been featured in many exercise magazines and newspa-

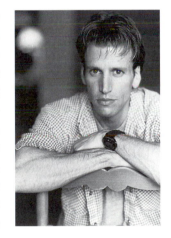

pers, and has appeared on numerous national talk shows. Kurt has trained a wide variety of clients ranging from athletes, actors, and models to businessmen and -women and senior citizens. He is a member of Strength Advantage, Inc. His body appears on the cover of this book and on the cover of *The Complete Book of Abs*.

Mike Brungardt is on the board of directors of Strength Advantage, Inc. He is strength and condition-ing coach for the San Antonio Spurs. As a member of Strength Advantage, he has given seminars at clinics for fitness educators in schools and health clubs throughout the country. He has worked with such pro-fessional athletes as ski racer Beth Madsen (1990 Rookie of the Year) and basketball all-star David Robinson. He specializes in the mental and motiva-tional aspects of sports performance and is also coau-thor of *The Strength Kit*. He has been involved in the consulting and design of a wide range of fitness facili-ties. Mike graduated from Central State University of Oklahoma, where he wrestled and played baseball. He has nine years of coaching experience at Northwest High School, in Grand Island, Nebraska, one of the most successful athletic programs in the state of Nebraska during the eighties.

Brett Brungardt, a former strength and conditioning coach at the University of Houston and at the University of Wyoming, is on the board of directors of Strength Advantage, Inc., a fitness consultation firm that advises professional and college athletes, coaches, and corporations in designing fitness programs and facilities. Brett is the coauthor of *The Strength Kit*, a manual for planning strength and conditioning programs for all levels: scholastic, collegiate, and professional.

He is the author of numerous publications in the area of fitness. He has an M.Ed. in exercise science from the University of Houston and is a certified strength and conditioning specialist with the National Strength and Conditioning Association.

Andrew Brucker is a New York photographer. He specializes in portraits and nudes. His work has appeared in numerous art journals, magazines, and books, including *Interview, Details, Rolling Stone, New York Woman,* and *Männer Vogue,* to name a few. He also did all the photographs for *The Complete Book of Abs.*

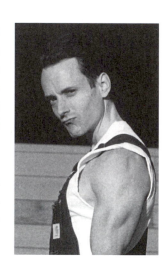

CHAPTER CONTRIBUTORS

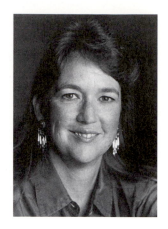

Becky Chase is a registered dietitian. She currently maintains a private practice through her business, Alpine Nutritional Services. Becky specializes in sports nutrition and eating disorders. She consults through the Aspen Club and MidValley Sports Medicine and Fitness Clinic, Inc. Becky lectures regularly to students and consumer groups about nutrition and programs she has developed: Market Smarts (a grocery-store tour) and Stop Dieting, Start Thriving (a program for compulsive eaters).

Becky has written many articles for newspapers, magazines, and hospital publications. She is currently working on a book based on her Market Smarts program. Becky has a B.S. and an M.S. in clinical dietetics from Texas Woman's University.

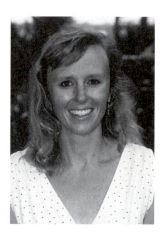

Deborah M. Holmes is the coordinator for the adult fitness program at San Diego State University. She is also the founder of Holmes Personal Training, which provides in-home training in the San Diego area. She is a member of the American College of Sports Medicine and I.D.E.A. She has her B.S. and M.S. in health science and education from the University of Florida and she is the founder of *The Living Well News Letter.*

Bryon Holmes is director of programs for Muscular Skeletal Evaluation and Rehabilitation at the University of California San Diego, Department of Orthopedics. As a member of the Holmes Personal Training team, he also does private fitness consultation for individuals and corporations. Bryon

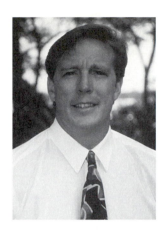

specializes in preventive care and rehabilitation of the lower back. He is a member of the American College of Sports Medicine. Bryon has a B.S. and an M.S. in exercise physiology from the University of Florida.

Dave Johnson is a writer and personal trainer in New York City. He was assistant strength coach at Wake Forest University. He holds a B.A. in writing from Wake Forest and an M.F.A. in writing from Columbia University.

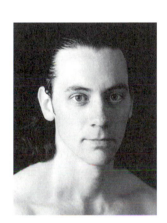

Joe Brown is a fitness enthusiast and restaurant owner in Snowmass, Colorado.

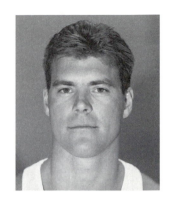

Peter Buener is a personal trainer at New York Health and Racquet Club in New York City.

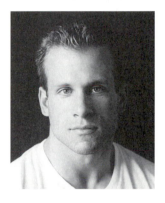

Sandra Brucato is a model living in Snowmass, Colorado.

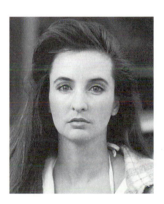

MODEL CREDITS

Coulter Bright— Biography on pages 258–59.

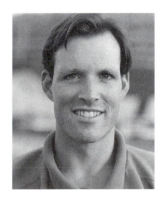

Charles Chand is a personal trainer living in Aspen, Colorado.

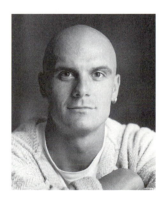

Charisse D. Layne— Biography on page 261.

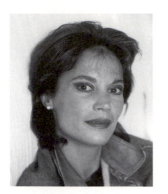

Charlie McArthur is a snowboard and kayak instructor in Aspen, Colorado.

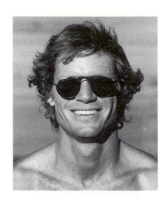

Rhonda Foley is assistant director of the Snowmass Athletic Club and studies Tae Kwan Do.

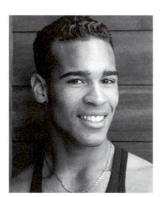

Eugenie Tartell— Biography on page 273.

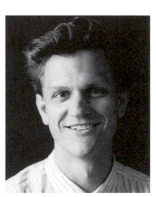

Darren Schnase is a fitness enthusiast and model who lives in Aspen, Colorado.

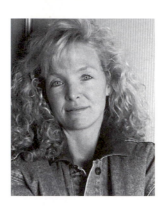

Lawrence LaRose is an assistant editor at Random House and a marathon runner.

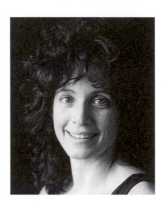

Jaclynn Parks— Biography on page 258.

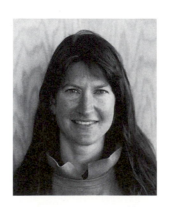

Kumiko Yamashita— Biography on page 265.

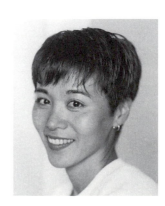

John Olson is a former professional model, now a stockbroker living in Aspen, Colorado.

Dave Osborne is a rugby player in Aspen, Colorado.

INDEX